Devices & Desires

Studies in Social Medicine

Allan M. Brandt and Larry R. Churchill, editors

Devices & Desires

Gender,
Technology,
and
American
Nursing

**Margarete
Sandelowski**

The University of
North Carolina Press
Chapel Hill and
London

© 2000 The University of North Carolina Press
All rights reserved
Manufactured in the United States of America

Designed by Jacquline Johnson
Set in Joanna
by Tseng Information Systems, Inc.

The paper in this book meets the guidelines for permanence
and durability of the Committee on Production Guidelines
for Book Longevity of the Council on Library Resources.

Library of Congress Cataloging-in-Publication Data
Sandelowski, Margarete
Devices and desires: gender, technology, and American nursing /
Margarete Sandelowski.
p. cm. — (Studies in social medicine)
Includes bibliographical references and index.
ISBN 0-8078-2579-4 (cloth: alk. paper) —
ISBN 0-8078-4893-X (pbk.: alk. paper)
1. Nursing — United States — History.   2. Medical technology —
United States — History.   I. Title.   II. Series.
[DNLM: 1. History of Nursing — United States.   2. Technology,
Medical — History — United States. WY 11 AAI S214d   2000]
RT42 .S26   2000
610.73′0973 — dc21   00-032588

04   03   02   01   00   5   4   3   2   1

Writing nursing history is no easy task. Those attempting it have not only to read between the lines to find nurses, but also to write against the prevailing view in nursing of worthy scholarship as exclusively "scientific." I therefore dedicate this book to all nurses engaged in these difficult and subversive acts of reading and writing and, most especially, to the eminent nurse historian, Joan Lynaugh.

All history is written backwards. . . . We choose a significant event and examine its causes and its consequences,
but who decides whether the event is significant? We do,
and we are here; and it and its participants are there. They
are long gone; at the same time, they are in our hands . . .
[and] under our thumbs. We make them fight their battles
over again for our edification and pleasure, who fought
them once for entirely other reasons.
  Margaret Atwood, *The Robber Bride*

The past was not . . . a chain of seemingly inevitable
events. . . . It was a multitudinous, simultaneous chaos
of choices made or not made by each human being alive.
Sometimes these choices were made for you and some
you made for yourself. . . . Even the choices you didn't
know you were making . . . would set the future.
  Rita Mae Brown, *Riding Shotgun*

You have to remember . . . you are your history. If you
cut any of it off, you're an amputee.
  J. Kogawa, *Obasan*

And, indeed, I do believe that it is important to know
about things, as well as to know things, which is different.
  Victoria Glendinning, *Electricity*

CONTENTS

ILLUSTRATIONS

In the course of the twentieth century, Americans have come to regard the explosive growth of new medical technologies with both profound hope and fear. The remarkable expansion of our ability to treat many previously fatal diseases effectively is closely tied to the omnipresent machinery that now fills our hospitals. These machines have helped to create boundless expectations in our ongoing attempts to alleviate disease and delay death. And yet, a deep sense of alienation and mistrust is engendered by these very apparatuses. This ambivalence to the rise of techno-medicine, argues Margarete Sandelowski, is crucial to our understanding of the complex role and identity of nursing over the last hundred years.

Investigating the implementation and impact of medical technologies is a critical aspect of the task of social medicine as an interdisciplinary field. As Sandelowski shows so effectively, the new machinery of medicine has had implications far beyond the effective diagnosis and treatment of disease: it fundamentally shapes professional responsibilities, relations among health care providers, and especially the relationship between these individuals and their patients. During the last century, the intensification of new technological interventions in medicine radically altered both the experience of illness and bodily experience itself.

Of course, the rise of these technologies was accompanied and supported by a dramatic rise of hospitalized care and the new bureaucracies and administrative structures this required. The growth of hospital beds, specialization, and biomedical research augmented the dilemmas raised by technology in subverting the traditional notions of nursing as dedicated to humane bodily care of the individual patient.

For nursing these technologies often proved especially problematic. At the same time that a new technology—like the thermometer—

appeared to give nurses new professional responsibilities, it also had the effect of reducing patients to simplistic and reductionist "readings," transforming subjective judgment and affective relations to new metrics of surveillance and monitoring. Further, Sandelowski demonstrates, as technologies passed from the primary responsibility of physicians to nurses, they have been simultaneously disparaged, marking a critical aspect of the traditional gender hierarchy characterizing hospital-based medical care. Technologies from which the doctor had derived considerable status soon became "easy enough for a nurse" to implement. In this way, technology was deployed in ways that defined the social boundaries of authority, knowledge, and practice, mirroring the historically gendered relations of medicine.

Would the new technologies ultimately transform the field of nursing from the care of the patient into the practice of a narrow set of technical skills? Nurses have consistently and conscientiously debated the impact of machinery on their mission, even as nursing was swept up in the unprecedented rise of new apparatuses throughout the twentieth century. In the identity of the nurse we see the essential questions of medical care and the patient: is medicine about care or cure, suffering or science? Although our immediate response might be both, as this book so clearly indicates, navigating this path has proven to be no simple task. As we evaluate the complex costs and benefits of a medicine in which technology is so deeply embedded, we often speak of a technological imperative that seems to eviscerate human agency. But as Sandelowski shows, these technologies are the work of men and women and they are given meaning in the day-to-day contextual interactions of caregivers and their patients. If nurses have been subject to the powerful impact of technology, so too they have a crucial role in the process of remaking technologies to serve professional needs—as well as the needs of their patients. The meticulous and thoughtful discussion of the nursing-technology nexus offered here reminds us that technology is inherently neither good nor bad, but rather, its impact depends on its timely, effective, and humane application.

To understand the often subtle but powerful impact of technologies on medical practice and professional roles, we need to return to a close reading of how machinery is utilized in specific historical and social contexts. In this way we can see how technologies shape the professional boundaries between doctors and nurses, as well as their implications for the care of the patient. We may see, reflected in these machines, the nature of professional identity and the social world of medical care. Only when we understand these relationships and their significance will we be able to, as Sandelowski suggests, "fit technology to care."

Allan M. Brandt
Larry R. Churchill

ACKNOWLEDGMENTS

First I wish to thank all of the nurses who participated in the interviews for Chapter 6. The nurses who gave me permission to include their names are listed here in alphabetical order: Carol Anderson, Louise Beasley, Sheila Bogan, Robin Britt, Mary Brodish, Brenda Carroll, Shari Chapman, Barbara Eucker, Patricia Gambill, Cynthia Garrett, Mary Ann Hulme, Cathy James, Linda Kapinos, Kathryn Koches, Marilyn Lapidus, Mary Loreto, Nancy Lowe, Dana Mochel, Jane Montgomery, Michelle L. Murray, Wanda Oakley, Judy Schmidt, Anita Webb, and Betty Wright.

I also gratefully acknowledge the Center for the Study of the History of Nursing at the University of Pennsylvania for awarding me a Lillian Sholtis Brunner Fellowship, which allowed me access to its excellent resources; my academic home, the University of North Carolina at Chapel Hill, for awarding me a Kenan Leave to finish this book; and Ruth Schwartz Cowan and Christopher Crenner for their thoughtful and helpful reviews of a draft of this book.

I thank my doctoral students, Donna Bailey (also my very able and energetic research assistant), Cydney Mullen, Patricia Pearce, Vivian West, and Diane Yorke, for helping me clarify, gain new insights into, and derive more enjoyment from exploring the nursing/technology relation. Benjy and Nellie thank you, too!

Finally, I thank my parents, Heinz and Amalie Sandelowski, who have always supported me and whose history set their future, too.

Devices & Desires

I Troubling Relations

In a critical essay on the close and class relations between women, servants, and machines, Alexandra Chasin cited a newspaper article in which the author listed the things human beings had invented to make their lives easier. These inventions included the wheel, fire, tools, servants, and computers. Chasin found the servant in this list "troubling" because including the servant "troubles" the distinction between human beings and the things human beings use—between using and being used. As she asked, "Is the servant . . . in the list . . . one of us or one of them, human or thing, subject or object?"[1] The relationship between nursing and technology has been similarly troubled, and this troubling link is the subject of this book.

Nursing and technology have been "inexorably linked" since the beginnings of trained nursing in the United States in the late nineteenth century.[2] Whether or not they thought of them as technology, nurses have necessarily always used a variety of tools, instruments, and machines, including thermometers and cardiac monitors, enema cans and respirators, and beds and infusion pumps, to appraise, treat, and comfort patients. Indeed, it would be difficult to conceive of nursing practice without these tools of the trade. Although nurses have typically appeared (if they have appeared at all) as no more than footnotes in the history of medicine and medical technology, they were indispensable to the early-twentieth-century scientific and technological transformation of health care and medicine in the United States, putting new technologies for diagnosis and treatment into use, including clinical thermometry, laboratory and x-ray diagnosis, antisepsis, anesthesia, and hospitalization itself. The hospital became the "carefully established space [where] rituals and ceremonies [were performed that] centered upon the conspicuous display of new tools and equipment."[3] Nurses made hospitals hospitable to both patients and the new machinery of care housed there.

Nurses have served as the primary users of machines and as "machine-body-tenders" in health care, responsible for the proper application, operation, and maintenance of health care devices and, increasingly after 1950, the interpretation of the rhythm strips, digital readouts, and other displays of information that new instruments and machines produce.[4] Nurses have been charged with enlisting patients' acceptance of technology. A significant component of the "sentimental work" of the nurse has entailed educating patients about new devices, getting patients to accept and comply with their use, and alleviating patients' fears about them.[5] Nursing has thus been the soft technology that has ensured the safe, effective, efficient, and even compliant use of the hardware of health care. Nursing roles, such as the intravenous nurse, the scrub nurse, and the "nurse equipment specialist," have been built around technological devices.[6] Specialty fields of nursing practice, such as critical care, nephrology, obstetric, and home care nursing, have been defined or transformed by the infusion pumps, kidney dialysis machines, cardiac and fetal monitors, and ventilators increasingly populating hospitals and homes. Technology has become a way to differentiate nursing specialties as high or low technology.[7] Technology has also become a way to differentiate nurses; in "telephone nursing," a new field of practice built around an old technology, nurses offering triage, consultation, and primary care services by telephone are "telephone nurses."[8]

By the end of the 1930s, when most nursing practice and patient care was occurring in hospitals, nursing became not only inexorably (or necessarily, fundamentally, and materially) linked to technology but also "inextricably bound" to it.[9] That is, the line between nursing and technology became harder to discern, and therefore the link between nursing and technology became more problematic and perplexing. Nurses began to worry that technical procedures were becoming synonymous with nursing and thereby eroding the essence of nursing. Indeed, it became more difficult to disentangle nursing and technology, as nursing was depicted both as a technology itself and as an antidote to technology. The ontological, conceptual, and representational boundaries between nurse/human/subject and machine/not-human/object, and between true and technical nursing, became increasingly blurred.

In early-twentieth-century campaigns to promote hospitals to an American public used to caring for the sick in the home and with a view of hospitals as places to suffer and die, both nursing and technology were sold together as life-saving services that could be obtained only in hospitals. "The rustle of the nurse's uniform," in addition to "the bell of the telegraph, the rattle of the hydraulic elevator, the hiss of steam, and the murmured ritual of the operating room," sounded the promise of the new technological hospital.[10] Charged with showing off new x-ray and laboratory equipment to hospital visitors, nurses were like the women hostesses and "spokesmodels" of today who show off cars and boats in commercial shows and who "tempt" consumers to buy.[11] Nurses displayed technology and, along with that technology, were on display.[12]

For most of the history of nursing, nursing and technology have been represented as servants to physicians and to the general public in their fight against disease. From the beginnings of trained nursing, physicians conceived of nursing as a component of the therapeutics of medicine, not as a complementary but independent profession. Physicians thought of nurses much like stethoscopes and surgical instruments, as physical or bodily extensions of physicians. One late-nineteenth-century surgeon referred to both "the amputating knife" and the "nurse" as "instrument[s]" surgeons used to realize their goals.[13] A resident physician in the 1950s implied an identity between nurse and object by commenting that "both instruments and nurses have to be worked with for a couple of years before you know them."[14] Nurses have been regularly referred to as the physician's eyes, hand, and "operational right arm."[15] Both nursing and fetal ultrasonography have been described as the "third eye" of the physician, while the operating room nurse has been conceived of as the "third hand" of the surgeon.[16]

Nurses have also been depicted as part of the homey room decor in print advertisements for hospitals (see fig. 1-1). They have been photographed alongside patientless and seemingly redundant machinery, often appearing redundant themselves[17] (see fig. 1-2). Inanimate objects have been conceived to perform the functions of a live nurse. For example, a nineteenth-century drawing (fig. 1-3) from the Bettman Archives in New York shows an example of "mechanized nursing." A patient is shown lying in bed attended to by the Larkin's "nursing table" (an invention patented in 1869) containing a funnel device and several bottles, which dispense medicines to the patient, suction his mouth, and provide a receptacle for vomitus and other body wastes. Nineteenth-century French physicians thought of the incubator for premature infants as a "mechanical" or "thermostatic nurse."[18] This mechanical nurse was to provide needed warmth to the infant without the expense and complications of human labor. Concerned with the sacrifice of direct nurse supervision for privacy, as hospital wards were increasingly being replaced by private rooms, early-twentieth-century hospital planners sought to provide "nurse substitutes," or mechanical or electrical devices for calling the nurse to the patient's bedside.[19] In the 1950s and 1960s the vital function monitor was to be the "constant finger on the pulse of the patient." The "lens of the television camera [was to] replace . . . the eye of the nurse."[20]

In order to garner respect for their work, nurses have described themselves as thermometers, barometers, monitors, information processors, and human/machine interfaces.[21] One nurse observed in the 1930s that both "nurses" and "roads" had allowed physicians to extend their professional reach and double their practice.[22] Nurses have used objects, such as stethoscopes, sphygmomanometers, thermometers, and pulse oximeters, to signify nursing as a scientific profession in promotional and recruitment displays. These objects have served as an "aesthetically less complicated" and culturally more resonant way to promote nursing for a "technologically literate audience" than, for example, the feminine hand or Florence Nightingale's lamp.[23] As Australian scholar Kim Walker proposed, symbols of science are more real and more prestigious than symbols of caring and have "semiotic primacy" in Western cultures. Caring "resists" such simple "representation."[24]

Alternatively the figure of the nurse has been used to stand for medical science and technology. In Robbie Davis-Floyd's description of the "technocratic model" of American childbirth, a female nurse holding what appears to be an elongated test tube is shown—along with a male physician (who is drawn with a fetus inside him) and a hospital building in the background—to represent the "American core values" of "science," "technology," "patriarchy," and "institutions." These values are, in turn, depicted as in conflict with the "American core values" of "nature," "individuals," "families," and "women," which are shown as a man and woman holding an infant with a house in the background. (See fig. 1-4.) Here technology is associated with something negative—namely, the male domination of women—and the nurse is depicted as colluding with the physician to deploy technology in the service of maintaining that domination.[25]

Accordingly, the signal link between nursing and technology was created early in the history of nursing, with the nurse variously and

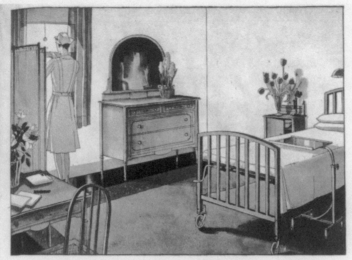

Figure 1-1. Nurse in homelike hospital room. (From Bulletin of the American Hospital Association 1, no. 2 [1927]: 121; courtesy of The Simmons Co.)

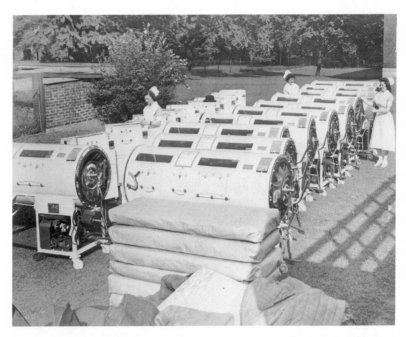

Figure 1-2. Nurses with iron lungs, 1942. (By permission of Temple University, Paley Library, Urban Archives, Philadelphia)

inconsistently depicted as embodying both sympathetic care (and thereby mitigating the effects of unsympathetic technology) and scientific care, in the form of technology.[26] But what exactly did the nurse signal or embody? Like the servant listed with the wheel and fire, was the nurse separate from the x-ray machine, stethoscope, and thermometer nurses and physicians used to care for patients, or was she herself an object that physicians and others used? Did nurses use thermometers, hypodermic syringes, and monitors, or were nurses themselves thermometers, needle bearers, and monitors? Did nurses use the new machinery of care in order to care, or were they component parts of the machinery—indeed, not even the "whole wheel" but, rather, the proverbial "hub in the complex machinery" of health care?[27]

The signal links tying nursing with technology still trouble nurses and nursing. While drawing from culturally valued entities, references to both nurses and machines as monitors and information processors have tended largely to reduce the labor of the nurse to machine labor and thereby to efface the distinction between nurse/human and machine/not-human. Although we are increasingly recognizing, especially with the advent of the computer, that human beings are "con-

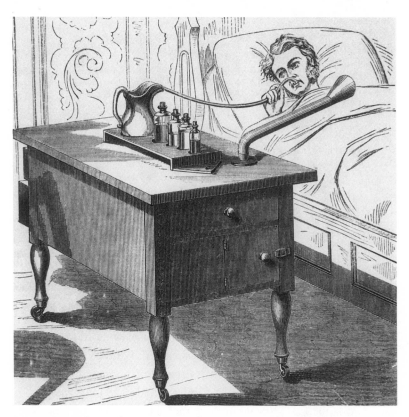

Figure 1-3. Mechanized nursing, 1869. (By permission of Corbis/Bettmann, New York)

tinuous" with the tools they use and the machines they create, and that the same conceptual scheme explaining the workings of a machine can be used to explain how human beings work, human beings still constitute something different from tools and machines.[28] But that difference is often minimized in depictions of the nurse as functioning like a machine.

Moreover, because technology is still often naively viewed as nothing more than the simple, unknowing, and even robotic application of science, defining nursing as a technology reinforces the idea that nursing is nothing more than manual labor and the mindless application of medical science on orders from physicians. The definition of nursing as a technology perpetuates the view of nursing as an applied field that owes its existence to medicine. By reference to Western cultural hierarchies that rank science above technology, and mental above manual labor, the depiction of nursing as a technology reinforces the

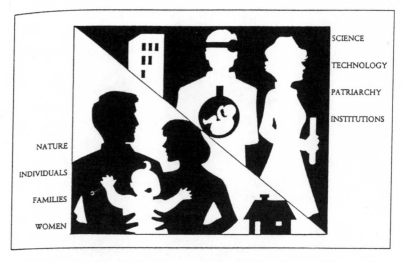

Figure 1-4. Nurse as symbol and purveyor of technology. (Original drawing by Janice Van Mechelen; by permission of University of California Press)

unequal social relations between nurses and physicians. As historian of technology Ruth Schwartz Cowan proposed, in Western culture, technology is science's Other, as female is Other to male. That is, technology is to science as manual is to mental and as female is to male, with technology, manual, and female in these metaphoric pairs in subordinate positions.[29] Only when technology is paired with nature does it occupy the superior position by reference to the ideological system in which nature is female and technology is male.[30]

The metaphoric link between nursing and technology, whereby nursing signifies instruments or means, also troubles by virtue of the cultural referent system that defines machines and females as servants that/who happily serve and willingly relieve their owners or employers of physically arduous, time-consuming, dull, dirty, and other work they need or want to have done but which they do not want to do themselves. Although there is an important Western dystopian tradition of fear that machines will take over as masters, there is a stronger utopian tradition in Western health care of lauding machines as servants or slaves.[31] Accordingly, when nursing is viewed as a technology, nursing signifies servant by reference to the ideological system that ties technology to servitude. Moreover, since servants tend to be invisible and to do work that is "immediately consumed or exhausted," the metaphoric link between nursing and technology "abets the forgetting of labor" and the historic invisibility of nursing.[32]

References to nursing as technology also trouble the association nurses have sought to create between nursing and genuine and selfless care. Chasin described her encounter with an automated teller machine that (or who), after she had completed her banking transaction, advised her that it had been a pleasure serving her. This machine was programmed to care for her. Accordingly, do nurses care like machines or like human beings? Are the nurses historian Susan Reverby described as "ordered to care" like machines programmed to care?[33] The depictions of nursing as a technology, and especially as a technology of care, trouble the distinctions among different kinds of caring and between caring and technology.[34] Indeed, in part to offset the blurring of technology into caring, nurses began in the 1970s to depict nursing and technology as in opposition to each other, with nursing as the humane antidote to technology. To position nursing as a female culture at odds with masculine technology, nurses wary of technology drew from ideological or referent systems that linked female/nurse to nature, nurturance, and caring, and technology to male/power and control over nature. Nursing/touch and technology were represented as two opposing paradigms of care.[35] Depicted as a force for the dehumanization of both patient and nurse, technology now signified Other to and even enemy of nursing.[36] Nursing has thus been identified both with and against technology and thus, in an ironic way, with and against itself.

Significance of Studying the Nursing/Technology Relation

Despite (or perhaps because of) the fundamental but confusing link between nursing and technology, it has yet to be the subject of much formal exploration. Technology can be seen in long-standing debates concerning the relative dominance of the hands, mind, and spirit of the nurse and whether nursing is an art, science, and/or (woman)craft, but it has rarely taken center stage. The nursing/technology relation has been the subject largely of anecdotes and speculation rather than the focus of formal research or critique. Although technology has been "a common doctrine of historical and causal primacy"[37] that nurses and others have used to explain events in nursing history (especially since World War II), we know little about how technology has shaped the nature and definition of nursing practice; how nurses have perceived and used new technologies; how new technologies have contributed to (re)negotiating the sphere of influence of the nurse and to the social relations and division of labor between nurses, physicians, patients, and others; and about what choices nurses had concerning these new technologies. If technology alone has not driven nursing history, it has, at the very least, shaped it, illuminating, intensifying, dramatizing, and telescoping persistent dilemmas and contradictions in nursing. But we have yet to see what the history of technology looks like when nursing is placed at the center of inquiry, and what nursing history looks like when technology is placed at the center of inquiry.

Significance for Nursing

The study of the nursing/technology relation is important for nursing because it can illuminate what Australian scholar Jocalyn Lawler described as the cultural "problem of the body" in nursing.[38] Nurses, alone among health professionals, tend patients' bodies. As nurse Cortney Davis poetized in "Touch," nurses "bathe all those bodies, wash urine from skin thin as paper . . . soothe skin that drinks up lotion. . . . [They] lift patients [and] hoist like farmers."[39] Nursing knowledge is also distinctively somological; that is, it is knowledge gained from the body.[40] But while nursing has historically been legitimated by this body work, it has also been tainted by it. Body work is "sacred" work that allows nurses to share with patients intimacies unknown to other health care providers. It is also "profane" work.[41] In Western cultures, body work is often considered dirty work, and body workers (largely women), as dirty workers.[42] Nurses have sought to resolve the problem of the body, in part, by turning away from using their "bodies as tools"[43] and toward technology, which seemed to promise a cleaner, less visceral, less intimate, and more scientific form of caring. With technology nurses no longer had to encounter their patients "bare handed," and they could "scientize and sanitize nursing."[44] Technology allowed nurses to replace or, at least, to mitigate the intense body intimacy of nursing with the "technical" and "measured intimacy" of medicine.[45]

A study of the nursing/technology relation can illuminate also what French scholar Marie Francoise Colliere described as the cultural problem of invisibility in nursing.[46] As woman's work, nursing is "deleted work," historically subject to a "technology of silence" by which nurses' work is either not seen as skilled work or is appropriated by others as their work.[47] Nursing "work that is done disappears into the doneness."[48] Nurses have turned to diagnostic and treatment technologies as one means to resolve the problem of invisibility, since the use of devices is a more overt and visible manifestation of nursing work and existence. As a "covert" aspect of nursing, caring remains persistently difficult to see.[49]

A study of the nursing/technology relation can illuminate, too, the cultural problem of handwork in nursing. Typically conceived of as nothing more than the physician's hand, and persistently caught in the Western cultural dichotomy between merely manual and highly prized mental, or intellectual, work, nurses have struggled to show that nursing is largely brain work. In the process, however, they have inadvertently complied with the prevailing cultural practice of denigrating the very "body-knowledge" that is the forte of the nurse.[50] In part to resolve the problem of handwork, they have also chosen to "flee [the] technique and technology" with which manual work is associated.[51] The paradox is that nurses have turned to technology, in part, to flee the body, yet they have also sought to resolve the problem of handwork, in part, by fleeing technology. These flights have moved nurses farther from fulfilling their desire to practice and to showcase nursing as a distinctive endeavor.

A study of the nursing/technology relation can also illuminate contemporary debates concerning the appropriate use and, more specifically, appropriate users of health-related technology. As the U.S. health care system is increasingly characterized by a blurring of provider roles and functions and by more open access to technology, the question of in whose hands to place various technologies becomes more important to answer.

Significance for Gender/Technology Studies

The study of the nursing/technology relation is important not only for nursing but also for gender studies of technology. Gender/technology studies comprise an interdisciplinary field of scholarship that emerged in the late 1970s from the social science critique of Western science and technology and the feminist critique of the academic disciplines and professions that began in the 1960s.[52] Drawing primarily from history, sociology, and, later, cultural studies, scholars in this area have taken on several projects, ranging from the liberal feminist goal of ensuring women's equal access to technology fields to the more radical feminist agenda of exposing the negative effects on women of technological innovations. More recently, gender/technology scholars have sought to theorize the Western cultural association between technology and masculinity. The increasing use of the term "gender studies" (as opposed to "feminist critique") of technology signals a more serious effort to examine gender as a cultural construction implicating both women and men (as opposed to studying only women). Contemporary analyses that problematize the gender/technology relation, however, remain informed by largely feminist, or pro-woman, liberatory goals.[53]

Gender/technology scholars have emphasized not only the underrepresentation of women in technology fields but also women's misrepresentation as only users, but not inventors, of technology. They have shown that women were more than footnotes in the history of technology by documenting their contributions to agriculture and food production, health and medicine, sex and reproduction, and machine and computer technologies. They have also examined the structural, psychological, and sociocultural factors that have impeded women's inventive capacity, motivation, and opportunity, including educational, occupational, and economic barriers to women in technology fields and their access to public and commercial rewards for invention. Gender/technology scholars have exposed the often negative effects not only of technologies used largely or exclusively by women, such as household and reproductive technologies, but also of ostensibly gender-neutral technologies, such as computers. Current efforts in the field are directed toward explaining the nature, ethics, and politics of the Western cultural association between technology and masculinity. Scholars increasingly seek to understand how gender and technology are constitutive of each other; how Western technology embodies or consolidates masculine identity, practices, and values; and how technology can be an equalizer in societies characterized by gender, class, and race inequalities.[54] Viewing gender itself as a technology, technology as engendered, and both gender and technology as cultural constructions, gender/technology scholars see gender as a "versatile tool" for studying technological change.[55]

Nursing is an ideal subject for exploring the gender/technology relation. As one of the most sex-segregated and exploited domains of female work, nursing is an important and heretofore largely ignored venue in which to examine gender as "both a determining cultural condition and a social consequence of technological deployment."[56]

Nurses and others have viewed technology as alternatively furthering and impeding the struggle for autonomy, visibility, and equality in nursing vis-à-vis medicine, thereby illustrating the "contradictory possibilities . . . technology can contain."[57] Technology has been credited with advancing the power, influence, and "leverage" of nursing by enlarging nurses' skills and sphere of influence and creating new opportunities for practice.[58]

Yet technology has also been charged with reinforcing the subordination of nursing to medicine, impeding its development as a valued province of knowledge and practice, and undermining its very essence. Barbara Koenig, for example, found that the incorporation of a new technology into practice only temporarily equalized the nurse/physician relationship, which reverted to its typically unequal character once that technology became routine.[59] Anselm Strauss observed that nurses were linked subordinately to medicine via technological innovations in medicine that precluded the development of nursing.[60] David Wagner described nursing as having been stripped of its prestige by virtue of its association with medical technology.[61] Marianne Lovell proposed that the transfer of technology from physician to nurse was "medicine's subtle way of reinforcing deceptive ignorance on the part of nurses: paternal medicine's promotion of female mind sedation."[62] For these scholars gender has persistently undermined the democratizing potential of technology.

As a "gender-marked" profession that shares many of the same technologies with another gender-marked discipline (namely, medicine), nursing is an ideal empirical site to study the different relations of women and men with the same technologies.[63] Nurses may use the technologies they share with physicians (and others) differently and also be seen as using them differently.[64] Although both nurses and physicians employ many of the same technologies, technology remains symbolic of medical science and progress. Western physicians have drawn much of their cultural authority and rewards from science and technology, but nurses appear not to have been similarly authorized or rewarded. Nurses still draw whatever authority they have largely from gender (including idealized notions of womanly caring and self-sacrifice), even while working more and more with new technologies in the hospital and, increasingly, in the home.[65] Nurses are often not reimbursed for performing the same services as physicians (who are reimbursed) and for performing services for physicians, which are then claimed as medical services.[66]

Nursing is an important empirical site also for the recovery of women's contributions to technological change and for the discovery of women's inventions. Like other women, nurses have remained hidden from history as inventors, or contributors to the invention, of health and medical technologies. From the earliest days of trained nursing, nurses have shown their inclinations and talents for altering the material world of practice to enhance patient comfort, reduce nursing labor, and maximize nursing efficiency. Nurses worked to make the best of what was available to them by transforming everyday and familiar objects into implements for comfort and healing. After World War II, nurses became important contributors to the design of many devices and technological systems. Yet few nurses themselves are actually listed as patent holders or have received public recognition as inventors or for their contribution to invention. Nurses exemplify how people "work around" the limitations of technology to make them work.[67]

Nursing is a valuable site also to explore the Western cultural association between technology and masculinity. Nursing offers students of the gender/technology relation the opportunity to explore whether and under what circumstances this cultural association is ideological or empirical. As the primary machine-body tenders in health care, nurses are hardly the technophobic or technically inept females alienated from technological society feminists have often described. Nurses have been eager, active, and competent users of complex technologies. Indeed, when they have noticed nurses at all, some feminists have criticized nurses for this eagerness, charging them with colluding with physicians in the deployment of technologies harmful to women.[68] Nursing offers an important site for gender/technology scholars to break the gender and technology "stereotypes" and to avoid the "twin dangers of technological determinism and essentialism," upon which they have often based their analyses.[69] Adhering to these stereotypes, these scholars have largely ignored nursing as both a scientific and a technological domain of women's work.[70] Nursing offers scholars the opportunity to avoid simplistic conclusions about the gender/technology relation and "camouflaging or essentializing" technology, gender, and nursing.[71]

Nursing also provides an important venue to study the transfer of technology between cultures, that is, the cultures of medicine and nursing. The study of the transfer of technology between historically male and female subcultures can be explored for the problems such transactions often entail. That is, the technology transferred is not simply the hardware component but also values, norms, and practices that may be in conflict with the receiving culture. Receiving cultures may, in turn, alter technologies to the extent that they are no longer the same as that which was transferred. Technologies are what they are, to a large extent, because of what they become in various user contexts.[72] Nursing offers gender/technology scholars an opportunity to study ostensibly the same technology in various gender contexts.

Reading between the Lines, Writing at the Margins

Anyone embarking on a history of nursing is soon confronted with the problem invisibles pose, that is, with how to study the relatively unseen.[73] Nurses looking in histories of medicine, hospitals, and health care will typically not find themselves there. Moreover, as Judith Parker and Glenn Gardner observed, the "nursing tradition is that of an oral culture and its transmission is private and transient."[74] Because there are fewer traces of what everyday nurses thought and did, a history of nursing requires special acts of reading and writing.[75] Alberto Manguel observed that there are at least two kinds of reading that occur in "segregated" groups.

> In the first, the readers [are] like imaginative archaeologists, burrow-[ing] their way through the official literature in order to rescue from between the lines the presence of their fellow outcasts, to find mirrors for themselves in [existing] stories. . . . In the second, the readers become writers, inventing for themselves new ways of telling stories in order to redeem on the page the everyday chronicles of their excluded lives.[76]

Accordingly, I have used whatever resources were available to me to rescue nursing from and redeem nursing for the pages of history and technology studies. I have tried to be mindful of the unique nature of the different sources I have used, and I have sought not to make inferences from them that they do not permit. Like the activities of nurses themselves, located "in between" patient and illness, patient and physician, patient and machine, and other "classificatory divides," this rescue and redemption effort requires reading between the lines of existing histories and "writing at the margin[s]" of several disciplines.[77] Nurses are used to crossing disciplinary boundaries to look for ideas that will illuminate and enhance their care of patients as well as to look for themselves.[78] I am used to crossing boundaries, not only by virtue of being a nurse but also because of my education in American studies, an interdisciplinary field. Crossing, blurring, and even ignoring boundaries is also the order of the postmodern day. Especially notable for this history is the "technoscience" merger created by scholars who are attempting to erase traditional divides among science, technology, medicine, and culture.[79]

Although the in-between location offers new spaces for inquiry, it also exposes inquirers to charges of an unscholarly eclecticism, of not adhering to the rules of any one discipline. For example, one guideline that has emerged in the history of medicine is that patient records of a period are better as primary sources of information about medical practice than medical literature of that period, as the former are assumed to be closer to actual practice and the latter to contain largely prescriptions for practice.[80] Indeed, medical historians have successfully used patient records to refute prevailing notions from medical literature of technological change in medicine.[81]

A growing and diverse constituency of scholars have also noted how inadequate and even misleading patient records are in representing nursing practice.[82] As the work of these scholars indicates, we obtain no better purchase on historical reality concerning nursing practice from patient records than we do from other sources, such as nursing literature of a period. Until relatively recently, nurses' notes from archived patient records were routinely discarded. Early-twentieth-century observers of nurses' writing habits indicated that nurses themselves were reluctant and, therefore, poor recorders of their work; they found the chore too time consuming, and they were too tired from their work with patients to do it.[83] Charting was also a way to exact conformity and discipline among nurses, as evident in the attention given to strict rules for charting, the nurse's penmanship, and the use of the proper pens, stamps, and other devices.[84] In addition, prescriptive literature directed toward nurses concerning charting indicates that nurses were to chart primarily to support and document the physicians' work, not their own.[85] Nurses were to use charts to record observations physicians needed to do their work.[86]

Moreover, nurses learned early to document by exception, that is, to document only what was deemed special or out of the ordinary. Since most nursing work was considered ordinary and routine, it was typically not represented in the record.[87] One precept for nurses was never to record "non-essentials," or that which constituted "good nursing care." Although back rubs and baths were essential to the patient's well-being and the essence of good nursing care, they were deemed of "minor importance" in the chart.[88] The nurse was thus to be the "keeper of the chart," but she and her work were typically not in the chart.[89]

Contrary to the prevailing and false view of the patient record as a mirror of clinicians' work is the more accurate view of the chart as part, and as a tool, of that work. Indeed, the "good" record is not the complete record, which ostensibly contains everything that was done for and thought about patients and comprehensible to anyone reading it, but, rather, the record that is comprehensible to and supports the work and agendas of the diverse constituencies using it, including clinicians, hospital administrators, insurance companies, and lawyers.[90] In addition, by virtue of what it typically allows to be recorded, the patient record tends to reinforce the invisibility of nursing and the unequal power relations between physicians and nurses.[91] There is typically only the "briefest trace" of nursing work in the patient record.[92] For example, all of the effort involved in ensuring adequate fluid intake and output may only be represented by a number on a flow sheet or a physician's progress note. Nursing work also appears as medical work in the patient record. Physicians, for example, often copied nurses' notations of patient conditions into their own summaries. Nurses' suggestions to physicians on a course of action tend to appear in the record as physicians' orders to nurses to take that same course of action.[93]

Accordingly, the patient record is better understood not as a source of information about clinical work but, rather, as an actor in the (re)production of work and social relations. There is no one historical reality against which the patient record can be compared and evaluated.[94] The historian is no safer drawing inferences from patient records than from medical literature of a period on the frequency, typicality, and typical performer of clinical work.[95] Although it may be viewed as of lesser value than patient records, nurses' published literature is an excellent source of information about nursing practice, as everyday nurses—not just elites—often described their work, with great detail and passion, through case anecdotes, clinical vignettes, photos, drawings, and sketches.

Thus I considered any data available to me that might illuminate two typically elusive subjects: nursing and technology. For this study I used a combination of techniques and sources commonly associated with social history, including archival sources of information (such as student lecture notes, hospital procedure manuals, and medical trade ephemera, photo, and instrument collections); professional literature (including medical and nursing textbooks and journal articles and other printed materials, such as advertisements); (auto)biographical literature; hospital histories; and interviews with nurses. Social history is generally concerned with recovering the world of ordinary people as they encounter both the everyday and the extraordinary events in their lives. Nursing has been described as the quintessence of "everyday-ness," and studying its past epitomizes "history from below."[96] Social history also tends to be informed by perspectives, concepts, and theories from the social sciences. I have drawn most heavily from social, cultural, and gender studies of technology but also from scholarship in the history and philosophy of technology and the history of medicine and nursing, and from my own experiences as a nurse in relation to technology.

A social history of technology, in turn, is based on the assumption that "objects have affected the ways in which people work . . . [and] live" and that people, in turn, "have affected the objects that they invent, manufacture, and use."[97] My orientation to technology emphasizes the material and social world of the nurse around "equipment-embodied technologies," as opposed to any process, system, or other means to achieve desired ends that might also be defined as technology.[98]

"Technology" has come to mean virtually anything a writer wants it to mean and is, therefore, in danger of meaning nothing at all. Although it will be evident in this book that I am fully aware that technology encompasses more than physical objects, and that the line between object and not-object is itself contested, physical objects are my starting and focal point. I want to maintain an analytic distinction between the material nature of technology and the human encounters with and around it, between the material devices nurses have used and the desires those devices have been used to satisfy or thwart. The essence of nurses' historical concerns with technology has resided largely in its physical thingness. Moreover, the contribution of thingness to technology is often trivialized in the fervor not to be seen as too narrowly oriented to technology in its mode of manifestation as physical object. Having a concern with objects is synonymous with neither technological determinism nor a trivialization or ignorance of the social, cultural, or symbolic significance of technology. Indeed, although nonphysical entities such as gender and language are now increasingly conceived of as technologies, it is often an object — typically an electronic and/or imaging device — that has engendered that conception.[99]

Organization of This Book

I have chosen events in the history of nursing that illuminate, exemplify, and/or dramatize key moments in the development of the nursing/technology relation. Some of these moments actually span broad sweeps of time, but I found them especially useful for showing the continuities, contradictions, and ironies of this relation. I focus on neither nursing nor technology alone but, rather, on the nursing/technology relation. As Ruth Schwartz Cowan observed, ideas about technology, whether that word is used or not, are ideas always "in relation to something else."[100] I refer to the nurse throughout this book as "she," since nurses were and remain envisioned largely as women, and nursing, as woman's work. In addition, most nurses were and are women.

This book begins by providing an overall understanding of key issues and practices relating to technology and to technology in nursing. Then the focus shifts to one domain of nursing work — observation and its relations to technology — followed by concentration on a specific technology of observation in a defined practice area: electronic fetal monitoring. Finally, I offer a wider vision of historical continuities with contemporary debates in nursing and health care. I emphasize observation because it was an activity that historically legitimated the existence of trained nurses, and it continues the stress placed on diagnosis in contemporary histories and social studies of medical technology, thereby offering a valuable interpretive context. Observation is also a domain of activity that has been contested between nurses and physicians and that can be studied over time. The practice of obstetrics is characterized by long-standing tensions between technology and nature and between doctoring and nursing, and it is a particularly good site to study the rise of surveillance practices in medicine. Electronic fetal monitoring, in turn, embodied these tensions and the move to technological surveillance, and it was largely deployed by nurses.

The chapters in this book thus move the reader backward and forward in time while maintaining a thematic focus. Each chapter can be read alone but is also thematically linked to the other chapters. In Chapter 2 I introduce the reader to key concepts and debates about Western technology that inform the study. In Chapter 3 I consider the period between 1873 and 1950, in which the nursing/technology relation was largely an embodied one occurring "behind the screens."[101] In Chapter 4 I explore nursing and the diagnostic revolution in medicine during the same time period. In Chapter 5 I consider the post–World War II period through the 1970s, a critical interlude in the history of nursing when nurses began seriously to address and experience the conflict between "true" and "technical" nursing. Nursing in this period moved from being a largely embodied practice behind the screens to a hermeneutic practice in front of screens.

In Chapter 6 I explore the entry of the electronic fetal monitor into nursing practice during the 1960s and 1970s. For this chapter I interviewed thirty-one nurses (between 1995 and 1998) from across the country who had practiced in labor and delivery in the late 1960s and 1970s in a range of community, university, and medical center hospitals. I placed an advertisement in a local North Carolina nursing newsletter (*Nursing Matters*) and a national publication (*Lifelines*) of the Association of Women's Health, Obstetric and Neonatal Nurses requesting contact from nurses who had been working in labor and delivery when fetal monitors were first introduced in their hospitals. The respondents ranged in age from 40 to 68 and had 8 to 35 years of experience in obstetric nursing practice at the time of interview. When fetal monitors were introduced into their work settings, 20 nurses had been practicing in labor and delivery for 6 months to 17 years: 1 nurse, for 6 months; 8 nurses, 1–2 years; 2 nurses, 2–3 years; 5 nurses, 4–5 years; and 4 nurses, 8, 11, 15, and 17 years, respectively. The fetal monitor had already arrived by the time the remaining 11 nurses began to practice in labor and delivery. I conducted most of these interviews by telephone; the interviews typically lasted about one hour. I mailed each nurse a draft of my interpretation of what she had told me and requested her review and further comment. Several nurses suggested minor revisions, which I incorporated into the final text. The burden of responsibility for the validity of this interpretation remains mine.

In Chapter 7 I consider historical continuities with contemporary debates in nursing and health care. In summary, I have sought to construct a history of the nursing/technology relation that shows its promise and paradox.

2 Object Lessons

Anyone embarking on a study of technology must soon confront its protean manifestations and "equivocal" meanings.[1] Students of technology dance in a minefield and are certain to provoke criticisms of having an overly material or, alternatively, too socioculturally determinist; insufficiently material or, alternatively, insufficiently social or political; and/or, generally, naive, narrow, or wrong view of technology.[2] In the case of medical technology, they are sure to be charged with paying too much attention to the physical "objects" of medicine—its "glass, plastic, [and] metal"—and not enough attention to the clinical and professional "objectives" of physicians, which may not have included any such objects at all.[3] Or they will be charged with paying too little attention to medical instruments and what their characteristics may or may not reveal about medical objectives.[4] In any event, the would-be student of technology is standing on shifting sands, trying to "seek a purchase . . . on the complex reality that is technology."[5]

Paradoxically, there is nothing more elusive and more tangible than technology. Technology most commonly brings to mind an array of tools, machines, and other hardware that engage us by their physical presence.[6] We can see and touch them; they take up space and time. Yet artifacts such as the ultrasound machine and glass have dissolved the usual spatial distinctions between inside and outside.[7] Modern computer technology increasingly entails a virtual reality neither accessible to direct sensation nor comprehensible by commonsense notions of space and time. As Alexandra Chasin observed, "The materiality of electronic machines is so elusive . . . it's as though there's no there there."[8]

We usually conceive of technology as comprised of inanimate things, yet pacemakers implanted near human hearts, artificial hip and knee joints, genetic engineering, and artificial intelligence systems confront us with the reality of and potentiality for living artifacts, vital machines, and cyborgs who/that blur the line between animate and inanimate.[9] "Bodies" have become increasingly "uncertain" as new media/medical technologies have made them more "plastic," "bionic," "interchangeable," and "virtual."[10] Bodies themselves are now "technological artifacts."[11] Corpses, experimental animals, fetuses, and brain-dead-but-otherwise-alive organ donors are components of medical technology that also confound and contest our notions of person and object, natural and artificial, and living and dead.[12] Monica Casper located the fetus "at the margins of humanity," neither human nor non-human but, rather, in the "spaces between . . . this conceptual dualism."[13] Technological (photographic and ultrasonic) displays of the fetus contribute to its marginality. Indeed, several scholars have noted the irony that the fetuses shown to the public as exemplars of life are often actually dead.[14] Lennart Nilsson's pictorial narrative of life before birth was constructed from photographic renderings of fetuses obtained from pregnancy terminations.[15] Contested objects, such as the fetus, exemplify the continuing effacement of the "fourth discontinuity" between human and machine.[16]

We talk about Technology as if it were a monolithic It separable from—that is, fundamentally different from and/or in opposition to— Nature, Culture, and ultimately, human beings, or Us. In fact, English language customs make it difficult not to essentialize as Technology all of the different ideas and things this term has signified throughout history.[17] These linguistic practices favor talking about Technology as if it were a historically changeless entity in a cause-and-effect relation with Nature or Culture (also frequently essentialized, or viewed as fixed and immutable), rather than talking about technologies as historically situated entities in continuous and mutually changing relations with natures and cultures. Although they all comprise Technology, the manual technology of the ancients and the dynamic technology of the Europeans are wholly unlike the computer technology of the modern world and the media/imaging technology of the postmodern world. David Rothenberg observed that no "successful explanation of technology would . . . blur saxophones and motorcycles, or nuclear power plants and ballpoint pens."[18] Yet when we talk about technology as Technology, we persistently blur the distinctions among these objects and forget that the concept of technology itself is subject to historical change, with people in different places and times having different names for what we now think of as technology.[19] Indeed, postmodern scholars conceive of language itself as a technology, thereby effacing the distinction between Technology and talk about technology and thus further complicating the definition of technology.[20] Ruth Oldenziel described technology as a "narrative production of our own times."[21] A "keyword . . . deeply idiomatic in American culture" and having enormous "evocative power," technology has been used as a "weapon" to include some groups and exclude others from its province. As she concluded, the "story" of technology is at least as much the story of the "term" "technology," as it is the story of human creativity, invention, and the production and application of useful knowledge and useful things.[22]

Technology has been variously linked to the arts, crafts, and sciences. Technology has been defined by its hardware and as a set of activities (such as making, designing, and using), as a way to organize labor and social relations, as a typology of knowledge (of making, designing, and using), and as encompassing human choices (concerning what to make, how and/or why to make it, and for whom). Technology has been depicted as both an instrument and a product of culture and nature, as both "social fact and sociological subject," and as both a means to satisfy desire and a stimulus for desire.[23] Arguably, when people consent to use a device, they are also consenting, in part, to the manipulation of their desires. Countering the view of necessity as the mother of invention is the view of invention as the mother of necessity. Accordingly, the technologies we human beings invent to achieve our goals, in turn, reinvent us—the way we think about ourselves, what we do, how we do it, and what we want to do.

In short, technology is inarguably "context dependent" in both "speech and in the world," functioning semiotically as cultural sign, as cultural artifact, and as culture itself.[24] As Bryan Pfaffenberger observed, technology is a "mystifying force of the first order . . . rivalled only by language in its potential . . . for suspending us in webs of significance that we ourselves create."[25] To think about and through technology is to think about and through history and culture, that is, to engage technology as both "fact and symbol" and as constituting both devices and desires.[26]

The Thingness of Technology

For most of the history of Western technology studies and American history, the essence of what we now refer to as technology has been found in its things, that is, in what Carl Mitcham described as its "mode of manifestation" as physical "object."[27] The "electronic technology" at the turn of the twenty-first century increasingly entails a virtual reality essentially devoid of the "robust physical presence" of the tools and machines associated with "industrial technology."[28] But in the minds of most Americans, technology still belongs to the material world at hand's end. Electronic technology still entails electric and telephone wires and the machines they link and power.[29] Indeed, the very materiality, or thingness, of technology has reinforced our belief in the "historical or causal primacy" of technology—that is, to see technology as a determining or driving force of history or, at the very least, as contributing to the "kind of society that invests technologies with enough power to drive history."[30] Even persons (most notably, social science, gender studies, and cultural studies scholars) most concerned that technology not be defined by physical objects nevertheless emphasize these objects (most notably, computers, medical visualization devices, the camera, and film) in their studies of technology.[31] Indeed, these very objects seem to have engendered the postmodern view of, for example, matter as immaterial and language, bodies, and gender themselves as technologies.

As material object, technology entails something physical, but not all physical objects are necessarily technological objects. There are objects of art, such as a sculpture, and objects in nature, such as a pebble on the beach or a stone on a mountain trail. An object becomes a "technological object" largely by virtue of being made, refashioned, or used to perform an activity for some purpose.[32] A stone may remain a stone—an object in nature—with no perceived usefulness, or it may become an implement in the technologies of warfare, hunting, or building. A stuffed animal is a toy to a child, but it becomes a tool in the therapeutic armamentarium of nurses when they use it as a chest splint in breathing exercises.[33] A rocking chair is a homey piece of furniture to sit, nurse a baby, and dream in, but it becomes a pain-relieving agent when nurses use it to ease postsurgical discomfort.[34] Similarly, the bedside table is a piece of furniture in patients' rooms used to hold meals and other necessary items, but it becomes a symptom-management or assistive device when nurses use it to alleviate shortness of breath or to help patients out of bed.

Moreover, as indicated by my inclusion of rocking chairs, toys, and tables in the category of technological object, technology is not just about cars, bombs, or computers. Feminist critics of technology observed that we have tended to see as technology only those devices of primary interest to men, to ignore devices of primary interest to women, and to define and categorize technology in ways that exclude women.[35] Menstrual hygiene products, baby bottles, and washing machines are as technological as cars, bombs, and computers in the sense that they are object means to ends. Moreover, beds, bedpans, and enema cans have been as significant in the care of patients as cardiac monitors, heart-lung machines, and computerized-tomography (CT) scanners.[36] A nurse using a bedside table to help her patient breathe is "no more or less technological" than a nurse using a ventilator.[37] As Autumn Stanley noted, "When technology is no longer just what men do, but what people do, both the definition of technology and the definition of significant technology must inevitably change."[38]

The User Context

Objects thus become technological and components of particular technologies not only by virtue of how they are defined and classified, but also by virtue of how they are used. Indeed, because they are usually conceived of as inanimate things, technological objects are often viewed as value-free or neutral and as acquiring value or non-neutrality only by virtue of how human beings use or abuse them. A popular manifestation of the belief that devices are neutral is the idea that guns do not kill people but, rather, that people do, or in a medical context, that the impact of the ultrasound machine depends solely on how it is used rather than on any inherent feature of the machine itself. Here the nonneutrality of a technology is seen to be derived not from the things themselves but, rather, from what philosopher Don Ihde referred to as their "use-contexts," and from what social scientists have described as the interpretive flexibility of technology.[39] Contrary to the determinist notion of technology as first cause is the view that society and culture determine what technological objects will be and do. As Stefan Timmermans summarized it in his study of resuscitation technology, the "potential and power of a technological device to shape an interaction is not pre-given but is realized in practice."[40] If a technology has any "power," it is "mediated" by social interactions and cultural constraints.[41]

Accordingly, the gun and the ultrasound machine are seen to exert little or no force by themselves in interaction with their users. When obstetricians use it, the ultrasound machine becomes a diagnostic device for monitoring fetal development and detecting fetal impairments. When expectant parents use it, the ultrasound machine becomes an acquaintance device for getting to know their baby.[42] When advertisers use it, the ultrasound image of the fetus becomes a device to sell cars.[43] When entrepreneurs use it, the ultrasound picture itself becomes a highly marketable entertainment commodity.[44] And when pro-life advocates use it, the ultrasound image of the fetus becomes propaganda material for promoting an antiabortion position.[45] Both nurses and physicians use the electronic fetal monitor to detect fetal distress, but when nurses use it to help women maintain control and stay ahead of their contractions, it becomes something other than a mere detection device. In the use context or culture of Western obstetrics, the electronic fetal monitor is an object in the technology of medical surveillance and diagnosis. In the use context or culture of nursing, it is an object in the technology of nursing comfort.

Indeed, the user context can influence the very design of devices. Physician and medical historian Jeffrey Baker showed how the late-nineteenth-century incubator was designed in France to promote the maternal involvement French physicians favored in the care of premature infants; by the early twentieth century, however, it had been redesigned, when it was transferred to the United States, to foster the nutritional and environmental approach to care American physicians preferred.[46] Arguably, there was not one device — the Incubator — but, rather, two devices: the French incubator and the American incubator. Similarly, nineteenth-century sewing machines for home use were designed to look more like furniture and less like machines as a way to resolve the cultural problem of bringing a machine into the home. As Diane Douglas argued, the sewing machine might have been ornamented to "dramatize" its presence. Instead, the favored design hid the sewing machine by encasing it in furniture, which served to reinforce the Victorian ideal of home as a refuge from technology.[47] In a similar vein, a prosthetic arm can be designed primarily for functionality or for looks.[48] The incubator, the sewing machine, and the prosthetic arm illustrate that physical artifacts are also cultural artifacts; artifacts embody cultural ideals, norms, and conflicts.

The Gender Context

For most feminist and, more recently, gender studies scholars, gender is a fundamental feature of the user context of technology and a key analytical tool for understanding it.[49] In contemporary critiques of the gender/technology relation, both gender and technology are viewed as cultural performances that women and men enact.[50] Like technology, the meanings of which are made in use as opposed to given, gender is conceived of as an "emergent feature of social situations" rather than as a stable attribute of women and men.[51] Like technology, gender signals something that is socially, culturally, and historically contingent. Like technology, gender is considered a product and mediator of, as well as an explanation for, various social arrangements. And like technology, gender must therefore always be understood in the context of, and "in relation" to, something else.[52] Encompassing ideas about human relations and what is possible and desirable, gender and technology have been variously regarded in relation to humans, animals, nature, culture, science, and most important to gender studies scholars, each other. Accordingly, gender and technology are practices and devices that are both socially and culturally constructed and mutually shaping; they are inextricable from each other. Gender is "both a determining cultural condition and a social consequence of" technology, and technology, in turn, "functions culturally as a frame or . . . stage for the enactment of gender."[53]

Technologies are thus thought to exert their influence, in part, by virtue of being engendered, and gender exerts its influence by virtue of being literally embodied and/or figuratively embedded in technologies. That is, technologies are discursively (that is, materially and linguistically) engendered by virtue of the Western cultural association between technology and male identity, work, and values; the activities, purposes, meanings, and expectations associated with individual technologies; and the material design features and ergonomics built into technologies.[54] The height, weight, and overall physical dimensions of a device may betray its designers' notions of who its primary user will be and toward what end it will be used. The baby bottle is a female technology by virtue of the fact that primarily women use it in what is perceived culturally as a feminine user context, namely, child care.

Technologies once previously considered masculine have been feminized. Richard Butsch described the "domestication strategy" whereby the "radio's gender" was transformed in the 1920s from exclusively masculine to feminine. The radio was redefined as, and redesigned to become, a "domestic appliance" featuring women, the family, and the home.[55] Sherrie Inness described how mass media were used in the early decades of the twentieth century to "feminize" or alter the once exclusively masculine "gender-coding" of transportation technology (including automobiles and airplanes) to increase their appeal to women.[56] Clinical thermometry became feminized in the late nineteenth century as nurses and mothers became its primary users.[57] In contrast, anesthesia became masculinized as anesthesiology by the 1930s. Because anesthesia was widely viewed in the late nineteenth century and the early decades of the twentieth century as only a "handmaid of surgery" and thus woman's/nurse's work, physicians sought to recode anesthesia as work only a physician ought to do.[58] Even ostensibly gender-neutral technologies, such as computers, are subject to engendering by virtue of the social relations and work processes surrounding them.[59]

Although technologies, whether originally coded or recoded as feminine or masculine, have helped women overcome gender constraints, they have also (or according to many feminist critics and gender studies scholars, more often) served to reinforce them. Butsch described how radio advertising appealed to but also exploited women to show how easy it was to use a radio; that is, "even" a woman could do it. In women's hands the radio became a domestic appliance, like the refrigerator and the stove, not the new, exciting, and masculine communication technology it had been just a few years earlier. As Butsch proposed, the domestication of the radio "reaffirmed the boundaries between masculine technology and feminine domesticity"; it did not transcend them.[60] Indeed, as Butsch further argued and as historians of women and technology have recurringly demonstrated, the domestication of technology, often achieved through advertising and other mass media, has been a key strategy for "feminizing technologies" and reinforcing gender norms and expectations.[61] Inness concluded that although girls' serial novels appeared to challenge stereotypes about women's relationships to technology, they ultimately reinforced the idea that men were inventors but women were only consumers of technology.[62] In short, as gender/technology studies have shown, not only do "artifacts have politics," but they specifically have "gender politics."[63] Technology is "saturated" with gender.[64] And whenever it reproduces existing gender expectations and relations, technology freezes rather than transcends gender.[65]

It is misleading, however, and even naive to think of technological objects as wholly dependent on their user contexts, as having unlimited interpretive flexibility. Historian Ruth Schwartz Cowan warned that tools are "not entirely passive instruments . . . [and] not always at our beck and call."[66] Although flexible to a certain extent, they are not wholly plastic to our will. As much as scholars may want to avoid the "black-box view" of technology, they must still contend with black boxes.[67] As Alan Prout concluded in his study of the metered dose inhaler, objects have agency separate from their inventors and users. Medical devices are not "merely props for social action" but, rather, like human beings, are "actors in social processes."[68] As Julian Orr observed, "Machines are a social presence through their participation in the social world."[69] They motivate human action and stimulate notice. Like human beings, machines have their own individual characters, histories, and quirks.[70]

Technological objects are what they are, not only by virtue of how and why they are used but also of what they physically are. What technological objects physically are certainly reflects human design choices concerning style, shape, color, materials, the availability of materials, and desires to achieve certain ends. But once devised, these objects acquire a "life of their own."[71] By virtue of both form and function, technological objects have what Corlann Bush described as "valence"; that is, like atoms, they are charged. David Rothenberg referred to the "latent language" of devices, and Don Ihde pointed out their "latent telic inclinations" and "implicit rhythms."[72] These objects "push" or "pull" their users in certain directions.[73]

The gun is "valenced to violence"; that is, it raises the likelihood of killing simply by virtue of its presence.[74] Because guns permit fast killing, they allow users to kill on impulse. In contrast to the hands or other devices used to kill, the gun does not permit users to change their minds. Once discharged, a bullet cannot be stopped. Persons using their hands or other implements often retain the option to restrain themselves before they have killed. Similarly, electronic mail (e-mail) is valenced toward impulsive behavior, as it permits us to respond immediately (often with disastrous results) without pondering what the best response would be. Unlike a letter we can tear up or retrieve after venting our emotions into it, an e-mail message—once sent—cannot be recalled. Like the bullet in a well-aimed gun, the sent e-mail message will hit its mark.

Devices such as ultrasound machines, cardiac and fetal monitors, and CT scanners change not only what we see but also how we see. Indeed, they require us to learn to see in new ways, as they produce images unnatural to the eye. Barron Lerner, for example, pointed out that CT images are not visual representations of the body but, rather, products of multiple x-ray projections of a cross-section of the body fed into a computer, which, via a mathematical algorithm, reconstructs the internal structures scanned.[75] Such technologies do not entail seeing in traditional ways, since they involve an optical display of properties (such as density or mass) initially conceived in terms other than optical; that is, they offer optical renderings of nonoptically computed data.[76] The viewer sees with these technologies, but it is a seeing no longer dependent on an observing subject, as these devices "separate the visual from an observing subject and from all those older modes of seeing that rely on perspective, or a fixed or mobile point of view."[77]

Fetal ultrasonography entails the paradox of "seeing with sound."[78] The image displayed—of the fetus "float(ing) disembodied in its amnesiac ahistorical representational space"[79]—permits the viewer to see the fetus as if it were independently viable and amaternal. Moreover, so-called real-time ultrasonic images are created so rapidly that a "cinematic view" of the fetus is produced whereby the illusion is maintained that the fetus imaged is—right here and now—in actual and natural motion.[80] The fetal sonogram itself is thus an actor that contributes to the process of signification that permits physicians to see the fetus as if it were a patient, parents to see it as if it were a baby, and entrepreneurs to sell the sonogram image as if it were a video of a baby.

Moreover, the features and style of a device may alter human work and behavior. Cardiac and fetal monitors "mesmerize" and "dramatize" simply by virtue of their physical presence and characteristics.[81] As one nurse observed, their flashing lights and bleeping sounds are "dramatic and exciting . . . attention-getters . . . [that] distract our eye from the patient" and demand notice.[82] Like television, monitors are valenced to "individuation" in that people are drawn to look at these machines instead of interacting with one another.[83] Indeed, clinicians and visitors at the patient's bedside must actively work to move their eyes away from monitors in order to counter the seemingly magnetic pull of the devices.

Technological objects also create a certain look, sound, and feel (like the machine-age atmosphere of the intensive care unit), and they are often sources of "aesthetic delight" or discomfort.[84] Indeed, technological objects are good examples of how things designed for other than aesthetic purposes can have an even greater influence on the "aesthetic consciousness" than objects typically considered works of art.[85] In U.S. culture, the car, the gun, the computer, and the ultrasound machine are important sources of aesthetic experience, variously stimulating the senses and emotions.

The aesthetic and work of writing is different depending on whether a pen, a typewriter, or a computer is employed. One can argue that we are not writing anymore when we use anything other than a pen or pencil but, rather, are engaged in typing or processing words. Suggesting that "handwriting is more connected to the movement of the heart," Natalie Goldberg, a teacher of writing, admonished would-be writers to "choose your tools carefully," as they "affect the way we form our thoughts."[86] In a similar vein, the replacement of the hand with a tocodynamometer to sense uterine contractions has altered clinical appraisal work. The clinician no longer palpates the uterus but, instead, sees contraction patterns on paper. In addition, while the hand entails direct tactile contact with a pregnant woman's abdomen, the monitor requires no body contact at all, as the "self" of the patient has been transferred to, and resides in, the screen.[87]

Technological objects also have purposes that can be usefully conceived of as separate from human purposes. The "device purpose" of the cardiac monitor is to sense and display the electrical activity of the heart.[88] In contrast, the clinician's purpose for using the cardiac monitor is to detect life-threatening cardiac events as they are occurring in order to prevent their morbid or lethal consequences. Although devices can be employed for purposes other than the ones for which they were designed, they cannot be used for infinite or any purposes. Cardiac monitors were designed to show heart activity. By virtue of their weight, they can also be used as door stops (although using them this way fails to make "sense" of these machines),[89] but they cannot be used to hold dressings in place. Human beings can appropriate, modify, and work around physical devices for their own purposes, but these artifacts themselves set limits for these activities.

Indeed, devices can also be usefully perceived as having purposes in opposition to human purposes. For example, Ihde described the tape recorder as an undiscriminating "sense-datum empiricist" for which all sounds are equally meaningful.[90] That is, the tape recorder is in-clined to record all sound available to it, even though its highly dis-criminating human user is likely to be interested only in certain sounds and to be overwhelmed by too many sounds. In an analogous vein, cer-tain physical features of fetal monitors incline them to over- or under-count signals, thereby misrepresenting the fetal heart rate. The "inclina-tions" of such monitoring devices challenge their human designers and users to recognize and even counter this implicit feature.[91] All moni-toring equipment obliges clinicians to separate factual from artifac-tual recordings — to recognize machine error. Texts on fetal monitoring interpretation, for example, typically contain information on "facti-tious" machine recordings and "dysrhythmias masked by instrument char-acteristics."[92]

The Second Self, Second Nature, and Secondhand Knowledge

Although the essence of technology may be said still to re-side in tangible things, thingness has tended, in turn, to overshadow the knowledge residing in technology. The word "technology" etymo-logically contains "thought" (logos) and thus connotes knowledge.[93] The definition of technology as "know-how" is much older than its association with machines. Yet know-how is often seen as an inferior form of knowledge. Especially in the health care arena, technology is commonly viewed as nothing more than applied science, that is, as the implementation of scientific knowledge with drugs and devices.[94] The definition of technology as the largely thoughtless application of medical science, when combined with a definition of nursing as a tech-nology, has served to undermine and undervalue the knowledge in both nursing and technology.

The ideas that technology is merely applied science and that it con-stitutes no knowledge itself have lost favor. Historian Eugene Fergu-son observed that the modern assumption that whatever knowledge resides in technology must be derived from science is "a bit of mod-ern folklore" that ignores "non-scientific modes of thought." The many artifacts around us are as they are because their makers have established their shapes, styles, and textures. These properties were thought about and visualized in the "mind's eye" but "cannot be reduced to unam-biguous verbal descriptions." As Ferguson noted, "Pyramids, cathe-drals, and rockets exist not because of geometry, theory of structures, or thermodynamics, but because they were first a picture—literally a vision—in the minds of those who built them."[95]

The close tie that now exists between Western technology and science is fairly recent, since what is currently referred to as technology used to be more closely linked to art and craft by virtue of an emphasis on design, aesthetic vision, utility, and skilled making.[96] The idea of the dependency of technology on science became entrenched only after the seventeenth-century revolution in Western science.[97] Emphasizing the actual practice of science, as opposed to its theoretical products, historians, philosophers, social scientists, and critical theorists have, since the 1960s, increasingly challenged the text(story)book image of the relationship between nature, science, and technology.[98] In this story, nature poses questions for and is subsequently explained by and mirrored in science, which, in turn, provides the basis for the technology that is used further to reveal and to control nature.[99] The narrative line in this image or story can be formalized as follows:

Nature → Science → Technology → Nature.

Although contemporary science and technology are so intertwined as to be often indistinguishable, many important technological innovations have preceded or owe nothing to science.[100] As James Maxwell argued, the telescope (which evolved from other technologies) made possible the discovery that the planets revolve around the sun. The invention of the steam engine led to the development of thermodynamics. The iron lung contributed to the enhanced understanding of respiratory physiology.[101] Although science has never been independent of technology, technology has been independent of science.[102] Indeed, technology may have a distinctive epistemology characterized by a practical-artifactual orientation, the central activity of which is design.[103] The relation between technology and art and craft is most visible in design.

One contemporary philosophical view of the science/technology relation that emphasizes human perception and practices is philosopher Don Ihde's conceptualization of "instrumental realism."[104] Instrumental realism prioritizes technology (over science) and emphasizes the transformation of nature (or reality or the world) by the technology employed ostensibly to reveal it. This view can be formalized as follows:

$\text{Nature}_1 \rightarrow \text{Technology} \rightarrow \text{Science} \rightarrow \text{Nature}_2$.

According to Ihde modern science is necessarily embodied in technology. The scientific reality intended to correspond to nature is, in actuality, a reality mediated by instruments, such as the telescope and the microscope. As Ihde argued, it is not technology that is the product or embodiment of science but, rather, modern science that is the product of technology and that is "technologically embodied. . . . Instruments form the conditions for and are the mediators of much, if not all, current scientific knowledge."[105] Technological objects permit scientists to see and shape (that is, to magnify or reduce) what they see. Science is largely visual by virtue of the instrumentation that enhances vision and the visual products of this instrumentation (such as photographs, rhythm strips, and graphs) that are subsequently seen and studied as nature.[106] Scientific activity is thus not about nature per se but about constructing nature.[107] This nature is, in turn, largely technologically constructed.

As the product of a technology-dependent science, nature is thus more made than found. Technology is a "practical engagement" with nature (Nature $_1$) that produces a new nature (Nature $_2$).[108] Rothenberg observed that the windmill reveals the power of the wind and the shovel discloses the nature of the soil. We grasp the significance of Niagara Falls (Nature) because of the tunnel (Technology) that brings us closer to it.[109] Yet the falls and our relationship with the falls are changed by virtue of the tunnel. Technology extends us into the world and, in the process, re-creates it. It is a recurring paradox that we use technology to reach nature but always lose it as it was because the very act of reaching for it changes it. Nature is thus always out of human reach because it cannot be what it was prior to our reaching for it. Allucquere Rosanne Stone noted how paradoxical it was that "the more we call 'that which becomes known' by the name 'reality,' the further we distance ourselves from it."[110] Our technology seems to make reality more intelligible and reachable, but it is a reality we no longer directly experience. Our understanding of the world or nature is increasingly technologically mediated and constructed; it is "secondhand" knowledge.[111] Not only is the nature that we—as part of nature and creators of artifice—strive toward altered by the things we use to reach it, but our very experiences of self are changed as well. We invent things, but they, in turn, (re)invent us, creating a new or "second self."[112]

Technology thus reveals and transforms nature, but it also conceals how it reveals and transforms. We are infected with a kind of "thought virus" that erases the evidence of its work as soon as it is finished, thereby blurring the boundaries between nature and what we do to perceive it.[113] The nature/technology dichotomy is thus an outmoded and even false opposition. Nature is not so easily separated from artifice, as instrument-mediated reality is nature in a new guise. Technology is "humanized nature."[114] Indeed, "what is natural is man's [sic] artifice."[115] Technology is second nature to us now, foreground and background to our lives and inside our bodies.

Instrumental Knowledge

As a practical engagement with the world accomplished through the making ("bringing into existence") and using ("putting into practice") of artifacts, technology is a kind of knowing of, in, and through doing and a kind of knowing that is different from knowing the world directly through the senses.[116] Ihde formalized this immediate and "in-the-flesh" knowing as follows:[117]

Human → World.

He also differentiated between four kinds of technological knowing, or human/machine, or human/technology, epistemic relations.[118] Indeed, as his phenomenology of the human/machine relation shows, different technologies entail different kinds of relations.

In *embodiment relations*, devices extend the senses. Indeed, in perfect embodiment relations, devices withdraw from notice to such an extent that they become almost transparent to the human user whose "I" is extended beyond body limits. Once users get used to them, and if they are properly matched to the user and functioning well, contact lenses allow users to forget that their vision is not immediate but, rather, instrumentally mediated. Ihde formalized embodiment human/technology relations as follows:

(Human − technology) → World).

Ihde used the example of the dental probe—a device that extends the user's tactile intentionality, or reach into the world—to illustrate embodied relations. Like the contact lens, the dental probe is experienced by the trained user as "quasi-me." The probe is an epistemic device; that is, it makes information about the tooth available to the user. Indeed, it amplifies knowledge, as it offers information about the tooth not available to the naked finger. Yet while the probe obviously amplifies knowledge, it also not so obviously reduces knowledge of the tooth only to what can be obtained through the probe. That is, while the probe provides information about the tooth that the unaided finger cannot provide (for example, pitting areas of decay), only the finger can provide information about the temperature and wetness of the tooth. According to Ihde it is a phenomenological principle of modern human/technology relations that with every amplification of experience made possible by an instrument, there is a simultaneous and generally unnoticed reduction of experience. We tend to notice technological amplifications or enhancements and thus perceive them as dramatic—hence our awe concerning technology. In contrast, we tend to overlook and even trivialize what we have lost as a consequence of these enhancements, which includes not only the tooth as it was before it was instrumentally probed (Tooth $_1$) but also often the skill of probing the tooth with only our fingers and the knowledge that can come only from this immediate probing.

While embodiment relations with devices extend our sensory capabilities and reach into the world, *hermeneutic relations* extend our interpretive capacities. In hermeneutic human/technology relations, not only is reality transformed by what instruments permit us to know of it, but the information produced is itself an altered representation of reality. Ihde formalized this relation as follows:

Human $\rightarrow$ (technology – World).

When clinicians appraise patient temperature with mercury thermometers or automated temperature devices instead of their hands, they are not engaging in the embodied activity of actually sensing variations in temperature (as when they touch a patient's brow to ascertain the presence of fever) but, rather, in the hermeneutic activity of reading or interpreting a text. Clinicians learn to interpret the height of a column of mercury in a glass thermometer or the digital display on an automated temperature device, both of which stand for— but which the clinician does not directly experience as—differences in temperature. Hermeneutic relations with devices involve relationships even more secondhand, or removed from the flesh or direct sensory experience, than embodied relations. Knowledge is not obtained from the senses directly or by extension but from interpretive readings of the texts machines produce, such as rhythm strips, numbers, and other visual displays.

Despite the fact that these texts often produce multiple and even conflicting readings among different readers, and artifactual (as opposed to factual) readings, there is a tendency to treat these displays as more real than direct experience. These texts of experience are taken to be natural traces and documentary evidence of the real things they represent and thus become real themselves. The line between the world and the devices used to perceive it is made increasingly contingent. For example, the fetus in utero is the fetus on-screen; the fetal heart is the electrical tracing of the heart on a roll of paper. Our knowledge of the fetus is amplified by ultrasonography and electronic monitoring, but in the process the fetus is reduced only to what we see on screen and on paper. Indeed, the fetus we know today is arguably what Ihde referred to as a technologically "carpentered" entity.[119] Historian Barbara Duden concluded that the human fetus is no longer the "creature of God or natural fact" it used to be for most of human history; it has become an "engineered construct of modern society."[120] This newly synthesized fetus is an entity that anyone can see; the historical fetus was a being accessible only through the "carnal knowledge" pregnant women alone possessed.[121]

In contrast to embodiment relations, where devices are experienced as quasi-me, in *alterity relations* they are experienced as "quasi-other." Ihde formalized alterity relations as follows:

Human → technology − (− World).

There is a stronger sense in alterity relations of interacting with something other than, albeit having some similarity to, oneself. Such relations can be said to lie on a continuum between I-It and I-Thou relations.[122] This quasi-otherness may manifest itself as quasi-animation or quasi-autonomy, where users positively or negatively experience a device as having a life and will of its own. Ihde referred to the computer as a strong example of the love-hate relationships often evident in alterity relations with devices and the tendency to animate and even to anthropomorphize devices romantically. As depicted in many (science) fictional treatments of human/technology relations, the machine can be experienced either as a friendly and helpful automaton or as a Frankensteinian monster gone wild.[123]

Background human/technology relations entail relations among machines, rather than with them per se. Ihde formalized these relations as follows:

Human → (machine
       World).

Technology is a pervasive feature of most human environments in the West; it is part of the general atmosphere, with behind-the-scenes technology (such as utilities) entering the home and workplace but remaining virtually unnoticed until a breakdown occurs. In background relations we do not experience ourselves relating to technology per se; instead, these relations comprise the environment we inhabit. Technological environments have become the natural habitats of most Westerners and of much caregiving in the home and hospital. Indeed, so natural are these habitats that the distinction between low and high technology seems less useful.

The Effects of Technology

Although technology is *of* and *in* nature, culture, and human beings, it can still be usefully conceived of as having effects *on* these entities. Moreover, although these effects are most often depicted in essentializing, binary, and oppositional terms that tend toward oversimplification, speaking about the effects of technology nevertheless captures some truths about technology. Two distinct but related debates about the effects of technology concern whether it serves as a force primarily for cultural stability or change and whether it serves as a force primarily for liberation or oppression.

The More Things Change . . .

Most Americans generally see technology as a force for cultural change. Few people would deny that cars, televisions, and computers have altered how we think about and live in the world and how we see ourselves in it. An illustrative case in point is the spectrum of reproductive technologies that have irrevocably altered the way we see and experience sexuality, conception, pregnancy, childbirth, and parenthood.[124] Even if we ourselves have never used them to manage our reproductive lives, these technologies have nevertheless altered our understandings of time, space, and social relations. They have also made the traditional biological role of the female in reproduction seem less unique and even less necessary, and they have made us revise existing notions of fetal viability and personhood.

For example, contraceptive and conceptive techniques have permitted the link to be severed between sexual intercourse and procreation. Engaging in sexual relations no longer necessarily entails conception, nor does conception necessarily require sexual intercourse. Conceptive techniques permit different women to be genetic, gestational, and social mother of the same child. Human pregnancy is no longer necessarily nine months long, as conceptive and neonatal technologies have permitted the embryo/fetus to spend less time inside a woman's body and still survive. In vitro fertilization has prolonged the experiential (as opposed to biological) process of getting pregnant, as women and men are now conscious of each step leading to conception. Techniques for early pregnancy diagnosis also make pregnancy seem longer, as they allow women to learn of their pregnancies within days of conception. Peri-conceptive, conceptive, and prenatal technologies together have contributed to the earlier parental, medical, and social recognition of the fetus as a baby and as a patient. Couples may, accordingly, become invested in their babies earlier in pregnancy, thereby deriving either more enjoyment or more suffering should the attempts at pregnancy be unsuccessful or the baby be lost. Prior to the development of external fertilization and early pregnancy diagnosis techniques, early pregnancy losses were likely to remain unnoticed.

Reproductive technologies have also been instrumental in the creation of new patients, new orientations to existing patients, and new definitions of pathology.[125] In addition to the creation of the fetal patient, reproductive technologies have allowed patient status to be extended to normally fertile and normally infertile women and to not-yet-infertile persons. Conceptive technology depends on the willingness of normally fertile women to donate eggs and wombs and to undergo infertility treatments on behalf of their infertile male partners. The very availability of conceptive technology for women in their forties, fifties, and even sixties has called into question whether the infertility associated with the (post)menopausal period is really normal. Practitioners are now encouraged to see cancer patients as potential infertility patients whose chemotherapy-induced infertility can be treated with conceptive techniques.

Although new technologies may contribute to many profound changes, they also often reinforce existing cultural values and social practices and arrangements. Technological change does not necessarily entail any cultural change at all. Fundamentalist feminist critics of technology, in particular, have observed how resistant to change existing gender norms and expectations are. In the case of reproductive technologies, they have argued that these technologies have largely perpetuated the cultural status quo, allowing gender, race, and class inequalities to remain unchallenged. For example, in vitro fertilization techniques reinforce the cultural emphasis on the importance of having a biological child and the tendency to treat women, even for male dysfunctions. Contraceptive techniques, which have been developed for and used by women almost exclusively, reinforce the cultural expectation that women are responsible for the outcomes of sexual relations. In the areas of race and class, conceptive techniques are much more available to white and economically privileged couples, while contraceptive techniques are more likely to be directed to minority and less economically privileged couples.

In a similar vein, household appliances have been commonly viewed as freeing women from housework. Yet although housework may now be physically less arduous, women continue to spend as much and even more time doing housework as they did before the advent of devices such as washing machines and vacuum cleaners. In fact, the very ease with which these devices can be used has raised the standard of cleanliness women must meet.[126]

Moreover, new technologies have actually or rhetorically de-skilled women. The early-twentieth-century introduction of artificial infant feeding actually de-skilled women in breast feeding and reinforced the role of physicians as experts in the care of children.[127] As women increasingly used technologies once reserved primarily for men, those technologies became easy enough even for a woman to use. Skill became "saturated with sex," as women's use of technology was rhetorically downgraded, even as it actually expanded.[128]

Accordingly, in the matter of technological change, the more things change, the more they arguably stay the same, as prevailing cultural assumptions and values are often hidden in new technologies. Diana Forsythe showed how the traditional social relations between physicians and patients and between physicians and nurses were incorporated into the design of a computerized information system intended to convey ostensibly objective information to and, thus, empower patients.[129] As she argued, this system failed to realize its democratizing potential by magnifying the voices of physicians while trivializing the voices of patients and wholly muting the voices of nurses. Similar concerns have been expressed that computerized information systems in hospitals will simply reinforce the invisibility of nursing work.[130]

Closely tied to the discussion concerning whether technology is chiefly an agent for stability or for change is the debate about whether technology is primarily a force for liberation or for oppression. The prevalent Western belief is that technological innovation means progress and thus constitutes a force for good. In the reproductive arena, for example, contraceptive techniques have given women the material means to control their lives, to pursue goals other than motherhood, and to protect themselves from the physical and psychic ravages of unwanted and untimely pregnancies. Contraceptive techniques have freed women to enter the mainstream of American life in equal partnership with men because they have allowed women to regulate a major biological function that has historically impeded equal partnership, namely, maternity.

In contrast to the belief that technology is a force for liberation is the conviction that it is an agent of oppression and a threat to humanity. Fundamentalist feminist critics of reproductive technologies have emphasized the iatrogenic harm caused by ineffective and/or unsafe devices and therapies. Moreover, they have argued that instead of expanding women's control and choices, these technologies have narrowed them. Indeed, the expansion of choice that proponents of these technologies promise is illusory. Reproductive technologies may permit unprecedented control over reproductive events, but unplanned pregnancies still occur, relatively few couples have a baby after undergoing in vitro techniques, and impaired infants are still born.

In addition, for every choice made available by a technology, another choice is made increasingly unavailable. The very existence of techniques such as amniocentesis to detect fetal impairment and in vitro fertilization to circumvent infertility makes the option not to choose these techniques less acceptable. Couples often find it difficult to turn them down. Because fetal ultrasonography and electronic monitoring have been incorporated into the standard of care, physicians have to defend why they may decide not to use them. The technological imperative is thus the imperative to choose. Opportunities become mandates as the freedom to choose becomes the compulsion to choose. Technological innovations also produce a chain of burden as one choice leads to other mandates to choose. For example, the couple that opts to have an amniocentesis will have to decide whether to terminate or to maintain a pregnancy in the event that a fetal impairment is detected. This mandate to choose did not exist before the advent of diagnostic techniques such as amniocentesis.

Technological innovations thus call into question the very meaning of innovation, progress, and choice. They dramatize the "deflective power" of technologies, not only to hide the old in the ostensibly new, but also to mask the limitations to freedom they often entail.[131] They also dramatize the extent to which we have become dependent on technology to achieve our purposes and satisfy our desires—to see technology as solution rather than as problem. Depending on one's vantage point, conceptive technologies, for example, may constitute a response to the problem of infertility, when it is considered the inability to have a biologically related child. Conceptive technologies themselves, however, may constitute the problem when they are seen to embody harmful patriarchal, pronatalist, and capitalist norms.[132]

Meaningful Technology

Technologies are what they are, become what they are, and/or exert their effects by virtue of their valences and inclinations, their user or cultural contexts, the epistemic relations they entail, and the way they use and produce culture.[133] Technologies also are and/or become what they are by virtue of the meanings they have and the meanings they hold for us. Any one technology leads a "double life."[134] On one hand, a technology is limited by virtue of its thingness; that is, there are hard(ware) limits to what a technology can mean, to what it can do, and for what it can be used. On the other hand, a technology is limitless by virtue of everything we can read into it, design it to be, use it for, and construe it as against. In the nineteenth century, physicians viewed the vaginal speculum as an instrument of female corruption. In the late 1960s, women's health activists viewed it as an instrument of female power.[135] Computer technology is an example of a technology whose meaning is further doubled by virtue of being not only a text itself but also by carrying texts in its programs and software.

As Alan Trachtenberg concluded about the Brooklyn Bridge, technologies function as "fact and symbol."[136] Tools can become metaphors that capture a zeitgeist. The computer, for example, is for David Bolter a "defining technology" of the Computer Age in that it "metaphorical[ly] . . . links . . . with a culture's science, philosophy, or literature . . . [and] is always available to serve as a metaphor."[137] A defining technology does not so much cause cultural change as it "collects and focuses seemingly disparate ideas in a culture into one bright, sometimes piercing ray." [138] The computer now serves as a "metaphor we live by" and a model for human intelligence. [139] By making a machine think like a human being, human beings re-create and define themselves as machines; the human brain, in turn, becomes an information system, like the computer. The computer is, as Sherry Turkle described it, like a "second self" and is only the most recent example of how technology has become the means by which we define and talk about ourselves; [140] it is also, paradoxically, the means by which we forget how technology serves to reinvent ourselves. As Bolter noted in the case of the computer, biologists and psychologists have so "thoroughly absorbed the technology" that they no longer see themselves as explaining the brain "in terms" of the computer but, rather, as comparing two " 'thinking systems,' " the human brain and the computer. [141]

The Duality of Technology

The conceptualization of technology that best captures the "object lessons" I have just reviewed, and the larger framework for this study of the nursing/technology relation, is Wanda Orlikowski's adaptation—for information technology and organization studies— of Anthony Giddens's theory of structuration. [142] Orlikowski proposed that a structuration model of technology allows scholars to embrace the various dualities of technology as material fact and social construction, as cause and consequence, and as trigger and mediator of change. The model also unites the design and use of technology, elements traditionally seen as separate. In the structuration model of technology, design and use come together, as users are conceived of as designers; users appropriate a technology-as-designed and modify it for their own purposes. Technology is envisioned as a medium of human action, as it variously facilitates and constrains human behavior (including design, development, and application) and human choice. These factors are, in turn, influenced by human engagement with technology, which can transform or reinforce structures of signification, domination, and legitimation or the shared meanings, power relations, and norms enacted and (re)produced in those engagements. The duality of technology thus lies in its recursiveness and in its existence as both objective, material force and as socially constructed entity, as separate from and continuous with human behavior, and as both device and desire. [143]

CHAPTER 3

The Utensils & Materials at Hand

From the appearance in the late 1870s of the first trained nurses, who practiced primarily in the home, through the 1940s, when nursing took place primarily in the hospital, nursing practice in the United States was almost exclusively concerned with the physical, that is, with the corporeal and the material.[1] Nurses observed, comforted, and treated the bodies of ailing patients and childbearing women, and they managed the physical environment (including people and physical objects) around them.[2] Nursing practice was largely body work, as the "object body" of the patient was the focal concern of the nurse and the object body of the nurse was the critical element in ministering to the patient.[3] Indeed, nurses would "lend their bodies as virtual prostheses for the ailing and inadequate bodies" of their patients.[4] The patient's body was the primary "site" of the nurse's work, and her body was the primary "tool" with which she accomplished it.[5]

Nursing practice entailed "in-the-flesh" techniques, such as observation, positioning, and lifting, which involved nurses' "trained" but unaided senses of sight, hearing, smell, and touch; deft and gentle hands; and strong back and limbs.[6] Nurses refined all of their senses for the close observation that would make nursing a scientific profession as opposed to merely a mechanical practice.[7] They developed the manual dexterity and sure, swift, and sensitive touch that would make trained nurses indispensable to patients and physicians, and they cultivated the physical prowess that would allow them to withstand the rigors of nursing.[8] Nursing practice was physically arduous and required nurses to push, pull, lift, and carry heavy patients and objects and, in the hospital, to walk "endless miles" in the course of a routine day to accomplish their duties.[9] Although nurses were cautioned to "use [their] eyes and ears, but not the tongue," they were to utilize their voices to soothe patients.[10] Indeed, nurses were initially viewed as ideal for administering anesthesia because, for one reason, the feminine voice was seen to calm the patient for an easier induction; nurse anesthesia was often referred to as "vocal anesthesia."[11]

Although in-the-flesh procedures were critical to nursing, the vast majority of nursing work included an increasing array of device-mediated procedures requiring the use of appliances, utensils, implements, mechanical devices, and other material objects. These procedures included feeding; bathing; medicating; irrigating; catheterizing; purging; administering heliotherapy, hydrotherapy, electrotherapy, and fever therapy; applying poultices, pads, and other paraphernalia to deliver chemicals, cold, or heat to the body; and setting bandages, splints, and other devices and contraptions to support or exert pressure or traction on various body parts. Even with the increasing availability, by the early twentieth century, of utilities that reduced physical labor, such as electricity and central plumbing, these aids relied for their use largely on the manual dexterity, manipulations, and/or muscle power of the nurse. The body of the nurse was still the most important tool in her growing armamentarium. The material world of the nurse in the late nineteenth and early twentieth centuries typically involved familiar and everyday objects, or the "common utensils and appliances" generally found in the home and not at all distinctive to nursing or medical practice.[12]

Indeed, nursing practice through the 1940s included a wide range of household and domestic work and, therefore, entailed cooking, housekeeping, laundry, and child care crafts. Examples of everyday objects found in both the home and the hospital were the beds and tables comprising the typical bed/sickroom and the materials, implements, and chemical solutions used for bed making, bathing, bandaging, feeding, and cleaning. Stopwatches (to count the pulse), safety pins, needles and threads, ice picks, and matches were included among the "equipment of the nurse's bag."[13] Early anesthesia, for which nurses were often responsible, involved no more than a "bottle and rag."[14]

Although there were relatively few objects in the nurse's world in the early decades of trained nursing that distinguished her work from that of other women, the trained nurse was to be distinguished from other women by the skillful use of these things. While women might arrange flowers, nurses cared for them as part of the management of the environment around the patient.[15] Women might make beds, but nurses used beds to comfort and treat patients. Indeed, the bed was an object that demanded the nurse's painstaking attention.[16] As the prominent nurse educator Bertha Harmer put it, the "greatest part of her work is around, about, and with the bed."[17] Patients suffering from enervating respiratory and gastrointestinal infections, fevers, and other conditions for which there were no treatments except the care of the nurse were often "condemned to weeks of imprisonment in bed."[18] Many kinds of beds were described in instructional texts for nurses throughout this period, differentiated by cases (such as surgical versus obstetric), therapeutic intent or purpose (for resting versus the pelvic examination), and the primary therapeutic modality employed (air beds versus water beds).[19] Nurses expressed preferences for what they viewed as the best materials out of which to make beds (including brass, iron, or wood) and bedding (linen, straw, or rubber) to achieve the various purposes for which beds were used and to facilitate maintenance, hygiene, and comfort. Several kinds of bandages, poultices, and other external remedies, as well as cleansing and therapeutic baths, were also important foci of didactic literature for nurses, with instructions including the materials and containers needed to make, apply, or provide the most functional, effective, comfortable, and aesthetically pleasing treatments.[20] When perfectly applied, a spiral bandage, for example, was beautifully symmetrical and provided the correct pressure or support.

Although late-nineteenth-century nursing practice usually entailed common household objects, twentieth-century practice increasingly required the use of items that signaled something more specialized than ordinary women's work. But again, nurses were not the only ones who utilized this special equipment. While they shared the use (albeit in unique ways) of common utensils and appliances with other women, nurses shared specialty objects—including implements such as thermometers, hypodermic syringes, and urinary catheters, and devices such as the incubator and the respirator—with physicians. In many cases nurses were the primary and, arguably, more proficient users of these special items because they utilized them more often than physicians and were better able than physicians to determine when and under what conditions special equipment should be used. Yet these objects were viewed as medical (as opposed to nursing) equipment, to be used only by order or under the direction of physicians. Physicians viewed nursing care in general as a kind of medical therapy and, therefore, largely subject to being ordered.[21] For example, the various kinds of baths that were central to the encounter between nurses and patients were also mainstays of late-nineteenth- and early-twentieth-century medical therapy and, therefore, had to be ordered by a physician.[22] The therapeutic bath exemplified how work performed exclusively by nurses was nevertheless conceptually located within medical treatment.

The devices nurses typically used in their practice generally extended their reach *over* but also *into* the patient's body. Most nursing practice through the 1940s involved ministrations to the outside of the body, including applications of heat and cold, poultices and dressings, and splints and bandages. But nurses also used techniques to enter body orifices. They instilled and removed air and gases, fluids, and substances for various cleansing, nutritional, and other therapeutic purposes. They used inhalers, tents, and other devices to deliver various kinds of respiratory and oxygen therapies, and they employed bottles, cans, and tubing to suction, gavage, lavage, evacuate, douche, irrigate, and catheterize body cavities. Bodily entries to remove excrement and other waste increasingly distinguished nursing from medical practice and emphasized the viscerality and "dirty work" of everyday nursing practice.[23] Such entries bound nurses and patients in the most intimate and often embarrassing and even repugnant human contacts.[24]

Fewer nursing procedures in this period involved "clean," or deep and, therefore, sterile, entries into the body. Although nurses gave hypodermic injections in the late nineteenth century and hypodermoclysis infusions in the early twentieth century (both involving the insertion of sterile needles in tissue just beneath the skin), not until well into the 1930s was the deeper intramuscular injection considered appropriate for nurses routinely to administer.[25] Intravenous instillations of blood and other fluids and removal of blood remained controversial as nursing functions until well into the 1960s.[26] Except in dire circumstances, such as the unavailability of a physician or conditions of war, activities that involved the deep/sterile penetration of the body with a needle or other implement were seen as largely in the physician's domain, with nurses assigned an assistive function. Assistance here, though, typically meant doing everything involved in the procedure except the discrete act of penetrating the body. Whether assisting physicians to perform a thoracentesis, paracentesis, lumbar puncture, or the deepest physical penetration of all—surgery—nurses were expected to have the knowledge to match the right equipment to both the procedure and the physician, prepare and arrange the equipment, ready the patient and the room, and care for the patient, room, and equipment after the procedure, which included watching the patient for untoward treatment effects and cleaning up.

Whether reaching over or into the patient's body, most of the devices nurses used during this period extended the nurse's hand and, vicariously, the physician's hand. Few devices nurses used extended either their senses or interpretive capacities. That is, nurses used few objects that helped them see, hear, or feel the patient's body better or differently. Except for minimal applications in the classroom, nurses did not use sense extenders such as the microscope. Taking the blood pressure with a stethoscope (a sense entender, in this case, of the ear) and with a sphygmomanometer (a device entailing the reading of a column of mercury) did not become part of routine nursing practice until the 1930s.[27] Indeed, few devices nurses used regularly entailed hermeneutic human/machine relations or demanded that nurses interpret texts produced by instruments or machines.[28] When the thermometer first made its way into nursing practice in the late nineteenth century, nurses were responsible only for reading and recording the number registered at the top of the column of mercury. Only physicians were obligated and even deemed capable of interpreting the meaning of that number and initiating clinical action on the basis of that interpretation. An argument offered for why it might be acceptable to delegate the use of this medical "instrument of precision" to nurses was that they would not be distracted by everything physicians knew about the science of clinical thermometry and, thus, make mistakes in reading the thermometer.[29] Although the mercury thermometer is a hermeneutic device, in that it requires the interpretive reading of a text to make full use and sense of it, the nurse was initially not expected to engage it hermeneutically. Indeed, nurses were to be not unlike thermometers themselves, which simply registered temperature.[30]

Out of Teapots, Enema Cans

One way nurses distinguished their specialized use from the common use of everyday objects was to transform them into implements for comfort and healing. They used bedside tables to relieve dyspnea (shortness of breath) by having the patient lean over the table in an upright position.[31] They fashioned bed supports out of broom handles.[32] A broomstick with the broom sawed off was wrapped in blankets and pillows and then placed under the patient's knees. A stout cord was attached to each end of the broom handle and then to the head of the bed. This innovative use of the broom not only provided comfort to the patient, but it also saved labor; nurses were spared the physical exertions of tugging and lifting patients who were constantly sliding down in their beds. As exemplified by how common items such as bedside tables and broom handles were used, many of the objects nurses modified in practice were not limited because of their design for one primary purpose. In the hands of nurses, everyday things often became "technological objects" in the domain of nursing and, therefore, served as material expressions of the specialized work of the trained nurse.[33]

Indeed, improvisation and invention were integral components of the work of the trained nurse. Nurses were encouraged to see the things around them in new ways. A prevailing theme in instructional and advice literature for nurses was the need to improvise and to use ingenuity in utilizing, fashioning, and transforming existing objects to provide nursing care.[34] Private duty nurses in the home, who were faced with "a deficient supply of things" available to hospital nurses for whom "everything is at hand," were especially encouraged to improvise and counseled on how to use the implements they had for a variety of purposes.[35] A nurse was considered "poor" indeed who did not have the "proper things to do with," but poorly trained if she could not make do without "complicated and expensive equipment."[36] Nurses apparently were easily seduced by new appliances. One student nurse, on a tour of her hospital in 1930, wrote in her log that the instruments in a sterilization room "took my eye immediately." She found the infant respirator, reportedly one of only four such machines in the country, "the most interesting part of the whole trip."[37]

As most of the care of the sick and of childbearing women had moved into the hospital by the 1930s, and the hospital became the standard for care, nurses were expected to use their skills to make the patient's home more like the hospital.[38] A photograph taken in the home of a patient of the Maternity Center Association of New York showed the nurse how to set up a bedroom or kitchen for a home delivery by making good use of articles normally found there. This improvised room featured a soft bed, newspapers, linens, jars, and basins. Although they stood in sharp aesthetic contrast to the hard metal furnishings and equipment characterizing the delivery room at New York Hospital (see figs. 3-1, 3-2, and 3-3), these rooms demonstrated how nurses could "imitate hospital conditions in the home" by using the "utensils and materials . . . at hand."[39]

Nurses were repeatedly admonished not to waste the resources or add to the expenses of their patients, whether economically advantaged

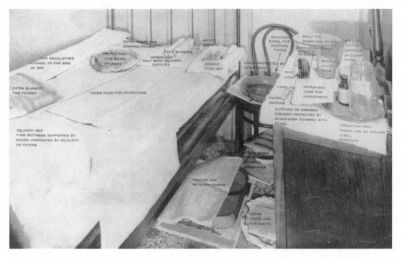

Figure 3-1. Bedroom delivery. (From Louise Zabriskie, *Mother and Baby Care in Pictures* [Philadelphia: Lippincott, 1935], 64)

or disadvantaged, by having them buy unnecessary implements. Public health nurses, who had limited access to the latest hospital equipment and for whom "tools [were] as necessary for doing a good piece of public health work as [were] the hundred and one mechanical appliances in a machinist's kit," were especially encouraged to use their ingenuity in making and adapting devices in the home.[40] As one nurse observed, nursing involved "making the best of things."[41] With "fire, water, salt, and newspapers, [the nurse] will seldom be embarrassed in any emergency."[42] Instead of forceps, a nurse could use a clothespin. Nurses could refashion teapots and flower sprinklers into enema cans and convert miners' pails into stupe kettles.[43] They could use paper bags as inhalers.[44] The fountain syringe, a staple of the nurse's bag, could be used for lavage and irrigation; its rubber tubing could be detached to serve as a tourniquet.[45] The fountain syringe itself could be replaced by a funnel with rubber tubing.[46] The nursing "appliances" and "devices" and new medical instruments exhibited at meetings and in journals demonstrated the interest nurses had in their material world and the value they placed on ingenuity.[47]

Nurses especially applauded labor-saving products and utilities, such as the electric pad to warm solutions to be administered internally to patients, beds and carts with rubber wheels to reduce noise, and a central water supply to fill bathtubs. As one nurse noted about the electric warming pad, "only nurses who have, quite literally, spent hours in

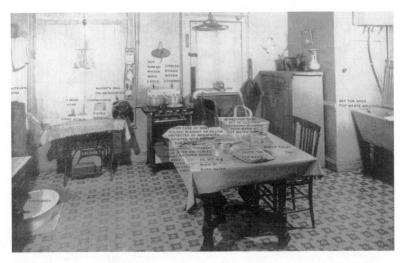

Figure 3-2. Kitchen delivery. (From Louise Zabriskie, *Mother and Baby Care in Pictures* [Philadelphia: Lippincott, 1935], 62)

filling and carrying hot water bags intended to keep solutions warm, can appreciate fully the simplicity of this carefully worked-out device."[48] Prior to the advent of central plumbing, a bath was a laborious, time-consuming, and at times uncomfortable affair for both nurse and patient.[49]

Nurses were encouraged to adapt ready-to-hand objects, to invent new kinds of devices themselves, and to publicize their improvisations and inventions. Indeed, nurses demonstrated somewhat of "a mania for adapting and inventing."[50] Professional nursing journals, such as the *Trained Nurse* (and, later, the *Trained Nurse and Hospital Review*) and the *American Journal of Nursing*, regularly featured articles, photographs and drawings, and brief written descriptions of the latest "remedies and appliances" either invented for use by nurses or fashioned by nurses themselves.[51] Although improvisation constituted an important and often unrecognized method of invention, nurses were encouraged to move beyond simply making do with what they had and to collaborate with manufacturers to place new inventions of primary usefulness to nurses on the market. In 1904 several hospitals adopted an improved medicine spoon that a nurse invented.[52] The New York City Board of Health adopted another nurse's invention of a new plug for infant bottles.[53] The invention and manufacture of the Good Samaritan Infusion Radiator exemplified a successful collaboration between a nurse-inventor and a manufacturer.[54]

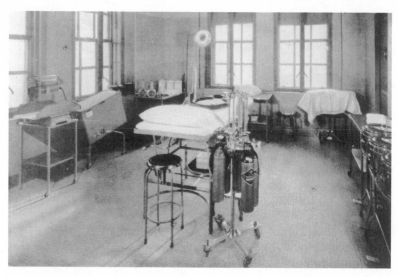

Figure 3-3. Hospital delivery. (From Louise Zabriskie, *Mother and Baby Care in Pictures* [Philadelphia: Lippincott, 1935], 65)

As one nurse argued, instead of "grumbling" about the inadequacies of hospital furniture, nurses needed to study this furniture with a view toward "chanc[ing] on a remunerative invention."[55] Nurses were intimately concerned with hospital furnishings and, therefore, in the best position to create equipment that conserved the time and energy of the nurses (and others) who had to use it. Patients could not be well served if the people around them were struggling with poorly designed equipment. Nurses were advised of the opportunities and even the obligation they had to participate in "original work in the improvement of hospital appliances."[56] There were no persons better suited to this work than the women who daily struggled with the problems and impediments to patient care these appliances presented. Indeed, one nurse lamented that in hospitals boasting complete operating rooms, x-ray departments, laboratories, and the latest equipment for hydrotherapy and electrotherapy, there was no satisfactory equipment for nursing. Although nurses often successfully used a single object for multiple purposes, this practice could also be harmful to patients and impede efficient practice. For example, infectious organisms were more likely to be transferred on basins used for both clean and dirty procedures, and the overuse of devices contributed to their early demise.[57]

Although "necessity [was] the mother of invention," nurses had to anticipate needs, rather than waiting for "dire necessity" to motivate them. Nursing invention might be impeded by too much improvisation (or too great a readiness to make do), but it was also thwarted by the lack of recognition of nurses' contributions to the design of equipment. As one nurse complained, the "individuality of the inventor [was often] totally lost." Either nurses were unaware of the commercial opportunities available to them, or manufacturers deliberately contributed to their ignorance by preferring that "royalties never [be] considered."[58]

Tools and Testimonials

Instructional texts for nurses emphasized improvisation (or making the best of things) and invention (or making the best things). Yet a third emphasis in these texts was on buying the best things. Instructional, but primarily promotional, literature advised nurses that the effectiveness of their work and their reputation in the eyes of physicians depended, in part, on buying the best equipment.[59] Indeed, as one text addressing the "ethics of nursing" promised, "The doctor will see at a glance if your instruments are just what they should be, that you know how to keep them, and the inference will be that you know how to use them."[60] One physician encouraged nurses in private practice always to buy the best thermometers, scissors, forceps, and dressing instruments. He also suggested adding to the nurse's instrument collection manometers (to determine the specific gravity of urine), litmus paper (to determine the pH of urine), and an eight-ounce graduated glass measure, as physicians could not carry all of these items from house to house, and it was easier for the nurse to include them as part of her outfit.[61]

The nurse's outfit, nursing bag, or pocket case was featured in both didactic and promotional literature.[62] For example, the Chicago Nurse's Case (made of the "best Morocco leather" and selling for $10), shown in a 1918 surgical instruments and supply catalogue, included vials, glass syringes and needles, forceps, thermometer, scissors, knife, probes and directors, baby scales, metal and rubber catheters, scarifier (for wet cupping), and razor.[63] Outfits including such items were promoted as suitable gifts for nurses (see fig. 3-4).[64] Indeed, implements such as watches with "sweep-second" hands, thermometers, and syringes, and even larger items, such as instrument sterilizers, were promoted throughout the 1940s as gifts that nurses would appreciate having and that would help them in their careers.[65]

Promotional literature also included testimonials by nurses on behalf of the thermometers and other implements they favored. In 1914, in the third edition of her popular nursing text, Clara Weeks-Shaw described the clinical thermometer as "this now familiar instrument [that] is indispensable to every nurse."[66] Becton, Dickinson and Company featured the B-D Clinical Thermometer as having "found much favor among the Nursing Profession."[67] The Judson Pin Company advertised the Capsheaf Safety Pin as "highly endorsed by trained nurses."[68] Meinecke and Company printed a nurse's testimonial for their Ideal Douche Pan.[69] The Lister Surgical Company claimed that nurses who used Lister's Towels preferred them to any other pads for women.[70] These ads made nurses aware of products to buy or to recommend to physicians and hospitals for purchasing. A note from the "Publisher's Desk" of the *Trained Nurse and Hospital Review* encouraged nurses to send for samples of the products they saw advertised in the journal. Assured that the journal permitted only advertisements of reputable products, nurses were encouraged to see these ads as equal in value to the other reading matter in the journal.[71]

These advertisements suggest that advertisers were aware that trained nurses were consumers of their products separate from physicians, and that nurses could influence physicians to buy their products in an increasingly competitive marketplace.[72] A 1927 Becton, Dickinson ad for asepto syringes featured "Nurses' Asepto Specialties," while a 1925 instrument catalog featured the "nurses' ice pick," the "nurses' hypodermic syringe," and the "nurses' training set," which included a baby scale, artery and dressing forceps, scissors, a bath thermometer, and a combination hypodermic syringe and clinical thermometer.[73] These ads appealed to nurses' professional aspirations. Some ad campaigns suggested that nurses were critical to maintaining patients' confidence in their physicians and even that nurses were more important to patients than physicians. The Denver Chemical Manufacturing Company's early-twentieth-century ad campaign for Antiphlogistine (a type of poultice used for a variety of ailments that was marketed through the 1940s) warned physicians never to leave its application in unknowing hands, as faulty technique would reflect badly on them.[74] Nurses were typically shown in their ads applying the poultices to patients or

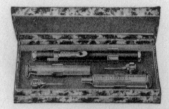
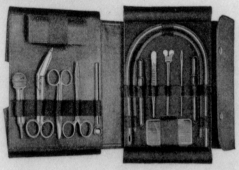
Figure 3-4. Commencement gifts for nurses, 1927. (By permission of Becton, Dickinson and Company)

holding the product. A 1904 advertisement for the poultice in the *Trained Nurse* rhapsodized,

> The Nurse who reads the Trained Nurse keeps
> Abreast of her profession; but
> The Nurse who knows how to apply Antiphlogistine
> Is of greatest value to the physician.

Moreover, "in the hand of the nurse, the spatula is more powerful than the surgeon's lance." The Denver company promised a spatula to every nurse who mailed in her name and address.[75]

Companies appealed directly to nurses by emphasizing in their ads the value of their products for both patient comfort and safety and nursing efficiency. Indeed, while doctors might "prefer" Antiphlogistine, and patients "appreciate it," it was the nurse who would find it "time and energy-saving," since she was the one who had to apply such treatments.[76] Moreover, the ads themselves offer clues about the problems various devices posed for nurses in practice. For example, a Becton, Dickinson ad for their clinical thermometers suggested problems with reading the markings, resetting the mercury, and preventing breakage (see fig. 3-5). A Taylor Instrument Companies ad showing a drawing of a nurse with a thermometer in a Tycos Safety Case pinned to her apron suggested that nurses often lost thermometers.[77] Judson Pin Company promised nurses a safety pin that "cannot catch in the fabric," suggesting that such pins often caused this problem.[78] The Lister Surgical Company promised a gynecological towel that was more absorbent, did not need to be washed, and in general saved "time, money, and annoyance," suggesting the labor expended and the displeasure associated with cleaning towels filled with gynecological blood and other discharges.[79] The Meinecke Company's douche pan was "ideal" because (by virtue of being "anatomically correct in shape") it did "not hurt," had a "capacious interior," and was easy to maintain "in a sanitary condition," suggesting both the patient discomfort and cleaning work to which nurses had to attend.[80]

Medical trade catalogs, although largely directed to the physician consumer, also promoted products that solved problems encountered primarily by nurses in promoting patient comfort and safety. These products also promised to make practice safer, less laborious, and even more aesthetically pleasing. Becton, Dickinson and Company, in their 1918 *Physician Catalog*, advertised the HY-JEN-IC thermometer as filling the requirements of nurses (and others) whenever "economy is a factor,"

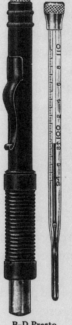
Figure 3-5. B-D clinical thermometers, 1921. (By permission of Becton, Dickinson and Company)

and the Olympian thermometer as popular with nurses (and others) "preferring strength, legibility, and 'easy shakers' to quick registration."[81] Greeley Laboratories promised to overcome common objections to administering medicines via hypodermic injection, including poorly designed syringes and needles that became clogged, stuck, slipped, leaked, and permitted breaks in aseptic technique.[82] In the Hospital Supply Company of New York's 1913 *Catalogue of Sterilizers*, ad copy acknowledged the "unjustifiably disagreeable duty on nurses" to make do with the "obnoxious prevailing method of emptying bed pans into open sinks." The Climax Combined Bedpan Sterilizer and Washer made this job less distasteful and reduced hospital odors. The same company advertised the Climax Dressing Sterilizer as preventing injury to the nurse because of poor design. As pictured and described in the ad (see fig. 3-6), the nurse was previously forced to "pass her arm past a hot Sterilizer and manipulate the valves in the constricted space between the apparatus and the wall." Their new design feature eliminated this potential hazard.[83]

Nursing the Equipment

As specialized devices became more prominent features of clinical practice after 1900, nurses began to discuss the many problems they encountered in using devices that were either minimized or ignored in the medical literature. These problems emphasized the vast, obstacle-ridden, but virtually invisible terrain that nurses traveled between the physician's order of a procedure and its proper execution at the bedside.

For example, physicians ordered oxygen therapy, but nurses had to administer it. That is, nurses had to find ways to maintain the appropriate dose or concentration of oxygen in a tent or chamber while simultaneously providing other kinds of care that allowed oxygen to escape, as when nurses bathed patients.[84] They also had to contend with the fear and claustrophobia these tents or chambers engendered in patients. Similarly, physicians ordered and initially applied Buck's extension traction to a fractured limb, but the nurse had to care for these "difficult patients"; that is, patient care was made more difficult by the device.[85] Nurses had to maintain the alignment of and weights applied to the limb, obtain the assistance of others to bathe and toilet the patient, take extra care to prevent the bedsores more likely to develop because of the inability of patients to turn over in bed, and alle-

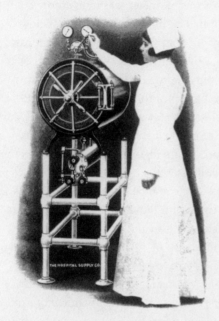

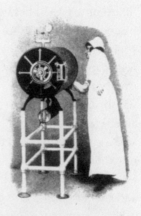

This illustration shows the awkward control of Sterilizers which have valves placed at the rear. The nurse must pass her arm past a hot Sterilizer and manipulate the valves in the constricted space between the apparatus and the wall.

Showing Ease of Control of "CLIMAX" Sterilizer.

The Hospital Supply Company's

"Climax" Dressing Sterilizer

. is

"Controlled From the Front
With One Lever
With One Finger"

Under U. S. Patent No. 916,611.

The Hospital Supply Company's "Four-way" Valve is the most notable improvement that has been made since the development of the Vacuum Sterilizer. It consists of a single insulated Lever which can be manipulated with one finger. It moves before a lettered dial and by simply turning it to the various positions indicated, the entire process of sterilization is controlled, including the entrance of steam into the jacket; the drawing of the vacuum; the entrance of steam into the sterilizing chamber and the drying of the dressings.

The simplicity of controlling the entire operation of "CLIMAX" Sterilizers, with a single valve in front with patented vacuum device places them in a class by themselves. Ours is the only Four-Way Valve made.

NOTE:—The Physical Laws of the movement of gases prove that the argument that a rear valve causes a continuous stream of steam through the Sterilizer is fallacious. The pressure of steam in closed vessels is the same at all points.

Figure 3-6. Climax Dressing Sterilizer. (Hospital Supply Company of New York, *Catalogue of Sterilizers*, 1913, Medical Trade Ephemera Collection, College of Physicians of Philadelphia, 10)

viate the discomfort from both the original injuries and confinement by the device itself.

Nurses assured one another that even the most complicated treatments were easy to learn, but they also recognized that simplicity in a device's construction or design did not ensure simplicity of use. As

Bertha Harmer warned, applying a compress to the eyes might appear simple, but the patients' eyesight was still at stake.[86] An ostensibly simple utensil such as the glass thermometer was much more complicated to use than it seemed. A thermometer in the wrong hands could injure or even kill because of broken glass or bacteria. A bedpan appeared to be a simple device, but selecting the wrong bedpan or misapplying it at the bedside would result in patient injury. A heating pad might appear uncomplicated, but if improperly applied to a patient, it could cause death. A newborn infant at Rex Hospital in Raleigh, North Carolina, died of burns she sustained when a nurse left her too long on an electric heating pad.[87] A procedure involving something so simple as the rubber tube used to administer an enema or colonic irrigation, or to enable the patient to pass gas, could be hazardous to patients and a problem for nurses. Hard tips could puncture delicate membranes, and rubber goods were difficult to clean and preserve.[88]

Moreover, the apparent simplicity of giving an enema belied the complex work nurses had to perform to alleviate patients' physical discomfort and embarrassment and to maintain cleanliness as well as the proper position of device and patient. As patients became more ambulatory by the 1940s, they posed additional problems for nurses charged with ensuring the safe and effective use of equipment. For example, one nurse noted the "considerable ingenuity" needed to devise ways for ambulatory patients requiring urinary drainage to be free of embarrassment while ensuring adequate drainage.[89] In the apparently simple matters of instilling fluids and removing them, nurses—not devices— ensured that liquids went into and left patients' bodies at the proper rate and/or temperature.

Formal analyses, including time studies, of nursing activities, which became increasingly common beginning in the 1920s in response to a national craze prior to World War I for efficiency and scientific management,[90] showed the complexity of even the most "elementary nursing procedures."[91] Not only did these procedures take skill, but they took time. In the early 1930s a cleansing bath averaged 41 minutes but could last up to 73 minutes (including the time required to prepare, administer, clean up after, and chart the procedure). An enema averaged 24 minutes but could take up to 45 minutes. A clysis averaged 57 minutes but could require up to 95 minutes. A catheterization averaged 15 minutes but could need up to 94 minutes.[92] The relatively little time needed to take a temperature or give an injection was offset by the increasing frequency with which these procedures had to be performed and the increasing numbers of patients requiring them. By the early 1940s the "four-hourly temperature" had become a "time-honored routine" adhered to more out of habit than necessity in the case of patients whose temperatures never varied.[93] Giving a hypodermic injection was much simpler by the 1940s than it had been in the early decades of the twentieth century, as the sterilization of needles and syringes became centralized in special departments of the hospital and as medications in tablet form that once required reconstitution were replaced by solutions ready to inject.[94] But the increasing frequency with which injections had to be given, a result of the development of new drugs such as penicillin, and the increasing numbers of patients to whom they had to be given offset these advantages and heightened the possibility of error.

On one typical day in the fall of 1935 at the Massachusetts General Hospital, nurses administered about 165 hypodermic injections; in the late 1870s they had administered none. On the unit where 60 of these injections were given, this one procedure alone consumed the equivalent of a full workday of about 1½ nurses. On a typical spring day in 1948, 454 hypodermic injections required the full-time effort of about 13 nurses, and 1,162 intramuscular injections demanded the full-time effort of 29 nurses. Together these two procedures required enough nurses to staff the equivalent of three pre–World War II 37-bed units.[95] In the early 1940s the nurses caring for one group of 473 patients in a 24-hour period at Strong Memorial Hospital in Rochester, New York, took 109 blood pressures (in intervals ranging from once every 15 minutes to once per day), assisted 60 patients to receive parenteral fluids, changed 230 dressings (not including the dressings removed simply to show the wound to the physician), and administered 1,500 medications by mouth or by hypodermic.[96]

Because devices were increasingly central components of the procedures nurses performed, "nursing the equipment" became as important as nursing the patient.[97] Indeed, the safe, effective, efficient, and finished care of patients depended in large part on the quality of nurses' care of equipment at and away from the bedside. Didactic texts typically emphasized the articles required for the many therapeutic and increasingly diagnostic procedures both the nurse and the physician performed that depended on the use of devices. Nurses were expected to match the correct instruments to both the procedure and the physician in surgery and other procedures that required nurses' assistance. They were also expected to perform or supervise the before-and-after care of equipment, which involved selecting and then arranging devices on trays; cleaning, disinfecting, or sterilizing apparatus; mending and otherwise maintaining the integrity of equipment; and preventing its destruction. A key feature of instructional literature and visual displays was the variety of specialized trays of equipment for the procedures nurses carried out themselves or assisted physicians to perform.[98] Nurses also held official positions as keepers of equipment, including as supervisors in central supply rooms in hospitals.[99]

Nurses were also expected to use supplies in ways that contributed to their professional mission of creating an environment most conducive to patient recovery. Devices were critical components of this physical environment. For example, to maintain a homelike atmosphere and to reduce patient fears, one nurse advised that medical and surgical appliances ought not to be visible in the sickroom.[100] Because light from a window or mirror could cause glare on the glass enclosure surrounding the patient receiving oxygen therapy, nurses were cautioned to be careful when setting up this kind of apparatus.[101] Nurses were also concerned with and invented ways to reduce the noise caused by various hospital carts and metal, glass, and enamel devices.[102]

Not only were nurses obliged to be technically proficient, but they were also to show their "appreciation of equipment."[103] A nurse could be judged extravagant and as misusing equipment. Breaking a glass syringe required a written incident report. In one hospital the need to preserve glass thermometers inspired friendly rivalry among wards as to which had the lowest incidence of breakage.[104] In an effort to "teach care of hospital equipment," some hospitals had bulletin boards displaying the number of various devices used and destroyed in a year, how they were ruined, and the cost to replace them.[105] Complex kinds of equipment, such as respirators, required special maintenance for proper operation.[106] In the era before the widespread and increasingly cavalier use of disposable devices, nurses had to develop a reverence for the things they used.

Handicapped by the Hand

From the beginning of trained nursing in the United States, physical objects and their use shaped both the content and the form of nursing practice. Much of nursing entailed the use of improvised and increasingly more specialized objects to diagnose, treat, and comfort patients, and the use of these objects eventually restructured the nurse's and the patient's day. Repetitive procedures such as taking temperatures and administering medications provided a new way to tell time, and they contributed to a new, more "functional" way to practice nursing. Instead of one nurse providing all the care that one patient needed, one nurse provided all the care that one thing required. By the 1940s, nursing care implied not just the care of the patient's body but also the care of the bed, the thermometer, the syringe, and the forceps.[107] The physical and moral order that trained nursing brought to the hospital was accomplished, in part, by the aesthetic order the nurse's use of these devices entailed.[108]

The devices nurses used or, in the case of the thermometer and sphygmomanometer, how they typically used them extended the hands as opposed to the senses or interpretive capacities of the nurse. As depicted on the May 1945 cover of the *Trained Nurse and Hospital Review*, the nurse's hand was "the instrument" by which nurses served their "fellow man." The implements nurses used at "hand's end" were material expressions of what most nurses and physicians viewed as the primary function of the trained nurse, namely, to serve as extensions of "the physician's hand."[109] Nursing identity and work were defined by what nurses did, which in turn was increasingly defined by the tools they used.

Although device-mediated procedures enhanced the importance of nurses to patients and physicians, they did not distinguish trained nurses from either lesser-trained or completely untrained women who also cared for the sick or from highly trained physicians. Nurses shared the use of common utensils and appliances with other women charged with the care of home and family, and they shared the use of specialized instruments and implements with physicians and under physicians' direction. As Rosemary Stevens observed, nurses were "handicapped" from the outset by appearing to be "all-purpose female service workers without a defined monopoly of scientific skills."[110] Nurses did whatever was necessary and what others did not want to do. Although the increased use of instruments and implements contributed to the scientific and socioeconomic advancement of medicine, it contributed to the "functional redundancy" of nursing in that no single activity distinguished nursing from other practices above and below nursing in the rigid "occupational hierarchy" of health care.[111] Although physicians were increasingly forced to share the use of new diagnostic and treatment devices with nurses and others below them in the occupational hierarchy, they managed to retain their functional indispensability, in part, by the way they used these devices and by the devices they used. When physicians used surgical instruments, they performed surgery; when nurses used surgical instruments, they handed them to physicians or cleaned them. When physicians used stethoscopes, they diagnosed disease; when nurses eventually used stethoscopes, they took blood pressures on orders from physicians. Physicians typically never handled laundry, feeding utensils, or bedpans.

Physicians also maintained their dominance by possessing and preserving for themselves special knowledge not readily available to nurses. Throughout this period, science training for nurses remained poor largely because of persistent concerns about overeducating the nurse and the use of student nurses as cheap labor for hospitals.[112] Moreover, even when nurses possessed greater knowledge than physicians, this knowledge was either not recognized or minimized, even by nurses themselves. For example, oxygen therapy rested, in part, on theoretical knowledge that physicians characteristically possessed of the physical properties of oxygen, its relation to health and disease, instrumental ways to deliver it to patients, and the doses required to achieve certain effects. But oxygen therapy also rested on the practical knowledge that nurses gained in actually delivering effective doses to patients in varying physical and emotional circumstances.[113] This practical knowledge of enactment and application was typically effaced, as nurses were perceived as merely carrying out the oxygen therapy physicians had ordered.[114] The carrying-out component of oxygen therapy was typically viewed as requiring only manual skills and no special knowledge—that is, no knowledge the physician did not possess.

Nurses themselves tended not to see the carrying-out aspect of nursing practice as requiring the development and possession of special knowledge. Although they understood the importance of what they did for patients, they did not see their doing as also knowing. The equation of science with scientific management, the relatively small amount of science content in the nursing curriculum, and nurses' lack of training in methods of scientific investigation, coupled with tenaciously persistent ideas about nurses'/women's place in the health care hierarchy and the need for cheap, trained hands (not minds) to perform the labor of health care, worked together to efface the practical knowledge nurses possessed and which they could have further developed and monopolized.[115] Nurses came closest to recognizing and treating the knowledge in their practice as practice knowledge in the

Teachers College studies of procedures, such as clinical thermometry, conducted in the 1920s and 1930s. More often, though, eager to do their part for hospital economy and to offset personnel shortages, nurses were oriented to "simplifying procedures," that is, to the time it took to perform a procedure, rather than to its content or outcome.[116] Engaged in the process of simplification, nurses inadvertently contributed to the view that nursing was simple.[117] In effect, nurses thereby de-skilled themselves.

The increasingly device mediated nature of nursing practice also contributed to the growing divide between nurses who saw their practice largely as a handcraft and occupation and nurses who saw it as an intellectual pursuit and profession.[118] While nurses at the bedside sought to make the best of things for their patients and were proud of their handiwork, nurses concerned with the scientific and social advancement of nursing sought to ensure that nursing not be wholly defined by handiwork or by their hands. The increasingly device mediated and technical nature of nursing practice was causing physicians, the general public, and even nurses themselves to view nursing strictly as work that extended the physician's hand. For nursing leaders, such as Lavinia Dock, Lillian Wald, and Annie Goodrich, nursing practice had to be understood as mental, not just manual, labor.[119] Although much of nursing practice was customarily initiated on orders from physicians, there was a world of difference between simply obeying a physician's order and intelligently carrying it out. As Mary Roberts observed, good nursing care was "not a mere series of procedures strung like beads on the wire of a doctor's orders [but] a carefully wrought fabric in which procedures stand out like a design against the less colorful but necessary background of understanding of personal, social, and psychological factors, intelligent observation of physical and mental symptoms and conditions." Good nursing was neither just "rote memory" nor "mechanical skill." [120]

Indeed, the increasingly procedural work of nursing contributed to further confusion about whether nursing was a science, an art, or a craft. In a 1929 editorial on the "science and art of nursing," Isabel Stewart sought to distinguish the "true artist in nursing from a mere technician or artisan." As she argued, "The real essence of nursing, as of any fine art, lies not in the mechanical details of execution, nor yet in the dexterity of the performer, but in the creative imagination, the sensitive spirit, and the intelligent understanding lying back of these techniques and skills." Without this imagination, spirit, and intelligence, nursing would only be a "highly skilled trade" and not the "profession" or "fine art" she and other like-minded leaders hoped it would become.[121]

While arguing for the individuality and subjectivity characteristic of the arts and crafts, Stewart also contested the individuality and subjectivity that allowed nurses to execute procedures any way they saw fit. Nursing leaders, such as Stewart, were concerned that the way a procedure was conducted was more dependent on which school the nurse had been trained in than on any rational principles. In one Teachers College study of nursing procedures, at least twenty-two different methods were proposed for giving a hypodermic injection. Other procedures showed similar variations.[122] Stewart lamented that while physicians studied which drugs produced the best results, nurses did not study which method of giving a hot pack or a footbath was most effective. Such nursing studies were critical not only to the understanding of nursing as a science but also to human welfare. There was an urgent need for nursing studies "of a practical type" that emphasized the "everyday work of nurses."[123] Yet a parallel but divergent concern was that nurses were becoming too machine-like, rigid, and invariable in their work. Quoting Lavinia Dock, who had criticized training schools for turning out " 'a set of machines all in the same mold with the same ideas and habits,' " Stewart also warned that "standardization . . . carried to excess . . . tended to discourage initiative and spontaneity and to make all nurses follow a set pattern."[124]

Accordingly, from the earliest days of trained nursing, nurses had an equivocal relation to the things they used in their practice. Nurses made the best of the things at hand, but there was always the question of whose hand it was and whether it operated like a machine or with a brain. As Clara Noyes, president of the American Nurses' Association in 1920, observed, "At one moment, the nurse's brain is [presumably] used, at the next, her hands only are required, at the next, both brains and hands, and, perhaps, at the next, neither brains or hands."[125] In the matter of nursing, it was arguable which body part prevailed.

4 The Physician's Eyes

If there was any part of nursing that could ultimately raise it above "mechanical, routine, nonintelligent practice and place it upon a scientific, professional basis," it was the "close observation" expected of the trained nurse.[1] If the hands of the nurse and the implements she held in those hands failed to distinguish trained nursing from other forms of female caregiving, her "trained senses" hopefully would not. As one hospital superintendent put it, as the "extra eye" of the physician, her careful observation of the patient and the immediate and accurate recording of the results of it would distinguish the trained nurse from the "mere trained attendant."[2]

Before the 1950s nursing observation was accomplished largely through the nurse's unaided but trained senses of sight, hearing, touch, and smell. Nurses used these senses to know their patients. In sharp contrast to the behaviorist cast that "knowing the patient" had in the 1920s and 1930s, the psychodynamic and interpersonal dimensions it acquired after World War II, and the phenomenological and narrative emphases it has today, knowing patients before 1950 meant knowing and getting to know them largely in the flesh.[3] Listening to patients, in the sense of eliciting and interpreting their deep motivations and, later, their stories in order to know them by heart (in addition to by sight, smell, and touch) was not an integral part of the rhetoric or fabric of the nurse/patient relationship until after World War II.[4] Indeed, Florence Nightingale viewed too much talking on the part of both patients and nurses as physically taxing for the patient and, on the part of nurses in particular, as intrusive and therefore indicative of poor nursing practice.[5]

Florence Nightingale and the
Observation of the Sick

Florence Nightingale had established observation as the habit and faculty that enhanced the utility of and legitimated the need for trained nurses. Nightingale believed that a woman who could not cultivate this habit ought to abandon the pursuit of nursing, even though she might be kind. In 1860, in the classic primer *Notes on Nursing*, she instructed, "The most important practical lesson that can be given to nurses is to teach them what to observe—how to observe—what symptoms indicate improvement—what the reverse—which are of importance—which are of none—which are the evidence of neglect—and of what kind of neglect."[6]

For Nightingale, acquiring the habit and faculty of observation was no simple feat. Speaking " 'the whole truth and nothing but the truth' " —whether in court or at the bedside—required "many faculties combined of observation and memory." There was no more "final proof" in the fact that a person had told the same story many times than there was in the fact that one story had been corroborated by many people. Nightingale had no patience with nurses who, albeit unknowingly, imparted false information about patients to physicians. False information often resulted from asking the wrong (that is, "leading" instead of "pointed") questions.[7]

Nightingale carved out an essential role for nurses in both the diagnosis and the treatment of conditions leading to poor health and sickness, even as physicians were increasingly claiming diagnosis and treatment exclusively for themselves. Moreover, in an era when most physicians were just beginning to understand the specific etiologies of disease and the importance of clearly differentiating one disease or disorder from another, and to adopt the view that specific treatments should be matched to specific diagnoses, Nightingale's ideal nurse was an expert in a kind of differential diagnosis not heretofore practiced by either nurses or physicians.[8] This nurse was able to discriminate among symptoms deriving from disease itself, from the therapies chosen to treat diseases, from deficiencies in the patient's life circumstances that might have initially contributed to the disease, and most importantly, from failures of the nurse "to put the patient in the best condition for nature to act upon him."[9] The trained nurse could differentiate, for example, among defects in cooking, choice of diet, choice of time for taking food, and appetite as causes of "want of nutrition" in the patient. The trained nurse also understood that each of these defects, in turn, required a different remedy. The remedy for the first defect was to cook better; for the second, to make other choices in diet; for the third, to offer patients food when they wanted it; and for the fourth, to show patients what they liked.[10]

Nightingale admired nurses who had developed a precision of eye virtually equal to the measuring glass, although she maintained that nurses' eyes could not fully substitute for the accuracy of this device. An observant nurse could tell at a glance how many ounces of food her patient had consumed, even if the amount was very small. Nurses also had to learn the "physiognomy," or look, of various diseases and how they appeared in combination with the looks of individual patients. Nightingale promoted nursing observation as the artful and idiographic corrective to the scientific "averages" that threatened to seduce nurses away from "minute observation" and physicians away from the particularities and peculiarities of individual cases.[11]

Nightingale's nurse cultivated the habit and faculty of observation to achieve the good nursing upon which good medical care depended. In the days before the development of specific pharmacologic agents or public health measures targeted directly at the causes of disease, and before the refinement of aseptic surgical techniques, medical care often entailed little else but nursing care. The trained nurse had knowledge only nurses could possess by virtue of their constant presence at the bedside, and it was this privileged knowledge that physicians needed for accurate assessment and management of patient conditions. Nightingale's observant nurse not only enhanced the comfort and promoted the health of her patients, but she often also saved their lives and saved the day for physicians who might otherwise be misled by the limited information available to them from their abbreviated contacts with patients.

The Powers of Nursing Observation

Nightingale's instructions concerning observation and its importance in nursing and medical practice were incorporated and developed in the earliest lectures to and instructional texts for students of nursing in the United States.[12] American instructors pointed to observation as a critical feature distinguishing trained nursing from uneducated womanly care of the sick. They emphasized the value of trained nursing and the shortcomings of medicine by constantly reminding students that it was nurses who provided accurate descriptions of patient conditions "to those who have had no opportunity for persistent observation."[13] The physician was completely dependent on the nurse for what only she could know and for what he had to know. As Clara S. Weeks, author of one of the most influential early textbooks of nursing, concluded, "The nurse, who is with her patient constantly, has, if she knows how to make use of it, a much better opportunity of becoming acquainted with his real condition than the physician, who only spends half an hour with him occasionally."[14]

Indeed, according to Weeks, the "very excitement" of (or agitation caused by) the physician's visit often so altered patients' conditions that they might look better or worse to the visiting physician than they really were.[15] In addition, patients often told nurses things they did not tell their doctors. Nursing observation was especially crucial in the cases of infants, delirious patients, and others who could not or ought not—in order to conserve their energy—speak for themselves. The trained nurse was the physician's eyes, but she did not so much extend the vision of a sighted physician as provide a picture for a virtually blind one. Indeed, he saw very little without her.

Authors, such as Weeks, who sought to establish nursing as a valued profession for women repeatedly reminded students of nursing of the responsibility and power that lay in the nurse's eyes and in the constancy of her vigilance at the bedside. The physician depended on the nurse's "powers of observation," and in that dependence lay her professional authority.[16] Accordingly, nurses were taught to take careful notice of their patients and the conditions surrounding them. Didactic texts emphasized the physical condition of the patient, the physical manifestations indicating aberrant mental states, and the physical environment of the sickroom. Nightingale's admonition to nurses to learn the laws of health and to observe the total life circumstances of their patients could be more closely adhered to in home and public health nursing, where nurses had the opportunity to see the larger family and other social circumstances that contributed to ill health in their patients. In the hospital, however, nurses were confined largely to observations of the physical and proximate causes of disease and discomfort—that is, to what they could immediately see, feel, smell, or hear from outside the body and to factors in the physical environment such as ventilation, lighting, and noise.

Symptomatology and Scrutiny

Nurses and their "relation to symptomatology" was a major topic of instruction from the earliest days of trained nursing.[17] Nurses were taught to differentiate between subjective and objective symptoms, between symptoms and signs, between real and feigned symptoms, between leading and misleading symptoms, and between symptoms and signs significant for nursing care and those significant for medical care. They were to note and record the degree, character, duration, frequency, time of occurrence, apparent cause, modification, and significance of an array of symptoms and signs, such as pain, palpitation, dyspnea, cough, expectoration, and vomiting. Nurses were to appraise the condition of every visible portion of the body, using parameters appropriate for that part. For example, they were to observe the color, volume, degree of moisture, coating, markings, motion, and manner of protrusion of the tongue. They were to note the rate, volume, strength, rhythm, and tension of the pulse.[18] Before technological intrusions into the living body were routine in clinical practice, learning the subtleties of symptomatology and of patient expression, posture, mood, and temperament was especially critical.[19] What could be discerned from the outside comprised virtually all the information available to the general nursing or medical practitioner.

Practicing close observation entailed not only cultivating the sensory faculties but also understanding and managing its effects on patients. Being under the constant scrutiny of professional strangers, whether in the home or in the hospital, was new to patients unused to either trained nursing in the home or hospital care. While being looked after was likely comforting to most patients, being looked at could be disturbing and even result in error. Nurses were admonished not to let patients know they were being observed, because this could generate misleading symptoms.[20] Nurses learned to observe patients while they were ministering to their needs; that is, they learned to take opportunities such as the bath to note conditions of the body. Indeed, the bath was an especially good occasion for covert observation. In contrast to physicians, who performed their physical examinations in a very public and even intentionally dramatic way,[21] nurses learned to disguise the assessments they performed.[22] They also learned to observe one patient while caring for another. Nurse trainee Mary Clymer noted the difficulty she had "trying to have my eyes in 13 while my hands make a bed in 11."[23]

The close observation expected of the trained nurse required knowledge of symptoms and signs and their various relations to disease, treatment, and environmental conditions; the cultivation of all the nurse's senses with an emphasis on the practiced and disciplined eye; savvy in patient relations; and the ability to communicate and increasingly record observations in a manner likely to be of most use to both patient and physician.[24] If the key to good nursing was observation, the key to accurate medical diagnosis and patient recovery was the close observation of the trained nurse. The trained nurse was to be all-seeing: to take all of the "visual opportunities" available to her and to maintain "visual control" of her patients and the sickroom.[25] Except for the stopwatch (to count the pulse), the candle, and the gas and, later, the electric light, nursing observation in the mid- to late nineteenth century was largely an in-the-flesh practice unmediated by technological devices.[26]

The Instrumental Eye

While nurses were learning the importance of observing the sick, medical practice in the late nineteenth and early twentieth centuries increasingly involved new technological means of observing patients—of looking into and through living patients in addition to looking at and over them. From the middle of the nineteenth century, physical diagnosis with and without sense-extending devices such as the stethoscope increasingly prevailed as understanding and monitoring the progression of disease replaced intervention as the focal point of the physician/patient encounter and professional medical identity.[27] After 1900 the primacy and value of physical diagnosis for understanding and surveillance were increasingly challenged by the x-ray and the analytic, graphic, and quantitative techniques of laboratory diagnosis, electrocardiography, and sphygmomanometry.[28] In order to harness the benefits of this new technology, physicians had to share its use with nurses (and eventually also with a host of new technicians whose jobs were created in response to it). These new "instruments of precision" and symbols of medical science complicated the work of the nurse.[29] Moreover, while they further distinguished the trained nurse from other women attendants to the sick, they also blurred the boundary line between nursing and medical practice.

Clinical thermometry became a routine part of American medical practice in the latter part of the nineteenth century. Although the mercury thermometer had been invented early in the eighteenth century, its initial design made it impractical as a clinical tool. Thermometers were originally rather large devices, about a foot long and bent at a right angle, and had to be carried in a holster under the arm, much as "one might carry a gun."[30] Moreover, because thermometers did not maintain temperature readings at their maximum level once they were removed from the body, physicians had to read them while they were still placed against the patient. The invention of portable and self-registering devices, the 1871 translation of Carl Wunderlich's scientific treatise on medical thermometry, and the 1873 translation of Edouard Seguin's manual on medical and family thermometry contributed to the virtually complete replacement in U.S. clinical practice, by the end of the nineteenth century, of the hand with the thermometer to discern patient temperature.[31] The glass or metal thermometer replaced the "hand-thermometer," or the hand *as* thermometer.[32]

In contrast to other diagnostic devices, such as the stethoscope, laryngoscope, and microscope, which nurses assisted physicians to use and/or only occasionally used themselves, the direct use of the thermometer was soon delegated to nurses. Indeed nurses, charged with taking and recording temperatures in the physician's absence and with maintaining the thermometers themselves, became the most likely and frequent users of this implement. As one late-nineteenth-century nurse observed, nurses' "acquaintance with . . . this well-known instrument" was formed early in their careers.[33] The thermometer was rather quickly incorporated into routine nursing practice and almost as quickly became associated with, and even to represent, nursing. The earliest American textbooks of nursing and lecture notes indicate that nurses were expected to use the thermometer in their daily practice; that is, at the very least they were to take and record the patient's temperature.[34] Advertisements for printed blank temperature charts appeared in the back of texts written for nurses, indicating that nurses were responsible for maintaining legible records of patients' temperatures.[35] The thermometer and thermometer charts were prominent features of what nurses, physicians, and advertisers considered to be part of the nurse's "uniform," "armamentarium," "chatelaine," and "nurse's case."[36] Companies manufacturing thermometers marketed them directly to nurses and as suitable gifts for nurses.[37] Early popular verbal and pictorial depictions of nursing, as well as advertisements for nursing itself, often presented the nurse with a "thermometer in her hand."[38] As Emily Bax noted about the "1930 model nurse," there was an "air of competence about the very uniform that, combined with the thermometer, [was] irresistible."[39] The thermometer was soon incorporated into the image nurses had of themselves and their functions. In her widely read 1893 textbook on nursing, Isabel Hampton encouraged the nurse to think of herself as the "ward thermometer and barometer [alert for] any change in the ward atmosphere."[40] Nurses not only used thermometers; they were to be thermometers.

Thermometry was depicted as a womanly "handicraft" and the thermometer itself as a means "second to none" in the practice of the womanly arts of mothering and nursing.[41] Edouard Seguin, who popularized "family thermometry," viewed the handling and intelligent reading of the thermometer and the accurate recording of the temperature as necessary to learning the "ABC of motherhood." The thermometer was requisite also to "that part of nursing which mainly consists in spying the subtle and bold invasion of disease, and of measuring . . . its deadly strides into the vitals of the innocent." Women were the sentries who would be first to detect and "measure the strength of the enemy on the stem of [their] thermometers."[42]

The earliest instructions that nurses received about the thermometer show varying detail and increasing complexity, with information ranging from the procedural (that is, how to take, read, and record the temperature in adults and children) to the scientific—the theoretical basis for clinical thermometry and the meaning of various temperatures and temperature profiles in the progression of disease. In Bellevue Hospital's 1878 *Manual of Nursing*, only one paragraph on the thermometer appears at the end of the book as an addendum, and it contains information on how to take an oral temperature, a reference to axillary and rectal temperatures, and what the normal axillary temperature is.[43] The Connecticut Training School's *Handbook of Nursing*, published in 1879, contains somewhat more information and a reference to Seguin's work.[44]

Fourteen years later, in 1893 in the first edition of *Nursing*, Isabel Hampton devoted a chapter to temperature, linking variations in temperature to variations in pulse and respiration and differentiating normal from abnormal temperatures, addressing diurnal variations in temperature and factors (such as the placement of thermometers and the temperature and nature of foods) that could raise or lower temperature. Hampton classified temperatures, ranging from the "temperature of collapse" at 95–97 °F to "hyperpyrexia" at over 105 °F, and she differentiated among continuous, intermittent, and remittent fevers. She included "specimen charts" showing temperature, pulse, and respiration in typhoid fever, pneumonia, and malaria.[45] Hampton taught nurses how to convert Fahrenheit to Centigrade and Centigrade to Fahrenheit; how to test a thermometer for accuracy; the differences between and the procedure for taking oral, axillary, and rectal temperatures; and how to clean and store thermometers. Reprising concerns raised by physicians about the dangers of substituting instruments for the trained senses of the clinician, Hampton advised nurses not to rely solely on the thermometer. As she observed, even though ascertaining temperature by touch alone could be highly misleading (as skin temperature was not a reliable indicator of body temperature), touching the patient was still an essential component of nursing observation that allowed the detection of conditions that might go unnoticed without it.

Didactic instructions for nurses concerning thermometry became more detailed over the years, providing more information on the scientific basis for clinical thermometry and its relation to the diagnosis and course of disease and detection of patient responses to treatment. Since many so-called medical treatments entailed nothing but nursing care (as in "fever" nursing),[46] the thermometer was as much an instrument of nursing—assisting the nurse to evaluate the effectiveness of her ministrations—as it was an instrument of medicine. As Bertha Harmer noted in 1922 in the first edition of probably the most widely read series of textbooks of nursing, it was not enough for the nurse merely to be able to take the temperature. She had to know what caused various temperatures to occur and the nursing measures that would lower or raise temperature to normal levels.[47] The nurse did not merely take the temperature; she used the thermometer to diagnose, monitor, and treat patient conditions.

As thermometry became routine in clinical practice and virtually the sole province—in the hospital—of the nurse, instructional texts for nursing included increasingly more information on caring for the thermometer and on "making temperature taking safe."[48] A "good nurse [was] known by the care she [took] of her thermometer."[49] The "safety work" of clinical thermometry included maintaining and disinfecting thermometers, ensuring the accuracy of thermometer readings, and preventing harm to patients.[50] Both instructional texts teaching nurses about thermometers and advertising texts promoting the sales of competing brands of thermometers indicate that breakage was a constant concern.[51] Nurses considered themselves fortunate if they were not required to pay for the thermometers they broke.[52] Since the same thermometer typically had to be shared among patients, nurses were also increasingly concerned with the best methods to clean thermometers. Clinical thermometry was one of the earliest foci of scientific investigation by nurses, as they evaluated the effectiveness of various procedures for disinfecting thermometers. Most notable in this area of research was the 1929 Erdmann and Welsh report of studies in thermometer technique conducted between 1927 and 1928.[53]

The safety work of clinical thermometry also included preventing situations likely to cause injury to patients from broken thermometers or from false temperature readings. Nurses were cautioned about hysterical or malingering patients who deliberately sought to elevate temperature readings by placing the thermometer against something hot while the nurse was not looking. There were also patients who did not or could not keep the thermometer in place for the length of time required to register its maximum reading. Nurses were warned never to leave a patient unattended with a thermometer in place unless they were certain that the patient was physically able, or could be trusted, to be left alone.[54] Although clinical thermometry did not create the idea that patients were often unreliable partners in restoring themselves to health, it reinforced and extended that view, since thermometry was a practice that depended on the cooperation of the patient.

Clinical thermometry also influenced the aesthetics of nursing (and of hospital nursing in particular), affecting the order and structure of work on the ward and the appearance of nursing care. As physicians became more interested in the scientific investigation of disease and in establishing patterns of temperature in various diseases, they ordered temperatures to be taken more frequently. Whereas temperatures might have initially been taken once or twice a day, increasingly they had to be taken four or more times in a twenty-four-hour period. Under ideal conditions, thermometers required about three to five minutes to register temperature in the mouth, but up to fifteen minutes to register temperature in the axilla, often a preferred mode of taking the temperature. Moreover, the normal diurnal variations in temperature required that it be taken at times when body temperature tended to be at its lowest and highest levels. Physicians also expected all temperatures to be taken and recorded before their scheduled morning and/or evening rounds. Accordingly, the practice soon arose of assigning one nurse—the "temperature nurse"—to take and record all the temperatures on a ward.[55] This early manifestation of functional nursing—that is, giving one task to one nurse to complete on all patients—stood in sharp contrast to the home or private duty model of nursing where one nurse provided all the care that one patient required. Temperature nursing was a by-product of clinical thermometry that represented an important departure from traditional nursing practice. Whereas "fever nursing" assigned one nurse to one patient, "temperature nursing" entailed one nurse to one technique.

Thermometers also figured prominently in the development of specialized equipment trays that became a characteristic feature of nursing care. These trays were a means for the nurse to be efficient and organized in gathering and arranging the materials needed to conduct procedures at the bedside and to give a finished appearance to her work. In instructional and advice literature concerning the thermometer and other trays, nurses were to consider not only functionality and safety in their work but also symmetry and neatness in presenting equipment to patients and physicians. Indeed, symmetry and neatness were essential to patient safety in clinical thermometry, as the rotating system nurses used to distinguish between clean and dirty thermometers on a tray prevented the nurse from inadvertently using a dirty thermometer.[56]

Accordingly, from the beginning of trained nursing in the United States the thermometer was both fact and symbol of nursing practice. If not originally designed as a female technology, the thermometer had nevertheless become feminized if only by virtue of its appearing more often in the hands of the nurse than in the hands of the physician. The thermometer was an instrument that helped the nurse to diagnose and monitor patient conditions and to detect and correct defects in nursing and medical care. As probably the first instrument of precision nurses used, the thermometer had an important place in nursing practice. When much of the nurse's effort was directed toward lowering the temperature in patients who often died from febrile diseases, taking the temperature was truly a vital component of the triadic activity of taking the vital signs (or the TPR—temperature, pulse, and respiration). Taking the temperature was hardly the perfunctory activity it became after World War II, when antibiotics and immunizations reduced the incidence of or cured these diseases and when devices more spectacular than thermometers became part of clinical diagnosis.[57]

As an instrument increasingly linked in professional, popular, and advertising literature with nurses, the thermometer in the late nineteenth and early twentieth centuries represented both the precision of science and the ministrations of the trained nurse. Indeed, in the earliest days of clinical thermometry some hospital patients were reportedly in awe of this new instrument and in awe of the persons using it.[58] The thermometer forged a link between nursing, technology, and science whereby nurses came to understand themselves not only as users of scientific instruments but also as functioning like them. But it was a tenuous link, as thermometers began to appear in hands other than the physician's or the nurse's. In the hands of nurses and, increasingly, in the hands of any woman and even patients themselves, the thermometer lost its wholly scientific veneer, appearing less like a scientific and more like a household device. The thermometer was thus an entrée for nurses into the world of science, but one that kept them on the threshold between scientific and womanly work.

Too Much Knowledge for a Nurse

In the case of the thermometer, the practice of taking and recording the temperature eventually fell to the woman or nurse in the home and to the nurse in the hospital. In contrast, scopic examinations, or physical examinations conducted with eye- and ear-extending instruments such as ophthalmoscopes, laryngoscopes, and stethoscopes, remained largely in the physician's domain through the 1940s. If nurses participated in scopic examinations at all, it was primarily to hold patients in position for the examination (see figs. 4-1 and 4-2), to ensure their cooperation, and to see to it that the proper equipment was available for the physician.[59]

Nurses' use of the stethoscope in this period was confined largely to listening to the fetal heart (often with a special fetoscope), although the practice of regular fetal auscultation, conducted with increasing frequency as labor progressed to delivery, had yet to become standard obstetric practice.[60] Nurses sometimes also used stethoscopes to take blood pressure, but taking the blood pressure did not become part of routine nursing practice until the 1930s. Nurses were instructed about blood pressure, but didactic literature and procedure manuals directed toward them indicate that taking the blood pressure was not something they were expected to do at all or on a regular basis.[61] Although

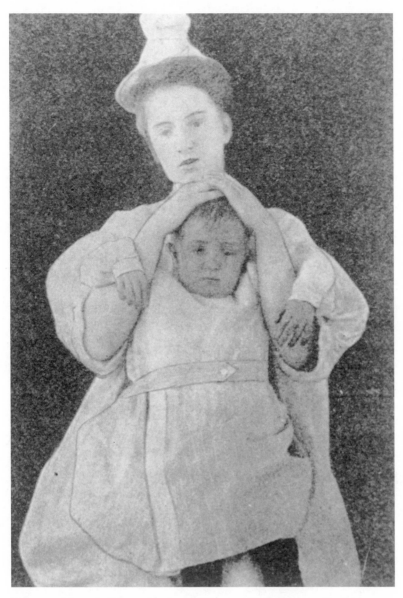

Figure 4-1. Nurse holding infant for examination. (From Minnie Goodnow, *First-Year Nursing: A Textbook for Pupils during Their First Year of Hospital Work*, 2nd ed. [Philadelphia: Saunders, 1919], 299)

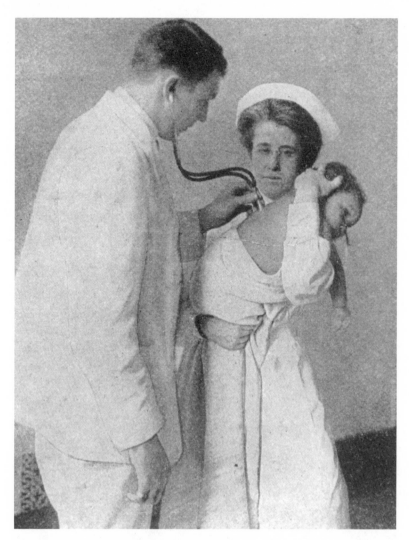

Figure 4-2. Nurse holding infant for stethoscopic examination. (From Minnie Goodnow, *First-Year Nursing: A Textbook for Pupils during Their First Year of Hospital Work*, 2nd ed. [Philadelphia: Saunders, 1919], 137)

there were physicians in the first decade of the twentieth century who still viewed blood pressure measurement as a dangerous substitute for digital observation (or palpation) of the pulse, blood pressure was typically considered a component of the physical examination of patients that only physicians could and should conduct.[62]

Indeed, the addition of the stethoscope to the cuff to ascertain blood pressure supported that claim.[63] Physicians had generally rejected using the cuff alone as a means to obtain the blood pressure,[64] since the cuff had initially been presented to them as a new device that nurses or orderlies could immediately be trained to use.[65] As physician and medical historian Christopher Crenner proposed, physicians may have been reluctant to pass a new device directly into the hands of non-physicians. Moreover, as he also concluded, the nurse's measurement of pulse pressure by obliteration of the pulse with the cuff likely undermined physicians' claims to special expertise in performing pulse palpation. The addition of the stethoscope to the procedure of taking the blood pressure made physicians more comfortable with replacing their fingers with devices, since the use of the stethoscope was conceived of as an unstandardizable practice that only physicians could master. The stethoscope more comfortably separated physicians from nurses, as it entailed special skills in perception and interpretation that nurses were generally neither taught nor perceived as able to learn.

In contrast to clinical thermometry, the labor involved in stethoscopic examinations was not so easily delegated. One user could not simply take and record scopically derived information for another user to interpret, as these instruments did not self-register any number or graphic analogue to the temperature. Anyone with reasonable visual acuity could read the temperature scale, but the user of scopic devices needed specialized scientific knowledge and perceptual skill to correlate device-mediated sights and sounds with an individual patient's anatomy and physiology, a subjective and interpretive skill apart from interpreting what those sounds meant for the diagnosis of disease. These interpretive talents were outside the sphere of anyone but the physicians who learned and practiced them. Indeed, the very subjectivity of the process of deriving information from scopic examinations, in addition to the ambiguity of the information itself, comforted physicians, as these features contrasted favorably with the simple readings nurses performed. The very subjectivity involved in scopic examinations legitimated the necessity for physicians and helped to offset their fears that new instruments producing "objective" information would undermine the distinctiveness of, and special need for, interpretive medical practice.

The stethoscope, especially, seemed to embody both the art and the science of medicine. Devices such as the thermometer ostensibly required no special knowledge or skill beyond the ability to read numbers. The stethoscope, however, demanded special knowledge and was thus a symbol for the doctor and the importance of the judgments only a physician could make.[66] Indeed, there was some concern that stethoscopic examinations were not appropriate for nurses to learn. One physician specifically excluded the use of the stethoscope as a topic for study in the ideal nursing curriculum.[67] Another physician reported in 1888 that he had been rebuked for teaching a nurse stethoscopic examination of the chest to detect heart complications in a case of rheumatism. Nurses, he was warned, would get into trouble for having "too much knowledge for a nurse."[68]

For Nurses with a Scientific Turn of Mind

In the first three decades of the twentieth century, patients were increasingly subjected to x-ray and laboratory examinations to diagnose and monitor their ailments or to detect diseases that had not as yet produced any discernible symptoms. In this period patients entered hospitals not only to receive medical treatment and nursing care for illness or injury but also to find out whether and why they were sick. Moreover, x-ray and laboratory tests were increasingly used to assign and confirm diagnoses already made and as ritual screening components of hospitalization. By the 1930s, admission to a hospital entailed being x-rayed, having blood drawn, and providing a urine sample.[69] X-ray and laboratory technology embodied the new scientific hospital, and x-ray and laboratory units and equipment were prominently featured in annual reports and other materials promoting hospitals.[70]

As a consequence of their increasing reliance on x-ray and laboratory testing, physicians in general practice became more dependent on specialist physicians, nurses, and others to use this technology. Roentgenographic and laboratory tests exemplified, perhaps more than any other technological innovations, the extent to which diagnosis became an interdependent and collaborative process involving (generalist and specialist) physicians, nurses, technicians, and patients, rather than a discrete moment in exclusively physician time. Unlike clinical thermometry and scopic examinations, these tests entailed many discrete activities that could be demarcated from one another and then delegated. Exactly what components of this new diagnostic process nurses performed depended on factors such as the extent of x-ray and laboratory testing conducted in the hospitals in which they worked and the availability of house physicians, specialist physicians, and technicians to do the work. For example, smaller hospitals typically offered less extensive in-house testing, but they also had fewer or no house physicians or other ancillary personnel to do this work. Shortages of personnel were especially acute after World War I.

Accordingly, nurses' work in x-ray and laboratory diagnosis variously included the before, during, and after care of equipment and of patients at the bedside or in the units in which the tests were conducted; the transportation of patients to these units; the collection, labeling, storing, and delivery of specimens; the creation and maintenance of written records of these examinations; and/or the conduct of the examinations themselves. Urinometers to measure the specific gravity of urine, litmus paper to determine its pH, and other devices to measure albumin and sugar were part of the nurse's outfit and responsibilities from the earliest days of trained nursing.[71] Nurses also performed a promotional function for hospitals, guiding touring visitors (during annual events such as Hospital Day) through laboratory and x-ray units and showing off the new scientific equipment housed there.[72]

In addition to carrying out the various tasks associated with x-ray and laboratory testing on the unit, nurses were employed as assistants in x-ray and laboratory departments, where they administered barium for fluoroscopic examinations of the gastrointestinal tract (see fig. 4-3) and maintained records.[73] Nurses were also employed as x-ray technicians and microscopists in hospitals and physicians' offices, where they obtained and developed x-ray pictures and conducted chemical assays of blood, urine, sputum, and other specimens. As students, nurses were rotated through x-ray and laboratory departments and had available to them elective training in x-ray or laboratory work in their last year of school and in postgraduate courses.[74]

There were both nurses and physicians who promoted x-ray and laboratory work as nursing specialties. Nurses advocating specialization saw this work as an opportunity to gain knowledge and skills that would make them more marketable to physicians and hospitals. In an era when most nursing positions in hospitals were still filled by student nurses, and when graduate nurses were increasingly competing with one another for decreasing positions in the home and in public health, the "needy" x-ray and laboratory fields offered employment to the equally needy graduate nurse.[75] The routinization of x-ray and laboratory diagnosis also legitimated the need for more science education in nursing curricula to make nurses more able assistants. The work that this new kind of diagnosis generated made even more essential knowledge of anatomy, physiology, physics, chemistry, and bac-

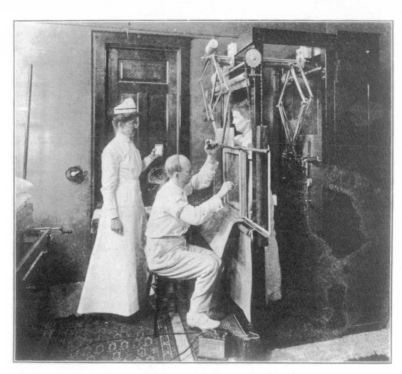

Figure 4-3. Nurse offering barium drink. (From Edward F. Stevens, *The American Hospital of the Twentieth Century*, 2nd rev. ed. [New York: Architectural Record, 1921], 225)

teriology. Moreover, by virtue of the association of x-ray and laboratory technology with the much revered science, nurses who were knowledgeable in these areas could further distinguish themselves, not only from untrained nurses but also from the trained nurses who knew nothing of these fields. Both nurse and physician advocates of nursing specialization promoted roentgen and laboratory work as especially fitting for nurses showing a "scientific turn of mind."[76]

For nurse and physician proponents of nurse specialization, x-ray and laboratory work offered an interesting departure from and often better working conditions than bedside nursing.[77] They argued that the hours of work were generally more regular and convenient, the pay was sometimes better, and the nurse won a reprieve from the daily complexities and physical exertions of caring for sick people that tended to shorten her working life. Although a departure from traditional bedside nursing, the work permitted the nurse to draw from her nursing background to alleviate the discomfort and fear that patients, especially children, experienced as they encountered these strange new tests.

Indeed, as nurse advocates proposed, this work demanded not only the skills associated with applying the technology but also the talents of the trained nurse in managing patients' emotions and in protecting the privacy specialized tests often threatened. Patients reportedly had many misconceptions and fears about these procedures and were embarrassed by having to remove their clothes for x-rays and other tests. Nurses' observations during these examinations were also critical to the accurate interpretation of test results and, therefore, to accurate medical diagnosis. X-ray and laboratory work was deemed especially suited to the nurse who wanted to keep in touch with nursing but who was less "adapted" by virtue of "physique or personality" to do continuous bedside nursing. Nurses were, therefore, considered "natural[s]" to assume the new work these tests generated, as they were already serving in hospitals, had a great deal of knowledge about patients and diseases, and were already trained to be assistants to physicians.[78]

Physician proponents of nurses in x-ray and laboratory fields viewed nurses as especially suitable to assume the work of busy, absent, and unavailable physicians. Physicians could not have large numbers of patients and the revenues they generated and also perform all the work the new method of diagnosis demanded. Accordingly, some of them turned to nurses as an available, cheap, and compliant alternative to house physicians. Lamenting the post–World War I shortage of interns in small hospitals, North Carolina physician Edmundson Boice advocated the delegation of "laborious" and "routine" tasks such as urinalysis, blood counts, and medical histories to nurses. Like other physicians, he had assigned these tasks to a "good nurse" and was very satisfied with the results. According to Boice, a good nurse could assume more and more tasks until she was "almost as much assistance as a well trained house physician."[79]

Boice acknowledged that by not having to compete for house physicians, hospitals risked lowering their standards and losing the new ideas these physicians brought with them. House physicians could also be paid less than nurses because they would not be performing their life's work. A house physician worked for the experience, not the $25 per month he earned. In contrast, a nurse worked for what she earned, and she had to make laboratory work her life. According to Boice, however, delegating these tasks to nurses was ultimately cheaper, since once nurses were trained, hospitals no longer faced the cost of training a new house physician every year.

Although x-ray and laboratory work was promoted in the immediate post–World War I period and the 1920s as good for both nurses and physicians, nurses appear not to have entered these fields as specialists in numbers sufficient to meet the demand.[80] By the 1930s advocates of nurse specialization promoted these areas to nurses for whom they were still "unknown land."[81] One physician reportedly lamented what he perceived as the timidity of most nurses, who lacked the "ability and thirst for progression" that becoming a "roentgenologist's assistant" could satisfy.[82] Some nurses apparently still feared the dangers to health and fertility that x-ray work entailed; roentgenologists were reportedly initially reluctant to permit nurses near x-ray machines because of these concerns.[83] Moreover, specializing was not always as interesting as advertised, as it typically involved routine and monotonous procedures. In addition, x-ray and laboratory tasks were often simply added to the nurse's ward work without any additional pay.[84]

Despite the difficulties of bedside care, most nurses seem to have preferred the intimacy of it to the science of laboratory or x-ray work. They were not schooled to pursue scientific work or may not have seen it as essentially nursing work. Indeed, there is some indication that nurses perceived x-ray and laboratory diagnosis as interfering with nursing work and the order of the ward. One nurse lamented that her colleagues often looked on a laboratory "test" as something that had to be done because the doctor ordered it, and they felt relief when it was over because the "routine" work of the ward could then proceed without further interference. But she also suggested that nurses were not being educated properly in this area; they would do this work with interest, enthusiasm, and accuracy if they knew the significance of these tests and the importance of the nurse in assisting with diagnosis.[85]

Multiplying, Dividing, and Denying the Labor of Diagnosis

Whether they viewed the new method of diagnosis as opportunity or interference, nurses acquired much of the labor associated with it. Instructional texts increasingly devoted more attention to the nurse's assistive role in medical diagnosis. By the 1930s "assisting [the] physician in examining patients . . . and [in] making diagnostic tests" was one of twelve "aspects of nursing skill" identified in a comprehensive activity analysis of nursing.[86] In successive editions of the classic Harmer (later Harmer and Henderson) textbooks on the principles and practice of nursing, tasks referred to in 1922 as "nursing procedures" used in the treatment of disease were, by 1939, described under the heading "assisting with diagnostic procedures."[87] The Ewald Test Meal, for example, was a nursing procedure used to treat alimentary tract diseases in 1922, but in 1939 it was a diagnostic procedure that nurses assisted the physician to perform.

Physicians increasingly depended on nurses to detect and act on problems early, since the nurse was likely to be the first person to discern an aberration in temperature or to find albumin in a patient's urine and, therefore, spare the patient dangerous delays in treatment. Yet as diagnosis was becoming a process to which nurses, patients, and others increasingly contributed, physicians sought to reserve the act of diagnosis exclusively for themselves. A recurring theme in instructional texts for nurses was that they were never to cross the line between nursing observation and medical diagnosis.[88] As one physician warned, "Outside of correct reports, the nurse has nothing to do with diagnosis or prognosis. And, beyond executing orders and recording bedside notes, [she] has no part in the treatment."[89]

Even before technologically mediated diagnosis characterized medical practice, physicians were ambivalent about what nurses needed to know and, more importantly, about what nurses should be taught to conduct the kind of close observation and reporting physicians required to prescribe treatment. On one hand, many physicians saw nurses as Baconian data collectors whose only job was to obtain the "raw data" the physician required. On the other hand, nurses were not just to report whatever they saw without interpretive comment; they should also discern the likely reason for a symptom, know what a symptom meant, and take the required action.[90] Nurses were in the bizarre position of having to be mindful of symptoms without speaking their mind about them. Nurses were to "know . . . as much as the physician about the meaning of symptoms," yet they were to have no "tendency to become medical women, or to set up their own opinions in practice."[91]

Physicians' ambivalence about nurses' powers of observation and the education required to cultivate them is evident in the vigorous debate about the "overtrained nurse." At times juxtaposed with the "under-trained" physician, the idea of the overtrained nurse emerged almost simultaneously with the appearance of trained nurses.[92] A general concern of physicians engaged in this debate was how much knowledge nurses should have for the good of patients and, perhaps more importantly, for the good of physicians. Arguing that both a little and a lot of knowledge were dangerous to both patients and themselves, physicians were especially concerned that nurses not assume that either diagnosis or treatment was in their sphere.[93] Especially troublesome to physicians most anxious about nursing education were examination questions for nurses that required answers only a physician should, and often did not, know.[94] As one physician argued, what patients required was not a nurse who could write a thesis about urinalysis or how to test for hydrochloric acid in stomach contents but, rather, one who could fluff their pillows, feed them, and report on their condition to the doctor. Indeed, advances in medical science and technology were causing both physicians and nurses to lose sight of the true and nonscientific function of the nurse.[95] As another physician summarized it: "We do not want a scientific person; we do not want a person with theories of her own, or with a smattering of other people's theories. . . . Of what use is it for [the nurse] . . . to hear lectures on the eye and the ophthalmoscope, subjects which occupy the earnest and constant study of highly educated men, and can be pursued to advantage by those only who give their whole time and attention to them?"[96]

Accordingly, nurses were recurringly admonished in didactic texts that diagnosis was not their business, even as they were increasingly being offered and sought more scientific knowledge about disease and clinical experience in various components of diagnosis, and as physicians were increasingly expecting them to perform de facto acts of diagnosis. Nurses were supposed to be able to distinguish between normal and abnormal conditions and to look for reasons for any abnormal findings. But nurses were never to use the words "normal" or "abnormal" in reporting or recording patient conditions, and they were to refrain from offering their opinions on etiology or diagnosis.[97] Nurses were not to use "diagnostic statements." As nurses were cautioned in a set of " 'don'ts' for nurses," it was not for the nurse to say that a patient was having "pain around the appendix." She was to say instead that the patient had "a dull pain in the lower right quadrant, radiating to the left side" and that it "seems less severe with knees flexed."[98] Nurses were to say (report and record) only what they saw, unlike physicians, who maintained the right to say what they knew.[99] Ethel Johns and Blanche Pfefferkorn summarized the paradoxical position of the nurse in relation to diagnosis by observing that "while the nurse is debarred from making a diagnosis, she is tacitly permitted to arrange into a pattern any significant symptoms upon which such diagnosis may be based."[100]

The new diagnostic technology reinforced the processual, as opposed to the episodic, nature of diagnosis and allowed this process to be divided into separate spheres of activity. As a consequence, technology both reinforced and blurred the line between the diagnosis that was supposed to be the physician's exclusive domain and the observation that was the nurse's shared domain.

A case in point involves clinical thermometry. When thermometers were first introduced into clinical practice, some physicians expressed concerns about whether nurses or family members could be entrusted with their use. Physicians soon discovered, however, that the kind of information they needed for the diagnosis, treatment, and scientific study of disease required a graphic record of temperatures taken regularly and at critical moments in the progression of a disease, and someone had to be at the bedside at the right times to obtain this information. Carl Wunderlich, whose treatise was so influential in persuading physicians that the thermometer was needed in medical practice, contended that a major impediment to the practical utility of the thermometer was that taking all the required temperatures consumed too much of the physician's time.[101] Seguin had also noted that there was no part of the physician's work that required so much help as thermometry. If only one or two temperature readings were needed, a physician could obtain these himself when he visited his patients. Indeed, if he could not, Seguin advised that the physician not take the case.[102] But if six or seven daily temperature readings were required, the physician needed help; it was not necessary that he take the temperatures himself, but only that he knew who took the temperatures and how they were taken. The physician's knowledge of pathological thermometry was sufficient to enable him to control or estimate the temperature readings obtained.

Moreover, anyone with good sight could be taught quickly to take accurate temperatures. Indeed, Wunderlich noted that persons unencumbered with the specialized knowledge of physicians were likely to make even fewer errors than the physician in obtaining an accurate temperature because they had no preconceived opinions to prejudice them.[103] In a similar vein, Seguin observed that "as astronomic observations are often better recorded by honest, attentive assistants than by astronomers, so a medical student, a nurse, [or] a relative can be made a useful assistant to the medical thermometrician."[104] Ignorance had its advantages, and it could be exploited to benefit the busy physician.

While Wunderlich noted the value and even necessity of assistance with medical thermometry, he also believed that the "mere reading of temperature degrees helps diagnosis no more than dispensing does therapeusis."[105] Physicians did not recognize or minimized the skilled safety work involved in obtaining temperatures from children or from delirious and fearful patients. Moreover, clinical thermometry was itself a technique that permitted the labor of diagnosis to be separated into unequal parts, with nurses increasingly assuming what were perceived as the largely mechanical tasks of taking and recording temperatures and of maintaining thermometers, and physicians taking on what was considered the higher-order interpretive task of evaluating what the temperatures meant. By placing the tasks of diagnosis in a hierarchy and reserving the label of diagnosis only for physicians' acts of interpretation, physicians could deny that nonphysicians played any part in thermometric diagnosis. If nurses interpreted and acted on temperature readings, it was because physicians allowed and needed nurses to engage in these "mental" activities, not because they were considered nursing work.

X-ray and laboratory technology also entailed an actual and rhetorical division and denial of labor. Nurses were seen as naturals to do much of the work of diagnosis without usurping the physician's preeminent role in the process. Physicians in general practice were especially worried about the encroachment of x-ray and laboratory physician specialists (such as pathologists and roentgenologists), who were competing for access to and revenues from patients by claiming the diagnostic act for themselves. Concerned over the abuse of medical specialization and the overuse of the new diagnostic technologies, rank-and-file physicians wanted laboratories and x-ray units to be seen as tools for the frontline, general physician—who knew the patient—to make diagnoses, not as diagnostic entities themselves.[106] Nurse specialization in these areas threatened neither physicians' access to patients nor, more importantly, their exclusive claim to diagnosis. The effect of this division and denial of the labor of diagnosis was to downplay the technical, interpersonal, and body-tending expertise of nurses and their frequently greater skill in these components of the application of the new diagnostic technology to the patient.

The delegation to nurses of tasks considered easy enough for a nurse to do belied the actual complexity of these tasks. An especially good illustration of the complexity of duties left to nurses was the Ewald Test Meal, which involved both technical and interactional skills. This test was commonly used to diagnose gastrointestinal ailments and included a carefully sequenced and timed orchestration of events, which could involve up to four patients undergoing the test at the same time. According to Elizabeth Connolly, superintendent of nursing at the North Carolina Sanatorium, fourteen student nurses had successfully conducted 365 tests between 1921 and 1923. In her description of the procedure, the test first involved patient preparation, which included instruction about the test and fasting.[107] On the day of the test, with the patient resting in a recliner, the nurse passed a rubber tube with a "bucket" (or tip designed to catch the gastric contents) into the stomach. This process often induced gagging in the patient, which the nurse reduced by spraying the throat with a 2 percent solution of cocaine. Once the tube was in the stomach, the nurse aspirated its contents with a syringe, taking care that the plunger not fit its barrel too snugly. Too tight a fit could cause the lining of the stomach to be damaged as it was sucked into the tip of the tube. The nurse then gave the patient the Ewald meal of bread and water, with or without the tube still in place. Removing it at this point meant that the nurse would have to reinsert it later rapidly enough to conform to the timing of events the test required. With a clock in full view, the patient was given four minutes to finish the meal. If the nurse was supervising four patients at 2:45, that meant that Patient #1 was required to finish the meal between 2:45 and 2:49; Patient #2, between 2:49 and 2:53; Patient #3, between 2:53 and 2:57, and Patient #4, between 2:57 and 3:01. Exactly eleven minutes after the patient had finished the meal, the nurse aspirated the stomach contents. Patient #1 would have her or his stomach aspirated at 3:00; Patient #2, at 3:04; Patient #3, at 3:08; and Patient #4, at 3:12. The nurse then placed the aspirated specimens into test tubes. She had to assure herself that the specimen was not tinged with bile, since that indicated that the bucket had passed out of the stomach into the duodenum, thereby invalidating the test. The nurse then removed the tube from the patient, taking care not to leave the bucket inside the stomach or esophagus and to avoid the laryngeal or pharyngeal spasms that often occurred during this process. Such spasms could greatly impede the tube's passage out of the patient. Tugging at the tube would both frighten the patient and further hamper removal of the tube.

The Diagnostic Revolution and the
Rhetoric of Diagnosis

The introduction of sense-extending implements, such as the stethoscope, the ophthalmoscope, the laryngoscope, and the fluoroscope, and of device-mediated techniques to measure, monitor, analyze, and record body functions, such as clinical thermometry, electrocardiography, and chemical assays of urine, blood, and other fluids, had an enormous impact on medicine.[108] This new diagnostic technology augmented physicians' abilities to investigate and diagnose disease; decreased their reliance on patients while increasing their reliance on instruments and specialist physicians, nurses, and technicians to accomplish diagnosis; and enhanced their prestige as the preeminent practitioners of science in an era when science was becoming the new religion. Indeed, physicians derived much of their cultural authority from their association with a technology that was seen to embody science.[109]

Many physicians were initially reluctant to use the new technology. They were concerned about "losing touch" with patients—that is, losing contact with them, losing their exclusive relationship with them, and losing their skill of "digital observation" and other largely embodied techniques for ascertaining what was wrong with patients.[110] Physicians also feared losing their authority and exclusive claim to the knowledge and skill that technology required and the knowledge about disease it offered. Physicians were concerned that reliance on technology would undermine their efforts to practice and to present medicine as an intellectual and independent (as opposed to manual and collaborative) pursuit. In the early nineteenth century physicians often associated technology with the manual labor, instrumentation, and barbarities of surgeons, from whom they were eager to disassociate themselves. By the end of that century, however, physicians were recognizing that the new diagnostic devices, like surgical instruments, allowed physicians not only to improve medical practice and advance medical science but also to be seen as actively and concretely doing something to earn the social standing, authority, and remuneration they sought. In an important sense the new diagnosis was visibly interventionist, thereby preserving physicians' long-standing professional identification with action.[111]

Moreover, although physicians differentiated medical from nursing practice, in part, by emphasizing the subjective judgment required to use instruments such as the stethoscope and sphygmomanometer properly, they were also eager to "purge subjectivity" from the practice of medicine by incorporating such instruments.[112] Physicians viewed temperature graphs, x-ray pictures, and electrocardiographs as material expressions of the science that ultimately distinguished medicine from other patient-oriented practices. Accordingly, physicians increasingly relied on what they perceived as more objective instrument- or machine-generated information. Physicians gradually became less comfortable with patient descriptions and their own unaided senses as the sole or even primary basis for diagnosis. Their increasing reliance on technology distanced them from patients in ways that both advantaged and disadvantaged physicians. Physicians were socially separated from patients by their acquisition of increasingly specialized and arcane knowledge not readily accessible to anyone but themselves. What the doctor heard and saw through the magic and science of the stethoscope and microscope could not easily be heard, seen, or understood by others. Physicians' new knowledge set them apart from and elevated them above patients and other professional competitors seeking access to the patient's bedside.

But physicians were also physically separated from patients, as medical diagnosis was increasingly accomplished at a distance and through the efforts of specialists, including other physicians, nurses, and technicians. The stethoscope had brought physicians closer to patients' bodies while maintaining a suitable space between the patient's body and the physician's ear. Rene Laennec, the inventor of "mediate auscultation" via the stethoscope in the early nineteenth century, was reportedly motivated by the desire not only to hear the sounds of body organs but also to avoid the close physical contact that placing an ear to the body entailed, but which patients' bodies made repugnant or social mores made suspect.[113] The microscope and the x-ray permitted diagnosis to occur without the patient's presence. Moreover, the new method of diagnosis increasingly required what the general practitioner typically or frequently did not have: the time and expertise of specialists to conduct these tests and to interpret their results.

The emergence of trained nursing in the United States in the 1870s and its capture in hospitals by the 1930s did not merely coincide with the diagnostic revolution that fundamentally transformed American medicine in this period; they were tightly linked.[114] During this time hospitals were increasingly sold to potential patients as sites for the sympathetic and scientific care embodied in the new trained nurse and the new diagnostic technology. Nurses played a crucial role in the technological transformation of medicine and hospitals, sharing with physicians the use of instruments such as the thermometer and often performing much of the physical, mental, and "sentimental" labor engendered by x-ray and laboratory tests.[115] Nurses made hospitals more hospitable, not only to patients but also to the new devices and device-mediated techniques that became the sine qua non of medical practice. Nursing was the soft technology that allowed physicians to use the new hardware of diagnosis.

Without making any claims to participating in diagnosis, nurses were expected to collect, record, and interpret information vital to the diagnosis—and, therefore, to the treatment and prognosis—of disease under the putatively watchful eyes of physicians. Both nurses and physicians had always conceived of nursing observation as the "third eye of the physician through which he sees his patient."[116] The physician required the "service of another pair of eyes that will be as alert in noting changes in the patient as his own eyes would be if he had the time to be with the patient continuously."[117] Nurses were encouraged to make and record observations that would enable physicians to evaluate a patient's condition "without having seen" the patient.[118] Physicians appropriated nurses' eyes as proxies for their own, just as they appropriated nurses' hands to carry out the work of diagnosis. The primary role nurses played in the technological transformation of medical practice was to put the new diagnostic technology into use.[119] Although nurses played no known part in the invention of the diagnostic devices discussed here, they did play a critical role in their application. Nurses performed key components of the work of medical diagnosis, variously obtaining device-mediated information from patients and recording, interpreting, and acting on this information. Nurses directly applied new devices and techniques to patients, and they provided the before-and-after care of patients and equipment. Nurses enlisted the cooperation of the patient for tests that could be uncomfortable, time consuming, and/or frightening. The new "medical gaze" of the physician, accomplished with the aid of diagnostic technology, was, in part, "articulated through and mediated by" the nurse.[120] The trained nurse's eyes and hands were the most critical instruments in the new diagnostic armamentarium of physicians in the United States.

Although nurses were essential to medical diagnosis, medical diagnosis was arguably not essential to nursing. For all of its revolutionary impact on U.S. medicine, instrumental diagnosis did not redefine nursing practice and the nurse/patient relationship as it did medical practice and the physician/patient relationship, where diagnosis replaced treatment in this period as the central point of the physician/patient encounter and the centerpiece of medical intervention. The central point of nursing practice and the nurse/patient relationship remained to minister to patient needs and to assist physicians to diagnose and treat patients. Nursing observation still entailed watching over patients for signs of disease or problems with treatment. Nurses did not see patients differently as a result of using or having access to implements that offered new ways and new things to see. With the possible exception of the thermometer, there is little evidence that nurses used the information derived from these instruments to alter nursing practice. Nurses continued to look at their patients, not through them. Nurses themselves did not use x-rays or electrocardiograms or the results of laboratory tests to initiate changes in the care of patients, nor did their views of patients and nursing substantially change because of these procedures.[121] The new diagnostic technology altered the material, but not the conceptual, world of the nurse. Nurses continued to observe their patients largely in the flesh, not through instruments. As the knowledge gained through instrumental observation was seen as more objective and scientific than knowledge obtained in the flesh, the powers once attributed to nursing observation were diminished.

Although the new diagnostic technology did not change the conceptual world of the nurse, it did complicate her work and ideas about what that work should be. Nurses had different tasks to perform. Patients entering hospitals for diagnosis were increasingly different from the traditional hospital patient in that they were not necessarily sick. As Clare Dennison observed, these patients did not require nursing "care" so much as nursing "services," which included not only diagnostic testing itself but also the work of meeting patients' new expectations for hospitals. These healthier patients expected hospital service to be much like hotel service; they anticipated being able to conduct their business and social activities in the hospital and wanted their desires for the size of and furnishings and decorations in their rooms to be met.[122]

Nurses also had more work to do, but nurses debated whether this work drew them away from their traditional ministrations. Nurses increasingly delegated traditional nurse/patient encounters, such as bathing, to ancillary personnel, in part to make time for their new medical duties.[123] Commenting on these "extra-nursing functions and the nursing load," however, Blanche Pfefferkorn and Marian Rottman implied that physician-to-nurse delegation of medical tasks did not necessarily require nurses to delegate traditional nursing chores to ancillary personnel. As they noted, it was often said that "technical and medical functions" were steadily being transferred to nurses, thereby interfering with nursing duties and greatly increasing nursing work. But, they argued, although this was likely true for graduate nurses electing that kind of work, the findings from a study at Bellevue Hospital in New York revealed "an almost negligible amount of time given to activities, other than those of a purely nursing nature." As they observed,

> If an assignment to take and record the blood pressure added two hours to a daily workload of 100 hours, the increase was not sufficient to burden the nursing service or to affect the quality of the nursing. It seems likely that the time emphasis placed upon new responsibilities outside the immediate field of nursing has been due to the fact that in most institutions, the required nursing load hours exceed the provided nursing hours, and, as a result, any addition to the already existing load is apt to be considered out of its right proportion.[124]

Less debatable was the fact that the new diagnostic technology was instrumental in both reinforcing the rhetorical and subverting the actual division between nursing and doctoring. Clinical thermometry and x-ray and laboratory diagnosis, by virtue of the physical operations they entailed, were "valenced" toward a division of labor that reinforced the usual invidious distinctions between manual and mental labor.[125] That is, they permitted tasks to be divided into a hierarchy of manual/physical/mechanical and mental/intellectual/interpretive components, which could, in turn, be easily matched to the existing social hierarchy in clinical practice. The standardization of devices such as the thermometer reinforced these distinctions, as it implied that there were procedures that could be performed independent of the mind of the worker. Certain tasks could be delegated to "lower-level" nonphysicians, while others could be reserved exclusively for physicians. Stethoscopic examination, in which tasks could not so easily be divided, remained largely the preserve of physicians through the 1940s.

Although the delegation to nurses of tasks physicians considered easy enough for a nurse to do degraded the knowledge and skill these tasks required, it also gave nurses an opportunity to advance their technical skills, obtain more scientific knowledge, and thereby enhance their social position. Physicians expected nurses to stand in for them as diagnosticians in their absence. By virtue of their absence and the constant presence of the nurse at the bedside, physicians had no choice but to depend on nurses. Nurses, in turn, had no choice—if patients were to be safe—but to perform de facto acts of diagnosis. Diagnostic technology did not so much create as it dramatized the advantageous position nurses were in by virtue of this spatiotemporal asymmetry between medicine and nursing.[126] In the language of measurement, nurses were the interval measurers for physicians, who were usually only nominally present.

There were several factors, however, that together offset both the advantage nurses derived from their constant presence at the bedside and the access to science and technology that the new method of diagnosis offered. Before the diagnostic revolution in medicine in the United States, the focal point of the physician/patient encounter was less on discerning the reason for an ailment than on alleviating its miseries, which meant primarily good bedside—that is, nursing—care. With the new focus on diagnosis, even in the face of a continuing absence of effective treatments for many of the diseases diagnosed, physicians gained power and control as the physician's diagnosis—not nursing care per se—was what increasingly brought patients into hospitals.[127] Indeed, new diagnostic instruments often played more of a "symbolic" role in the service of physicians than a therapeutic role in the service of curing patients.[128] Physicians could sell medical tests to patients as a new "medical commodity" that did not fail, as had so many of their treatments.[129]

In this era of new diagnostic techniques, nursing seemed less autonomous and more dependent on medical diagnosis for its existence. The new technology materially contributed to the idea that nursing was derivative, that it was comprised of no more than the manual work derived from the physician's mental work. As more nursing was being practiced in hospitals than anywhere else, the diagnostic revolution in medicine diminished the importance of nursing by subsuming it more firmly under medicine. Moreover, it reinforced the service, as opposed to professional, role of the nurse, as the new procedures meant assisting physicians to advance medicine and dealing with patients who were not sick enough to require the body care nurses were used to providing. If nurses thought that the move from home and private duty care to hospital nursing would help them escape being treated like servants, they often fared no better in hospitals, where they were still treated this way by both administrators and patients.

Moreover, by defining diagnosis as only what the doctor did, physicians were able to offset any threat that nurses may have posed to their command and dominance. For physicians with the authority to define it, diagnosis was quintessentially about ordering and interpreting tests; it was not about ensuring that procedures were properly done, or conducting the test, or gaining patients' cooperation. Nurses themselves never sufficiently protested this definition of diagnosis, and nurses never pursued specialization in x-ray and laboratory work in any organized way that might have advanced their standing. Instead, nurses maintained the "purity" of diagnosis for physicians, thereby assisting physicians to derive the cultural authority they gained from new diagnostic technology. That is, nurses relieved physicians of having to deal with the human complexities entailed in making sure that tests were properly conducted and anxious patients were assuaged. While nurses performed the "defiling acts" of diagnosis, physicians often had only to deal with interpreting test results, thereby maintaining the unequal social relations between nurses and physicians.[130]

Accordingly, although nurses shared many new diagnostic devices with physicians, they had different relations to them with different effects. They gained new knowledge, but they did not gain the prestige that using scientific instruments ought to have given them in a culture that revered science and technology. Once a "prestige tool" exclusively associated with physicians and science, the thermometer soon became feminized by association with women and nurses.[131] In the case of implements that both physicians and nurses used, the user context determined the prestige accorded to their use. Nursing continued to be legitimated not by science but, rather, by gender.[132] The nurse's use of a device depended on "skillful manipulation"; the physician's use, on "scientific training."[133] Nurses watched out for patients the way nurturing women did; they did not watch them the way scientists did.

The denial of nonphysician diagnosis was largely a rhetorical move that became well entrenched in social custom, the law, and the popular imagination.[134] Diagnostic technology further elasticized the sphere of the nurse. That is, this technology did not so much enlarge the sphere of influence of the nurse as permit her scope of responsibility to expand or contract according to whether physicians or others were available to perform the various tasks required by the technology. Whether a nurse did virtually all or very little of the work associated with a diagnostic procedure depended on the availability of other personnel, the drive to save money, and physician preference. Whether a skill was viewed as simple or complex depended, in part, on who performed it. Indeed, "simple" and "nursing" became virtually synonymous by virtue of their frequent association with each other. From the beginnings of trained nursing, the very definition of skill was "gender-biased."[135]

Although the nurse's scope of responsibility was not fixed, there were certain purification duties that were relatively constant. Nurses were always charged with gaining the cooperation of patients, and they always cleaned up. Accordingly, although nurses acquired new knowledge and skill, what they gained most of all was new and more work to do that advanced primarily medical goals. Like mediate auscultation, a specialized form of listening accomplished with the stethoscope, hospital nursing became mediate medicine, a special form of medical practice accomplished with nurses. The nurse was to the physician another device—much like his stethoscope and x-ray machine —in his new armamentarium of diagnosis. Indeed, she was hardly different from the standardized thermometers and manometers she was entrusted to use. Like these other-meters, she simply registered numbers.

5   Truly & Technically Nursing

The most important milestone in the history of nursing after World War II was the virtually complete hospitalization, "proletarianization,"[1] and "bureaucratization"[2] of nursing. At this time approximately 60 percent of nurses were employees of hospitals, as opposed to private entrepreneurs or agents of public health providing care in patients' homes and in work settings.[3] In addition to graduate nurse and student nurse, the category of "nurse" encompassed an array of diversely educated and skilled personnel, including the nurse's aide or assistant, the licensed vocational or practical nurse, the registered nurse educated in a three-year hospital-based program of study, and increasingly in the 1950s, the registered nurse educated in a four-year university school of nursing or in a two-year community college program. Moreover, nursing practice was increasingly characterized by "team nursing," whereby one registered nurse supervised the care of up to fifty patients by lesser trained nursing personnel, and by "mass nursing care," or functional nursing, whereby one nurse carried out one technique, such as the taking of temperatures and the giving of injections, for all the patients requiring it at one time.[4]

Nursing practice still included an array of devices and encompassed a variety of activities, which did not necessarily signal a distinctive professional domain. Nursing work, increasingly performed by any one of a cadre of diversely prepared but seemingly interchangeable nurses, continued to entail housework (including the housework itself and its management) and medical work. A 1945 pictorial rendering of nursing exemplified its ambiguous nature.[5] The implements of nursing pictured included common household items, such as mops, brooms, and vacuum cleaners, and medical paraphernalia, such as iron lungs and gastric suction devices. Nursing included dusting and flower arranging as well as caring for seriously ill patients in oxygen tents and respirators. The practice of nursing entailed the "menial" and "simple" and the "complex" and "technical."[6]

As registered nurses were increasingly charged with efficiently administering patient care (as opposed to ministering directly to patients), the telephone, the chart, the desk, and the clock competed with the bed, the bedpan, and the bandage as key implements of nursing. In one of the many function studies of hospital nursing conducted in the 1950s,[7] registered nurses reportedly spent approximately four times as much time on the telephone and on supervision and instruction and three times as much time with records, reports, and requisitions as they did providing direct patient care.[8] Similar studies also showed nurses to be "subjugated to time" and paper,[9] with the most highly trained nurses spending more time supervising patient care or executing medically delegated diagnostic and treatment procedures than ministering to patients.[10] When registered nurses appeared at the bedside, it was more often with a needle or a clipboard than with a bedpan, linens, or a "touch[ing]" hand.[11]

Now "intrinsically linked" to the hospital, the "embodiment of modern medical science" and "icon" of technological progress,[12] nurses in the post–World War II period through the 1960s became increasingly concerned about what the essence of nursing was and ought to be.[13] At the center of their concerns were the increasingly problematic relations between "true" nursing and "tenderness and technique."[14]

Body Work and Technical Nursing

Despite their long-standing focus on techniques—that is, on performing chores such as bathing, bedmaking, and toileting—nurses had always had a sense that the essence of nursing lay beyond technique. As one late-nineteenth-century writer observed,

Doctors may bleed and purge in one generation, feed and stimulate in the next; one may wrap a rheumatism patient in blankets and apply hot-water bottles, another will place him in an ice pack; snails, slugs, and dead men's bones may be gravely ordered by the faculty in one century, salicilate of soda, quinine, and anti-pyrine may be in vogue in the next; one generation of medicos may stifle a fever or small-pox case in scarlet blankets and hermetically sealed windows, the next will blow him almost out of bed with the most approved ventilators. . . . But always and ever will the sick man require to be nursed, to be gently lifted, his bed carefully made, his wants unselfishly attended to.[15]

For this writer, the work the nurse performed was in a larger sense more elemental and enduring than what the doctor did. There was a natural and unchanging core to nursing; "fashions in treatments come and fashions in treatment go, but nursing goes on forever."[16] For early-twentieth-century nursing leaders such as Isabel Stewart and Effie Taylor, the essence of nursing was not in the technical details of procedures or in the manual dexterity of nurses but, rather, in the knowledge that lay behind their skills and in the humanity with which they approached their patients. This larger intelligence and grace made nursing a profession as opposed to a skilled trade.[17] In mid-century Faye Abdellah observed that technical procedures were only the most "overt and visible" and least "unique" parts of nursing.[18]

After World War II, pharmacological, technological, and other treatment innovations, such as antibiotic and intravenous (IV) therapy, early ambulation, and earlier hospital discharge, called into question the meaning of technique in nursing and the value of the bed and body work that had comprised the natural core of trained nursing since its beginnings. Whereas bathing patients to reduce the fever from an infection used to be a life-saving activity, an injection of penicillin now eradicated the infection, and it did so faster, more effectively, more reliably, and with much less effort. Antibiotic therapy transformed many infectious diseases from potentially mortal to highly treatable and short-term conditions. Similarly, the IV infusion of fluids was a more efficient way to hydrate sick patients than coaxing them to take liquids by mouth.

Moreover, not only were patients staying in hospitals for shorter periods of time, but they were occupying their beds for less time while they were in the hospital. Between 1931 and 1951 the average general hospital stay declined from fourteen to ten days.[19] By the early 1950s bedrest was declining as a mode of therapy, and more patients were getting out of bed within two days of surgery.[20] No longer were patients "condemned to weeks of imprisonment in bed," nor was the greatest part of the nurse's day spent "around, about, and with the bed."[21] The traditional bed and body work of the nurse became literally less vital to patients and figuratively less dramatic than new drug and surgical treatments, even as more patients were being admitted to hospitals. In addition, despite the fact that nurses increasingly administered many of these new therapies to patients, the accolades went to the physicians who ordered them. Indeed, as "needle bearers," nurses became arguably more visible than physicians as the proximate agents of discomfort and pain.[22] Getting a shot became for the patient a fearful and disturbing experience tied to nurses.[23]

Accordingly, needle and other new therapies not only devalued traditional nursing work but also undermined the traditional comforting role of the nurse. These procedures reinforced the role of the nurse as physician's assistant: a person who appeared to have no important therapies of her own to offer patients and who even caused patients to suffer. Nurses not only gave injections; they also forced patients in pain to get out of bed sooner than they wanted after surgery, and they enforced the sometimes incomprehensible and even frightening rituals of hospitalization. With obstetric patients, for example, nurses attempted to assimilate "hospital routines" into personalized care, but they were still often seen by childbearing women as unkind.[24]

As nurses were increasingly charged with administering needle and other new medical therapies to patients and with supervising entire hospital units, much of the core bed and body work of nursing was transferred to practical nurses and nursing assistants, whose numbers increased much more rapidly than those of registered nurses. Between 1950 and 1970 the number of registered nurses almost doubled, from 375,000 to 722,000, while the number of practical nurses almost tripled, from 137,000 to 370,000. The number of nursing assistants more than tripled, from 220,000 to 700,000 in the same time period.[25] Nurses lamented the loss of what they perceived to be the natural functions of the nurse to lesser-trained personnel, and of the "unmediated relationship" they once had with their patients.[26] In their mid-1950s study of maternity nursing, social scientist Marion Lesser and nurse educator Vera Keane found that body care was a "major channel" through which nurses established relations with their patients.[27] Moreover, so closely did many patients connect body care with nursing that they viewed anyone who gave it as a nurse. Proliferating at a much faster rate than registered nurses and more visible to patients at the bedside, these lesser-trained persons soon dominated both the ranks and the general public image of nursing.

Yet what nurses increasingly described as "natural" in nursing in the post–World War II period was not bedside work but, rather, the continued acceptance of previously medical and more managerial tasks.[28]

Most nurses seemed to believe they had no choice but to accept these new tasks and to delegate what they had once conceived of as natural in nursing—bedside work—to others. While most nurses viewed the delegation to nurses of administrative duties and tasks once exclusively performed by physicians as inevitable, many nurses were also pleased to accept them and to delegate, in turn, the traditional bedside work of the nurse to lesser-trained personnel. Although still important to patients' comfort and well-being, bathing and bed making had lost their status as medical therapies and had reverted to being ordinary womanly or maternal functions. These and other core bedside functions of nursing had once been viewed as requiring special knowledge and skill, but they were now seen as simple tasks entailing largely common knowledge.[29] As shown in nursing function studies, even temperature taking, which had been the trained nurse's first entrée into precision-instrument patient care, was delegated to ancillary personnel as a commonly held skill.

Nurses' assumption of delegated tasks served medical, managerial, and nursing interests. Physicians were able to maintain their authority over patient care while relieving themselves of more of its mundane duties; nurses were an efficient and cheap supply of labor in hospitals; and many nurses saw the delegation of bedside nursing tasks to others as a step toward full professionalization. As nurses assumed responsibility for an increasing array of medical tasks and for managing hospital units, many perceived these new functions as more professional and saw themselves less as the virtuous lady with the lamp and more as hospital managers and physicians' assistants. Indeed, nurses were characterized or typed in the 1950s and 1960s by the many social scientists who studied them, in part, according to their affinity for or orientation to the new apparatus of care. Nurses who preferred technical and managerial functions were described as technicians, administrators, and professionalizers, while nurses with a high affinity for providing tender loving care were described as ministering angels and traditionalizers.[30]

"Scientifically inclined" nurses were less concerned about handing over such ostensibly nonscientific functions as bathing and toileting to others in order to move professionally closer to science.[31] For these "ironhands," the new technology of patient care made nurses more visibly active and nursing more important.[32] Nurses evaluated fields of practice, in part, according to how central devices were to practice in those fields. For example, obstetric nursing seemed much less important than operating room (OR) nursing, with its "glittering array of . . . intricate instruments."[33] On a surgical unit there were dressing carts, orthopedic paraphernalia, and other apparatus. In contrast, a medical unit had "little machinery to be pushed around." The nurse on the surgical unit was consequently seen as doing things of "recognizable importance," such as changing dressings and swinging orthopedic frames into place. On medical units, what the nurse did was less visible, as it often entailed no thing per se and, albeit important to patient care, nothing more than looking at or touching patients to observe their breathing, for example, or to palpate the pulse. The apparatus of care reportedly inspired confidence and pride in the nurse, and it reassured the patient.[34] Not only did it make the nurse visible and nursing tangible to the patient, but it made nursing more palpable to the nurse herself. Nurses often conceived of sphygmomanometers, stethoscopes, and other implements associated with physicians as "badge[s] of status" or, at least, as more tangible indicators of their value.[35]

As early as the 1930s, however, nurses had been worried that technical procedures were interfering with true nursing. As one nurse observed then, "Modern scientific methods required a nurse to weigh and measure, chart and test far more than was formerly demanded of her." Tying these modern methods to the growing problem of "hospital inhospitality," she asked whether nurses were not allowing "science and efficiency [to] rob us of humanity and personal touch."[36] In a landmark report on nursing published in 1948, Esther Lucille Brown observed that physicians more often expected nurses to perform procedures formerly carried out only by physicians. Moreover, she warned that physicians were not likely to take these procedures back and would probably hand over additional duties to nurses in the future. Nursing education had overly emphasized these procedures, preparing "skilled technicians" as opposed to health teachers.[37]

Five years earlier, prominent nurse educator Isabel Stewart had remarked that nurses were abandoning "health nursing," which involved the "prevention of disease, the teaching of hygiene, [and] the upbuilding of family and community," in favor of the more "dramatic" and "practical . . . sick nursing" practiced in hospitals. Yet, as Stewart recalled, Florence Nightingale had envisioned the trained nurse as both a health teacher and a minister to the sick. Stewart concluded that new diagnostic methods and treatments had increased the demand for the "nurse's skillful hands" and "crowded out" other central nursing functions.[38] These health supervision functions were even being crowded out in public health nursing itself, where they ought to have prevailed, as the implements of hospital care were invading the home. In one agency there had been a dramatic increase between 1947 and 1950 in requests for visiting nurses to give hypodermic injections. In 1945 fewer than half of nurse visits were for "morbidity cases," but by 1948 over 70 percent of visits were for morbidity cases, owing largely to the increased use of needle therapies.[39]

Hospital nurses argued that they had less time to perform true nursing, or the intimate bed and body work of traditional private duty nursing, and to a lesser extent public health nurses were concerned that new therapies would interfere with health supervision and teaching in the home. Hospital nurses, in particular, worried about the increasingly technical nature of the functions nurses had to perform and the machine-like performance these functions seemed to engender. Yet nurses' resolution of this problem was not to preserve the functions of the true nurse for the true (or professional) nurse but, rather, to transfer bedside nursing in hospitals to ancillary personnel and to a new category of nurse: the technical nurse or nurse technician. Paradoxically, this technical nurse was not to perform the procedures that were crowding out traditional bedside nursing but, instead, bedside nursing itself. According to Mildred Montag, the nurse educator who introduced the idea of community college education to train the nurse technician, technical functions were those activities that were repetitive and did not require much education or judgment. Montag divided the labor of nursing, envisioning nursing functions on a continuum from the very simple to the complex.[40] Believing that much of the nurse's bedside work entailed only simple to minimally complex functions, she proposed that they could be safely delegated to nurses with only a technical (as opposed to professional) education. In an ironic and fateful twist of words, which served further to trouble nurses' efforts to define their identity and work, the technical nurse now performed true nursing functions (or bedside care), while the professional nurse performed technical functions (or the execution of complex medical tasks and administration). True nursing did not necessarily require a true nurse.

Although motivated by the author's desire to emphasize the complexities of professional nursing and to resolve the nursing shortage, Montag's differentiation between technical and professional nursing, a polarization of nursing embodied in team nursing and later endorsed in the American Nurses' Association's 1964 position paper on nursing education, formalized the idea that nursing was largely a simple affair reducible to a set of discrete functions that were easily carried out by minimally educated persons.[41] Medical practice was never comparably subdivided into minute functions that were still considered medical practice and most of which were dismissed as simple. When doctors transferred functions, they were careful to delegate them to persons who would never be called, mistaken for, or trained as physicians. They thereby preserved their value in the health care delivery marketplace. No one had ever suggested brief training for a technical (as opposed to professional) physician to multiply the numbers of physicians, or that medicine could ever be practiced by anyone other than physicians.

The idea and actual proliferation of the technical nurse disparaged the traditional bed and body work of nursing as much as the advent of antibiotics and early ambulation had seemed to trivialize it. The fact that professional and technical nurses often still performed the same functions, despite their educational differences, made diversely educated nurses seem interchangeable and nursing seem comprised only of a set of tasks. In contrast, nurses who performed the same functions as physicians were never seen as interchangeable with them. Nurses might perform medical functions, but they were not practicing medicine, the central core of which was diagnosis, prescription, and treatment. Moreover, the fungibility of nurses reinforced the long-standing belief that nurses themselves — not assistants to nurses — could be trained in a very short period of time. Advocates for advanced education for professional nurses thus continued to find it difficult to convince physicians, the general public, and many nurses themselves of the need for expending more time and money on professional nursing education.

Venous Envy

One new and very visible medical procedure after World War II was IV therapy. Until World War II, venipuncture, or the piercing of the vein with a needle to draw blood for laboratory analysis or to administer blood, fluids, or drugs, was a procedure wholly in the physician's realm. IV therapy was considered highly dangerous because of the risk of introducing infectious agents in the course of penetrating the vein — an especially mortal danger in the pre-antibiotic era — and because of the rapidity with which any agent injected directly into the bloodstream could cause serious injury or death. As one physician commented, "Nature never intended that the human being be fed and watered by vein, and, therefore, the insult of such a procedure should be respected." Yet he also noted that by 1935 feeding and watering patients by vein had become an increasingly "popular" (as opposed to emergency) mode of therapy.[42] In the early 1940s, one in every eight patients at Strong Memorial Hospital in Rochester, New York, received IV therapy.[43] The use of IV equipment at the University Hospital of Cleveland increased by 177 percent between 1938 and 1953.[44]

Although nurses were neither formally taught nor explicitly legally permitted to puncture patients' veins before World War II, they were responsible for all of the before-and-after care associated with IV therapy.[45] They gathered and assembled the appropriate equipment for the procedure, prepared the patient, ensured or carried out the sterilization and maintenance of IV utensils, and observed the patient afterward for any untoward effects. Because physicians often declined to stay with patients for the time it took for large amounts of fluids to flow into the body, nurses were increasingly charged with ensuring and regulating the flow of fluids and with watching the patient for any signs of infiltration (the discharge of fluids into surrounding tissue caused by the needle penetrating the vein wall), allergic responses, or fluid overload (generally caused by instilling fluids too rapidly). Ensuring the correct flow was difficult for both patient and nurse, as any movement by the patient could dislodge the needle, and any drop in the rate or a temporary cessation of the stream could cause blood to clot, thereby permanently stopping the flow. IV equipment through the 1940s included inflexible metal needles and rubber tubing that were difficult to sterilize, manipulate, and hold in place. Patients had to have their arms (the usual site for IV therapy) restrained, which tended to cause discomfort and to interfere with their mobility. Accordingly, nurses bore the responsibility for securing the site of therapy while ensuring the comfort of the patient. As IV therapy expanded to include more drugs, nutrients, and blood products, they were expected also to know the uses and effects of the different agents prescribed for instillation into the vein so they could recognize the signs and symptoms of any local or systemic reactions and quickly notify the physician.

Although IV therapy entailed much more than just venipuncture, and the greatest danger to the patient was in the period after venipuncture, when the agent introduced into the vein was coursing through the body, it was venipuncture alone, or the discrete act of penetrating the vein with a needle, that initially defined IV therapy as a medical as opposed to a nursing act. One traditional legal test of what constituted medical (as opposed to nursing) practice was the "piercing or severing of human tissues," but nurses had been piercing human tissues since the late nineteenth century.[46] Nurses administered medications subcutaneously (right beneath the skin) by hypodermic injection, and they infused large amounts of fluid subcutaneously by hypodermoclysis injection. By the early 1940s more nurses were administering drugs by the deeper route of intramuscular injection, a practice that accelerated after World War II with the advent of penicillin and other antibiotics.

But it was during World War II that nurses also began to do venipunctures themselves, primarily to administer fluids intravenously to injured soldiers on the front lines. Nurses also performed venipunctures on the home front in hospitals, however, since there were not enough physicians available to continue to restrict this procedure only to physicians. During the war Hartford Hospital, for example, had instituted a six-month training program for nurses in which they learned about the management of blood banks and to prepare and administer IV agents. The program was so successful that it was continued and expanded after the war.[47] Accordingly, by the end of World War II, nurses were performing de facto, if not de jure, medical acts of piercing human tissues on orders and with instruction from, if hardly ever under the direct supervision of, physicians.

Yet venipuncture as a domain of nursing practice became highly contested after the war. Although there were physicians who had objected to nurses giving intramuscular injections, the transfer of this mode of piercing human tissues to nurses did not engender the controversy that nurses performing venipunctures did.[48] IV therapy carried more risk to the patient than other needle procedures, but the performance of venipuncture by the nurse also seemed to threaten more deeply the clean line of bodily penetration traditionally drawn between doctoring and nursing. For many physicians, venipuncture by nonphysicians was a serious incursion into medical territory, entailing an activity closer to surgery than to simply giving an injection. (Some IV therapy actually entailed surgical incisions, or cut-downs, to insert cannulas into veins.) For nurses, venipuncture exposed them to the serious risk of being charged with practicing medicine without a license. In 1943 the attorney general of New York had specifically declared venipuncture the illegal practice of medicine if performed by anyone other than a physician. In the late 1940s through the 1960s a debate ensued as to whether venipuncture was a medical or a nursing act and whether nurses ought to be allowed to continue to perform it, except in extreme emergencies, such as war or natural disaster. Whereas venipuncture was viewed before World War II as unequivocally a medical act, after the war it became a borderline procedure on the "fringe of medical practice," with nurses, physicians, hospital administrators, and lawyers debating how it should be defined and whether nurses should perform it.[49]

For nurse proponents of nurses performing venipunctures, the vein was an entry point into a new field of practice. In the late 1940s, articles began to appear in the nursing and hospital literature urging nurses to take up IV therapy as a way both to upgrade women already in nursing and to entice more women into nursing.[50] IV therapy was promoted, much like x-ray and laboratory work had been touted in the 1920s and 1930s, as a new nursing specialty that would advance nurses and their profession.[51] Like x-ray and laboratory work, IV therapy was presented as a nursing specialty built around a technology that for most Americans embodied advances in medical science. As IV therapists, nurses would relieve the physician shortage, improve hospital efficiency, and make IV therapy more effective and less painful for patients. Like the temperature nurse before her who took all the temperatures of all the patients on a unit, one IV nurse could administer all elective IV treatments within a given time period.[52] She could then more easily and closely supervise these patients, thereby allowing more efficient scheduling of other events in the physician's and the patient's day. Moreover, as a specialist the IV nurse therapist would have the current knowledge about blood and fluid products and the apparatus to dispense them that the average practicing physician lacked. Allowing a highly skilled nurse therapist to find and insert a needle into a vein on the first try was preferable to having rotating and unskilled house officers repeatedly piercing a patient in their efforts to find a vein. A cadre of IV therapists was invaluable in the event of major disasters with large casualties and in emergency cases where veins were difficult to find, such as in patients with burns or in severe shock. Indeed, the ideal applicant to be trained as an IV therapist was a registered nurse who was both technically capable and congenial.[53] Technical capability and congeniality were twin traits that the trained nurse had always been expected to show.

By the early 1960s, more hospitals were establishing IV therapy programs and teams largely comprised of nurses trained by and under the nominal supervision of physicians, typically anesthesiologists, surgeons, or pathologists. Citing the need for nurses to keep up with the demands of modern medicine, to free physicians from certain "bedside" procedures, and to end treatment delays for patients waiting for busy house officers to start their IVs, nurses and physicians called for more nurses to "enter [the patient's] vein." [54] Nurse proponents viewed IV therapy as yet another function that nurses had "inherited" from physicians and the venipuncture as the last in a line of needle punctures "ceded" to nurses.[55] These proponents were pleased to participate in yet another medical innovation that had not so long ago been considered daring and even dangerous but was now accepted and even taken for granted. To protect themselves, nurses worked to have venipuncture declared a legal nursing act. The 1943 New York state ruling that venipuncture was illegal if performed by anyone other than a physician was reversed in 1961 after the New York State Nurses' Association asked the attorney general to review that measure.[56] Nurse specialists learned how to use IV needles, what sizes and types of devices were suitable for different patients and different fluids, and other aspects of the paraphernalia and procedures for entering, drawing blood from, and instilling agents into veins. They helped design special carts to hold IV equipment. By 1973 nurse specialists had established the Intravenous Nursing Society and in 1975 published the *Journal of Intravenous Nursing*.

Yet not all nurses and physicians agreed that venipuncture was a procedure appropriately delegated to nurses, even with restrictions placed on the kinds of agents nurses could inject or on when nurses could do venipunctures (typically when there was no physician available or when physicians asked nurses to do them). In part because of the legal ambiguity surrounding IV therapy, nurse educators debated whether to teach venipuncture, and many refrained from instructing or permitting students to perform them through the 1970s.[57] There continued to be wide variation within and across states in whether professional nurses were permitted to do venipunctures and hang blood and in what medications they were permitted to add to an IV line already in place. According to a national survey published in 1962, twenty-two states reported no ruling covering the IV administration of medications by nurses in hospitals. Only Maryland required that physicians administer IV medications. Other states permitted registered nurses and/or medical technicians to administer IV medications under medical supervision. In Indiana nurses' authority to give IV medications was implied because it was not excluded, and in Virginia the definition of nursing practice was broad enough to include IV administration, as IV therapy involved giving medications prescribed by physicians. As the attorney author of this report concluded, nurses might administer IV medications, but they might do so "with qualms about their legal rights to perform this function."[58]

In addition to the legal ambiguity of performing IV therapy, there was the professional ambiguity of whether a practice built around a medical procedure was a nursing specialty. Early leaders in nursing had always sought to define nursing as more than mere doing and nurses as more than physicians' assistants.[59] But the nurse's assumption of IV therapy reinforced the identification of technical procedures with true nursing and the role of the nurse as the physician's hand. Moreover, it reified the one-nurse-to-one-technique approach to nursing at a time when nursing leaders were seeking to reestablish the one-nurse-to-one-patient approach. Indeed, some nurses became "so occupied with the technicalities involved" in IV therapy that they were cautioned not to forget the patient " 'on the end of the tubing.' "[60] As IV nurse specialists, nurses accommodated both physicians, who wanted to rid themselves of the work of IV therapy, and hospital administrators, who wanted to provide the most services for the least cost. Although by the mid-1960s nurses in some hospitals were performing IV therapy as part of their total care of the patient, the prevailing practice was to leave IV therapy to specially trained nurses whose contact with patients was confined to that therapy.[61]

For their part, physicians, who maintained the right to decide what medical and, by association, what nursing practice entailed, found ways to permit nurses to do venipunctures without defining the procedure as a component of nursing practice.[62] George Lull, physician secretary and general manager of the American Medical Association, argued that the administration of IV therapy constituted something more than just nursing practice. Accordingly, if the nurse administered it, she did so *not as a nurse* but, rather, as an agent of the physician.[63] Charles Letourneau, a physician serving on the Council on Professional Practice of the American Hospital Association, advocated the legalization of venipuncture and other procedures that nurses were already performing without legal protection but with physician consent, and he referred to venipuncture as a simple technique that could be taught to nurses and other nonphysicians.[64] Peter Terenzio, assistant director of

Roosevelt Hospital in New York, noted that IV therapy was becoming as routine as a backrub and was no longer an "awe-inspiring" measure. Moreover, in an emergency anyone could do a venipuncture. Indeed, since civilians in civil defense programs were already being trained to do venipunctures and technicians in blood banks did them routinely, the de facto performance of venipunctures by nonphysicians could not be illegal.[65]

In short, the argument for legally allowing nurses to do venipunctures rested on the fact that they and other nonphysicians had done them and were still doing them, and on the assertion that if nurses were doing them, they acted not as nurses but rather as physicians' assistants. Moreover, reprising an increasingly familiar tautology, if nurses (and others) were doing venipunctures, they must be simple enough for nurses to do. Although venipuncture itself used to exemplify the body piercing rule by which medicine was distinguished from nursing, what now distinguished medicine from nursing in the matter of IV therapy was the continuing right to prescribe it and to delegate its execution to others. Accordingly, what was ultimately ceded to nurses was not "full jurisdiction" over a domain of nursing practice but, rather, a "limited settlement" in a domain of medical practice.[66] Nurses were granted legal permission to do the work of IV therapy but not the authority to control that practice. Venipuncture was not redefined as an act of nursing, nor was IV therapy redefined as a nursing measure extending the traditional nutritional or comfort work of the nurse. Venipuncture and IV therapy remained medical functions that nurses were legally allowed to perform for physicians; thus the physician shortage was relieved without an increase in the number of physicians, and doctors continued to attend to the awe-inspiring work of health care while still maintaining control over the less awesome tasks they no longer wished to perform. The assumption by nurses of the work of IV therapy allowed, in sociologist Andrew Abbott's words, the "extension of dominant effort without division of dominant perquisites."[67]

The assumption of IV therapy by nurses mandated that they obtain new knowledge and skills, but it also permitted the "delegation of [the] dangerously routine work" that tends to undermine professional prestige.[68] As IV therapy became less mortally dangerous to patients and ostensibly as routine as a backrub, it became more professionally dangerous to physicians' dominance to continue to administer it. Although IV therapy as a specialty practice returned registered nurses to the patient's bedside, a space increasingly occupied by lesser-trained nursing personnel hired specifically to offset the shortage of registered nurses, IV nurses returned to the bedside not as nurses but as agents of physicians. IV nursing, as it was legally defined and commonly viewed in joint medical and nursing policy statements through the 1960s, extended doctoring, not nursing.[69] While it alleviated the physician shortage, the administration of IV therapy by nurses did nothing to relieve the much lamented post–World War II professional nursing shortage or to resolve the problem of what constituted true nursing. Indeed, the assumption of this task by nurses further complicated their efforts to define nursing work and to establish a distinctive nursing identity. Professional nurses were once again performing medical tasks, while the newly defined and rapidly proliferating technical nurses and nurse's aides were performing true nursing. The debate over IV therapy underscored how hard it had become to define nursing as well as how important it had always been — to physicians — to define nursing in ways that did not "encroach" on but nevertheless served medicine.[70]

The post–World War II assumption of IV therapy by nurses illuminates the dilemma they recurringly faced when new technologies, or the intensified use of old technologies, demanded new work, and when patients required services that physicians were never or no longer willing to perform or that were deemed too time consuming or too expensive for physicians exclusively to perform. Nurses were permitted to participate in a new domain that undeniably increased their knowledge, enhanced their skills, and boosted their value in health care, but at the cost of the continued subordination of nursing to medicine. IV nursing moved nursing further into the jurisdiction of medicine, thereby threatening the already endangered sphere of true nursing. Yet if nurses had refused to assume the work of IV therapy, nursing (and arguably patients) would have been endangered also by the proliferation of nonnurse IV technicians.

As a specialty nursing practice built around a technology that remained in the jurisdiction of medicine, IV nursing served the interests largely of organized medicine and hospitals. Nursing was rhetorically erased when nurses were permitted to perform the work of IV therapy but not as nurses. In the matter of IV therapy, skill was again not an objective entity but an ideological device used to maintain power.[71] Nurses performing IV therapy were not actually de-skilled; indeed, they were en-skilled. But nurses performing IV therapy were rhetorically de-skilled, as IV therapy was described as easy enough for the nurse to do and "skill [became] saturated with sex."[72] The vein was a portal of entry for nurses, but one with limited access. The debate over IV therapy demonstrates how technology can function both to create and to destroy jurisdictions, and why technology alone does not necessarily move an occupational domain closer to professionalization or overcome its gender coding.[73]

Requiem for the Instrument Nurse

During the same post–World War II period that IV therapy was emerging as a controversial new nursing specialty, OR nursing, one of the oldest specialties in nursing, was under "siege."[74] Like IV therapy, OR nursing was an area that in the early twentieth century became organized around a therapeutic technology, surgery. Nurses had assisted physicians at operations conducted in the home and in the hospital since the beginnings of trained nursing and modern surgery in the late nineteenth century. Nurses performed a variety of functions, including the preparation and care of the patient, room, and equipment before and after surgery. They also held patients in place, anesthetized them, and/or passed instruments to surgeons during surgery.[75] Nurses were the first specialists in anesthesia, and they were deemed especially vital to ensuring the aseptic conditions of the surgical environment and the " 'aseptic conscience' " of everyone in that environment.[76] As both surgery and nurses moved to hospitals and separate sterile operating rooms, and as more surgical procedures were performed, OR nursing became a distinct field of practice separate from surgical or anesthesia nursing. It was subdivided into two roles: the "sterile" instrument, or scrub, nurse whose job it was to pass instruments to the surgeon, and the "unsterile" circulating nurse, who was to ensure that the sterile physicians and nurses at the operating table had what they needed to perform surgery, that all sponges used in operations were accounted for outside the bodies of patients, and that aseptic conditions were maintained. OR nursing became confined to activities in and around the operating room, as nurses who assisted in surgery no longer also cared for patients before or after surgery. OR nursing was a well-established and room-based field by the 1920s and, through World War II, a respected area of nursing practice.

By the 1960s, however, nurses were increasingly debating whether OR nursing constituted true nursing.[77] For nurses who sought to emphasize the intellectual over the manual component of nursing, the comprehensiveness and continuity of nursing care over nursing procedures, the interpersonal nature of the nurse/patient relationship over the technical features of nursing care, and the independent role as opposed to the dependent functions of the nurse vis-à-vis the physician, the passing of instruments to surgeons and the keeping of a room were difficult to defend as true nursing. For these nurses, instrument nursing especially was strictly a technical role emphasizing manual skill and rote performance, and the scrub nurse was nothing more than the "surgeon's third hand."[78] Although OR nursing, set in a room with a surgeon and an array of dazzling equipment, might have appeared glamorous in relation to other fields of nursing, OR nurses were likely to remain unnoticed. In the popular renderings of operations that frequently appeared on television and in the movies, viewers were not likely to notice anything beyond the surgeon, the surgical lights, and the instrument table. If nurses were noticed, it was only because they passed a scalpel to, or mopped the brow of, the surgeon.

Moreover, for nurses who conceived of OR nursing as not truly but only technically nursing, OR nurses could hardly be described as providing nursing care to or interacting with patients, since patients were asleep or about to be put to sleep by the time these nurses encountered them. Their sole contact with surgical patients was for the relatively brief time these patients were in the operating room, and their sole interaction with patients was with their bodies and, even more narrowly, with that part of the body to be surgically incised. OR nurses were often asked by other nurses whether they missed patient care, as these nurse colleagues viewed OR nursing as not entailing any nurse/patient relationship at all.[79] After World War II and the rise of interest in the mental and emotional health of not just psychiatric but all patients,[80] the nurse/patient relationship increasingly required—to many nursing educators—talking with, as opposed to doing things for, patients.[81]

For nurses seeking to advance nursing in the intellectual and social order of professions, OR nursing epitomized everything that stood in the way of this goal. They conceived of it as a wholly technical and task-oriented field that reinforced the subservient role of the nurse as the physician's hand and the keeper of equipment. By the late 1960s OR nursing had all but disappeared as a distinct component from the basic curriculum in university schools of nursing, and it was quickly disappearing from hospital schools of nursing.[82] As many nurse educators argued, if nursing students did not have to take an x-ray picture to understand and meet their patients' needs, they certainly did not have to pass instruments to surgeons in operating rooms.[83] In one hospital school of nursing with an average enrollment of 230 students, trainees reportedly spent less than three weeks in the operating room, which was considered an extensive period of time relative to other schools of nursing. In 1966, of seventy-five nurses who graduated from this program, only twenty-six were employed in hospitals, and not one had chosen to practice in the operating room. Indeed, not a single graduate of this school had joined the OR staff in the preceding three years.[84]

The shortage of OR nurses resulting, in part, from a general shortage of professional nurses and the lack of exposure of student nurses to the operating room in their training programs led, in turn, to an increase in the replacement of nurses with nonnurse OR technicians who assumed the functions of the scrub nurse.[85] The scrub nurse was becoming a "dying species" as, in the words of one surgeon, the "quick-witted, dexterous, and devoted instrument nurse [who] cherished every instrument in the set" was quickly being replaced by, according to one OR nurse, "ex-hairdressers, farmers, and porters."[86] Whereas before World War II hospitals had required that scrub nurses actually be nurses, after the war increasing numbers of nonnurses were being trained on the job to be scrub nurses. The Joint Commission on Accreditation of Hospitals had defined the scrub nurse's function as a "mechanical position" suitable for delegation to a lower-level nurse or a nonnurse technician.[87] Although both OR nurses and surgeons lamented the "disappearing" OR nurse (one surgeon wrote a "requiem for the scrub nurse"), they were forced to accept nonnurses as substitutes.[88] Some surgeons eagerly accepted these technicians or hired their own nurse or nonnurse assistants to assist them in surgery. OR nurses, in turn, often resented these technicians but emphasized the importance of placing them under the training and continued supervision of OR nurses.[89]

OR nurses and surgeons also sought to counter the move to dismiss OR nursing as not truly nursing and to stem the tide of nonnurse technicians who were increasingly flooding operating rooms in the United States. For these proponents of OR nursing as a "professional specialty," nurse educators were making a serious mistake in eliminating OR training from the basic nursing curriculum and in treating this area of practice as a purely technical and not professional nursing field.[90] Nursing advocates, usually experienced OR nurses and supervisors, charged that nursing educators were so "traumatized" by their own OR experiences that they were willing to sacrifice an area critical for both nursing education and patient safety, a field of practice that was as old as modern nursing itself.[91] Nurse advocates allowed that the OR experience had too often been exploitive, and that students had been forced to spend their time cleaning instruments, folding sheets, and stacking supplies and to submit to the tantrums and ill temper of surgeons and even some OR nurses themselves.[92] They admitted that too much emphasis had been placed on "mastering the mechanics of scrubbing and circulating."[93]

Ideally, they argued, the operating room was the best and often the only place where students could learn and/or practice the principles of asepsis and antisepsis, anatomy and pathology, the technique and impact of different operations on the body, and teamwork. Although the operating room was the ideal place to develop manual dexterity and to learn about and to handle equipment, the major function of the OR nurse was not merely manual and mechanical but entailed anticipating the needs of the surgical team and ensuring the comfort and safety of patients and continuity of care before, during, and after surgery.[94] OR nursing was better viewed as it once was: as surgical nursing. The professional OR nurse—like the surgical nurse of the late nineteenth and early twentieth centuries who cared for her patients before, during, and after an operation—was confined neither to a room nor to instruments but, rather, committed herself to total and personalized patient care.[95]

Indeed, far from having no relationship with patients, OR nurses had a singular opportunity to cultivate special nurse/patient relations. The OR nurse was in the best position to provide patients with emotional support.[96] Interacting with the frightened patient, the OR nurse had to use her knowledge of psychiatric principles. Interacting with the sedated patient, the OR nurse had to cultivate nonverbal communication skills and finely tuned habits of observation. The fact that surgical patients were "without sensation, aseptically draped, and with [their] face[s] hidden from view" made them no less subject to nursing care than unconscious or comatose patients on the unit. In fact, such patients required more intensive nursing care.[97] Did anyone ask nurses practicing outside the operating room and caring for comatose or nonverbal patients whether they missed patient care?[98] Did anyone think that registered nurses, who supervised hospital units or instructed students and thus also spent very little time with patients, were not nurses?

In short, nurse advocates of OR nursing as true nursing sought to show that although much of OR nursing occurred in a specific locale and was organized around a specific therapeutic technology (surgery), it was not confined there. Indeed, OR nursing embodied true nursing. Nowhere else could nurses learn so much about the essence of nursing.[99] The OR nurse had so many skills, she could function anywhere in the hospital; other nurses could not. In addition, the fact that OR nurses were increasingly held legally liable for their own actions was testimony to the professional knowledge and skill required of the OR nurse.[100] Nurses arguing for the professional status of OR nursing observed that while OR nurses required excellent manual skills, they also needed excellent organizational and interpersonal skills, knowledge of anatomy and pathology, and the ability to react quickly in an emergency. Because technicians were incapable of responding to events beyond what they had learned in their limited training programs, the professional OR nurse became even more essential to supervise their work. By permitting nonnurse and lower-level nurse technicians to take over in the operating room, nurses were once again "abdicating [their] practice . . . [and] delegating [their] natural functions" to technicians in order to take on only "secondary functions."[101] Nurses were once again taking the nursing out of nursing and handing it over to others, without replacing what they had relinquished.

Reprising the metaphor of the dying species, William Monafo, chairman of the Department of Surgery at St. John's Mercy Hospital in St. Louis, lamented that the scrub nurse was "disappearing from behind a giant scotoma [a spot in the visual field precluding vision] that permit[ted] only her dexterous hands to be seen."[102] As he argued, if "scrub nursing" was viewed solely as comprised of hand activities, it made sense for nurses to be replaced by technicians. After all, hands were interchangeable. But if surgeons, who also worked largely with their hands, had to be physicians first, why was it not mandatory that the person passing instruments to the surgeons be a nurse first? As Monafo concluded, focusing exclusively on the handwork of OR nursing prevented the viewer from seeing the brain work behind it.[103]

Recognizing that many OR nurses were functioning like "automatons," nurse proponents of OR nursing as a professional nursing specialty sought to emphasize the nursing and deemphasize the OR in OR nursing.[104] Yet the organization of labor and geography in hospitals worked against the realization of this goal. There were too many tasks to be completed in the operating room itself to allow the few nurses in it to venture out to patients' bedsides. Moreover, the care of surgical

patients was confined to certain spaces, which reinforced the confinement of the OR nurse. Presurgical care occurred in the patient's room;
surgery, in the operating room; and immediate postsurgical care, in the
recovery room. Although some OR nurses managed to leave the operating room to visit patients before and after surgery, OR nursing remained confined to the operating room and burdened with the reality
and image of being too technical for true nursing.

From Ward Thermometer to Monitor

Although nurses had in some way always been preoccupied
with the technical—first with doing procedures and then with differentiating technical from true nursing—not until the 1960s did nurses
begin to think about technology qua technology, that is, as a unitary
force with potentially irrevocable effects on nursing identity and work.
Indeed, nurses did not generally perceive themselves as having been
engaged with technology at all until the 1960s. Some nurses reportedly
believed that the only tool nurses had used in the past was the thermometer.[105] Jo Ann Albers, a nurse pioneer in renal dialysis, noted that
"technology in hospitals was just beginning" in the early 1960s; as she
recalled, there were iron lungs, but there were no cardiac monitors.
Trish Maddox, at the vanguard of nursing in the intensive care unit, recalled that there was not "much technology" before 1960; there was not
"a lot of equipment, like monitors." The "most complex" equipment
included "oxygen tanks and chest bottles and catheters." Nursing was
not "with the equipment."[106] In her memoirs covering a half-century
in nursing, Stella Goostray compared the "complicated equipment" of
the 1960s with the "simple equipment" of her day. She described the
device used to administer saline by rectum: a thermos bottle with a
two-hole rubber stopper. Through one hole a glass tube was inserted
into the bottle, and a rubber connecting tube and rectal tube were attached to the glass tube. In the other hole was a glass tube to allow
air to escape. Another apparatus she described was a tent set up in a
patient's bed with a length of pipe inserted to introduce steam from a
kettle on an electric plate at the bottom of the bed.[107]

Prior to the 1960s nurses were typically preoccupied with the complexities and physical labor of manipulating and maintaining often
cumbersome, unyielding, fragile, and hard-to-clean items. Goostray
had worried about accidents with the steam tent apparatus. Florence
Downs recalled "the good old days . . . powdering OR gloves in a lung-

wracking haze of talc, swabbing the decks of the pediatric wards, filing burrs from needles, bruising my shins on exposed bed cranks, emptying water from the ice chests of oxygen equipment, and standing ankle deep in water that had flowed in tidal abundance from a forgotten sterilizer."[108]

With the advent of electric beds, alternating air mattresses, kidney dialyzers, computerized record-keeping systems, and, especially, electronic monitoring devices in the late 1950s and early 1960s, nurses believed they were entering a new era. Nurses began to view technology —or what they referred to in the 1960s as automation and the "new machinery"[109]—as "an explosive force" that was likely to change nursing forever.[110] The technology stimulating the most attention from nurses was machine monitoring in the form of cardiac and vital function monitors. As Ruth Edelstein observed, the advent of the "EKG monitor, perhaps more than any other piece of equipment," had prompted intensive study of changes in the nurse's role and her relationships with patients, physicians, and other nurses.[111] The cardiac monitor, more than any other device, heralded something new and explicitly technological in nursing.

The new machinery evoked optimistic responses from nurses on the front lines of patient care.[112] Imbued with the spirit of the New Frontier and fascinated by the space travel of the era, these nurses described the new machinery as promising adjuncts to nursing care.[113] In awe that "patient monitoring" was in 1961 "more than just a dream," Rita Chow, assistant editor of the *American Journal of Nursing* at the time, marveled at the "telemetering devices" hidden beneath astronaut Alan Shepard's silver space suit that had led to the use of monitoring machines in patient care.[114]

Nurses described cardiac and other vital function monitoring as more reliably and precisely extending the traditional observation functions of the nurse. Indeed, some nurses began to refer to the close observation that had been critical in legitimating the establishment of trained nursing in the nineteenth century as monitoring. As one Kansas nurse saw it, nurses had always "served as a form of monitor" for the physician. Monitoring equipment was, therefore, "simply a tool to extend human observation."[115] Similarly, Adeline Jenkins, nurse coordinator of a coronary care unit in Florida, proposed that if the ultimate goal of nursing was to care for patients who were sick and return them to health, then the cardiac monitor was "simply another tool in our hands for the achievement of our goals." As these nurses implied, although new and "dramatic and exciting," machine monitoring was in a larger sense also as old as nursing observation itself.[116]

For these nurses, monitors represented both continuity and a break with the past in nursing. The newly developing intensive care units were resurrecting the private duty model of nursing care, whereby nurses could again tend to only one or two patients and thus be able closely to observe each charge. Indeed, intensive care units were originally designed not to house new machines but to permit intensive nursing observation.[117] But the machine monitors that soon followed nurses into these units demanded a kind of observation wholly different from the largely in-the-flesh attention of the private duty nurse. Nurses using machine monitors now obtained information about their patients from screens.

Emphasizing the continuities between the new machinery and nursing practice, nurses described themselves in mechanical terms. In one of the best examples of the new technological self-understanding nurses were developing in the 1960s, an OR nursing supervisor observed that the intensive care nurse herself was a monitor. In a drawing accompanying the article, the head and hand of a female nurse were depicted as machine parts. The nurse's brain was likened to a high-speed data processor, capacitor, and information storage and retrieval system. Her eyes were light-wave receptors and emotional indicators; her ears were sound-wave receivers; her nose was an olfactory detector; her mouth was a gustatory collector and information discharger; and her hands were tactile input devices.[118] Photos of nurses interacting with large machines and drawings of nurses as robots (see figs. 5-1 and 5-2) accentuated the continuity between nurse and machine. In these depictions nurses appear to be one with, rise from, and be tethered to machines (see fig. 5-3). As shown in the photo in fig. 5-4, a nurse is auscultating a machine to check a patient's blood pressure. These visual displays and nurses themselves reinforced the link between nursing and devices first forged in the late nineteenth century. In 1900 the nurse had been encouraged to think of herself as a thermometer and a barometer. The nurse in the space age of the 1960s was encouraged to think of herself as an information processor and as a monitor who monitored monitors.

Nurses found that the new machinery not only illuminated the monitoring and other capabilities they possessed, but it also improved them. The electric mattresses and beds, oxygen tents, suction devices, and other automated devices that were replacing the manu-

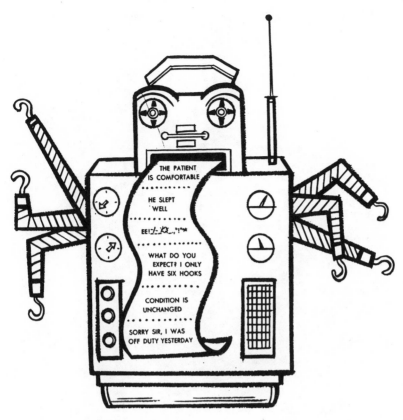

Figure 5-1. Nurse robot. (From *American Journal of Nursing* 63, no. 4 [1963]: 66; by permission of Lippincott Williams and Wilkins)

ally operated and individually crafted apparatus nurses had once used and/or fashioned made nursing practice easier. Moreover, machines allowed nurses to evaluate their patients faster and more accurately. Joyce George, an instructor at Bethany Hospital in Kansas City, where nurses were among the first in the country to use machine monitoring, observed that "conventional, manual methods" of taking the vital signs (that is, temperature, pulse, respiration, and blood pressure) required more nursing time than electronic methods.[119] In addition, conventional methods yielded inaccurate data and reinforced misconceptions about the stability of these vital indicators. Machines moved nursing forward from "intuitive care to intelligent care based on scientific knowledge," a goal toward which nursing leaders and scientifically minded nurses had always aspired.[120] Machine monitoring, in particular, taught nurses more about human functions, such as the

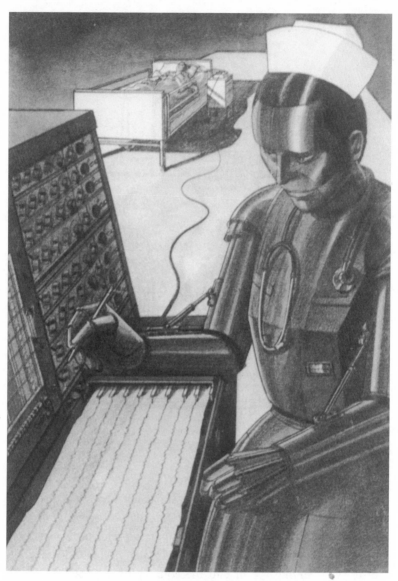

Figure 5-2. Nurse robot with vital function monitor. (From *American Journal of Nursing* 80, no. 9 [1980]: 1588; by permission of Lippincott Williams and Wilkins)

variability in temperature, blood pressure, and heart rates, and provided a compelling reason why nurses had to become more knowledgeable about the biophysical, physiological, and engineering sciences. Although nurses could not become engineers, they were still obliged to learn as much as they could about these machines to ensure

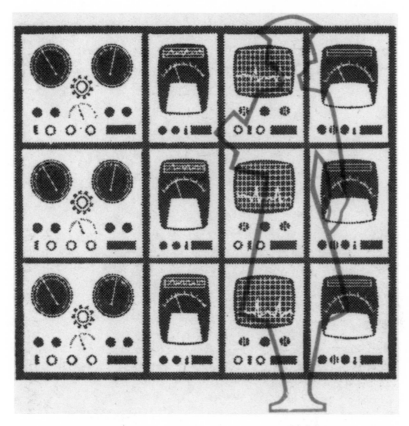

Figure 5-3. Nurse as one with machines. (From *American Journal of Nursing* 65, no. 2 [1965]: 68; by permission of Lippincott Williams and Wilkins)

their proper use with patients. They were not to remain "uninformed watcher[s]" of equipment.[121]

Nurses perceived the "marvels of machinery" as largely a "boon to nursing" and a "facilitator" of nursing practice.[122] As Barbara Schutt noted, "Hooked in with these machines seem to be vast opportunities to extend nursing practice, knowledge, and research." The new machinery promised improvements not only in nursing practice but also in the social position of the nurse and in nurse/physician relations. Whereas new technologies such as needle therapies and surgery had diminished the vital importance of bedside nursing care, devices that tracked and supported vital functions, such as electronic monitors and kidney dialyzers, reemphasized it. Physicians were even more dependent on nurses for their skills in using the new equipment of care, as machines and the patients tethered to them required constant atten-

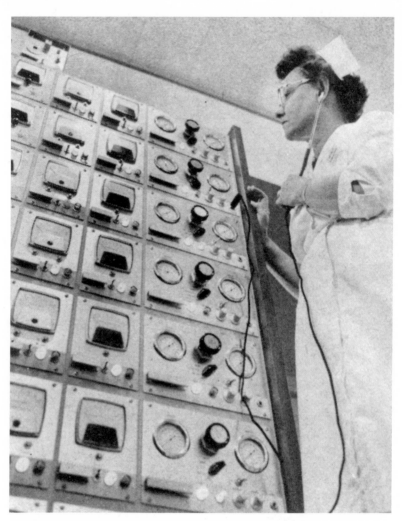

Figure 5-4. Nurse auscultating machine. (From *Nursing Outlook* 11, no. 8 [1963]: 575; by permission of Mosby, Inc.)

tion. As Schutt remarked, nurses might be "grumbling" that physicians were "pushing more and more of their functions over on" nurses, who were searching for their "own 'unique' place in health care." Nurses would likely be "quibbling over the propriety or legality" of nurses managing patients in coronary care units, but the nurses in these units were likely not complaining. They were smiling while discharging patients because they knew that it was a nurse who had "turned the pacemaker knob at the right time to bring [a] patient's heart out of cardiac arrest."[123]

The benefits of machine monitoring could not be fully harnessed without nurses who understood and could act immediately on the information monitors generated. The new equipment of care depended on the "watchful vigilance" and "technical observations" of the nurse.[124] Nurses were encouraged by what they perceived to be physicians' amazement at the expertise nurses had in using these machines. Not only did nurses perform functions once reserved only for physicians, but nurses' technical expertise in performing these tasks often exceeded that of physicians.[125] Nurses advised and worked with physicians and manufacturers concerning design improvements and ensured that expensive machinery was fully utilized to make it an economically sound investment for the hospital.[126]

Moreover, nurses were critical not only in ensuring the safe, effective, and efficient operation of devices but also in selling these devices to patients—that is, in ensuring patients' acceptance of, accommodation to, and cooperation with the application of these machines. The factor recurringly identified as vital to and even as a prerequisite for effective monitoring was having a cooperative patient.[127] And the factor recurringly identified as ensuring the cooperation of patients was the "reassuring presence of the nurse."[128] Ruby Harris, director of nursing at Bethany Hospital, which had established an intensive cardiac care unit in 1961, argued that if the nurse was "'sold'" on the use of machine monitoring, she was more likely to sell it to the patient—that is, to win the patient's confidence and acceptance. In fact, nurses' attitudes toward electronic monitoring were as important to its successful use as the absence of technical malfunctions. Accordingly, it was as important to "lay the right lines" with nurses as it was to properly wire the equipment itself. The "research-minded" nurse, able to maintain an attitude of objectivity and inquiry, was likely to secure the best results from machine monitoring, in part, because she was likely to be the best salesperson for it.[129]

Nurses viewed "mastering the mysteries" of machine technology as moving them closer socially and professionally to physicians, even as it moved them farther from nurses who could not or would not learn the secrets.[130] Nurses using this technology were seen as special, and they often received more pay and were perceived as more skilled than other nurses.[131] While the new machinery of care fostered inequality among nurses, it stimulated collegiality, collaboration, and a "more equal" relationship between nurses and physicians, if only because both nurses and physicians were often equally unfamiliar with it and harnessing its benefits required that nurses be allowed to diagnose and treat emergent life-threatening conditions. As nurse psychologist Ruth Edelstein put it, "Reading EKGs and operating a pacemaker . . . pushe[d] the [nurse-]submissive–[physician-]dominant balance out of kilter," and in a way that administering IV therapy and passing surgical instruments could not.[132] Nurses working in intensive care units felt they "were really good" and even "elite."[133] As one of these nurses noted, "We had information others didn't have, we understood the EKG, we could do things."[134] The new machinery also proved the value of nurses in their traditional roles of watchful observer and nurturant comforter. By mastering the mysteries of machines, these nurses believed they would, in turn, be seen by patients and physicians as more masterful. One nurse described colleagues who worked with this "awesome equipment" as "steering an uncharted course through a sea of [nurse, patient, and even physician] insecurity."[135]

Nurses who expressed largely optimistic sentiments about the new machinery of care located it within true nursing. Viewing the new equipment as the embodiment of advancements in medical science, these nurses saw monitors and dialyzers and other new life-recording and life-supporting technologies as offering better ways to see, hear, feel, care, and otherwise accomplish the purposes of nursing. For these optimists the new machinery was likely to have positive effects on nursing, as it filled the void left by bedside care, and filled it with scientific care. These nurses believed there was a harmony of interests between nursing and machinery, and as knowledgeable users, they could harness the benefits of technology for the advancement of nursing and patient health.

Bugs, Beeps, and False Alarms

Almost as soon as machine monitoring and other technological innovations were introduced into nursing practice, nurses noted the many technical problems, or "bugs," associated with them.[136] Although these machines had the potential to save nursing time and labor, ensuring the reliability of machine-generated information and the safety and comfort of the patients attached to them had actually increased the amount of time and labor nurses had to expend. These "machines looked wonderful," but there were persistent problems with placing sensors on patients' bodies, separating true from false alarms, restrictions in movement of both nurses and patients (caused by the size and paraphernalia of these machines and their tendency to record any patient movement as data), and maintaining the general function of these devices.[137] Indeed, nurses often had to resort to conventional, manual methods of checking blood pressure and heart rate, which were supposed to yield less accurate information than the newer electronic methods, in order to validate electronic data that looked wrong. In one case a patient reportedly looked pale and felt cold and clammy — signs of dropping blood pressure — but the monitor recorded his blood pressure as high.[138]

Nurses noted the increased work needed not only to maintain adequate machine/patient connections but also to provide psychological support for patients and families fearful of these machines. Automation had not only created a new kind of work for the nurse; it had also increased the need for what had always been the core work of nursing: to provide physical and psychological comfort. The new machinery engendered not only a greater need for emotional support of the patient, but its physical design mandated more physical care. Sensors caused skin irritations, and restrictions in movement required by the new equipment caused bedsores and respiratory complications.

Responding to suggestions that the new devices might eventually reduce the need for their services, nurses argued that automation increased the need for nurses and especially for highly educated nurses. Futurists' predictions that computers, monitors, and other technologies could offset shortages of nurses, and the advent of central monitoring systems located in nurses' stations, reinforced the idea that one nurse could care for a vastly increased number of patients. One writer heralded "nursing's electronic lamp" and the lone nurse monitoring twenty-two patients arranged around a central console. Florence Downs recalled a get-well card that pictured a mechanical servant caring for a bedridden patient and a newspaper article in which physicians and scientists forecasted a day when all patient care would be mechanized.[139]

Automation reinforced nurses' fears that patients would soon be "untouched by human hands." As one editorial writer warned, the new machinery was likely to devalue the human brain, much like the industrial revolution had devalued human brawn. Already, telephones in hospital rooms were substituting for the presence of nurses and physicians, radios were keeping patients' fingers off their call bells, and television was reducing the need for nursing attention. This writer worried that nurses, who tended to be too late in recognizing the negative effects of change, would again be among the last to realize the effects of automation on nursing care.[140] Accordingly, nurses repeatedly observed that equipment could never replace the critical judgment and care of the nurse. Having described themselves as the "most sensitive and reliable monitors," nurses were increasingly cautious not to describe machine monitors as "automatic nurses," and they were careful not to refer to the automation of nursing but, rather, to automation in nursing.[141]

Although nurses argued that machine technology required even more of the traditional services of the nurse, they were also increasingly concerned with how the drama and fascination this technology engendered were distracting nurses from performing and developing these services. Technological advances seemed to be causing the loss of true nursing and patients themselves. Technologies such as hyperbaric chambers, life islands, and kidney dialysis machines were fragmenting the "essential unity" of patients.[142] The new mandate to "preserve the machine" seemed to be undermining the mandate to preserve traditional nursing.[143] Like nurses before them in the age of ostensibly simpler equipment and simpler nursing, nurses in the age of the new machinery were concerned that nursing not be defined by the technical procedures that increasingly "filtered down" to nurses.[144] Indeed, nurses debated whether intensive care nursing was a special form of nursing, "junior doctoring," or "just nursing" as usual.[145] For many nurses the marvels of the new equipment were masking the persistent problem of nurses doing physicians' work under the guise of nursing care.

In a key paper concerning automation in nursing, Hildegard Peplau, an early nurse theorist and leader in psychiatric nursing, warned that the time had come for nurses to reaffirm the central mission of nursing: to assist individuals to use their capacities to become more fully human.[146] According to Peplau, who perceived the essence of nursing to reside in the interpersonal (as opposed to technical) relationship between nurses and their patients,[147] nurses had the distinctive obligation to determine whether and how automation or "cybernation" fit with this mission.[148] Although nurses assisted physicians in their central mission of treatment and cure, nurses were primarily obligated to counsel and teach—that is, to use the opportunities afforded by disease and treatment to enhance humanness. "Mechanization" of nursing care increased the tendency to treat people like "things." But nurses' distinctive interpersonal service could never be automated. Indeed, it was the special mission of nursing to develop "countervailing practices" to minimize the depersonalizing, distancing, and other deleterious effects of automation. In fact, mechanization held the potential to free nurses more fully to be nurses—to free them "for acts of tenderness, concern, and interest in the person who is the patient." Advocating less "cling[ing] to the traditional technical aspects of nursing" and a shift to more "sociopsychiatric content" in the education of nurses, Peplau tended to downplay the machine-body tending work of the nurse as rote, mechanical work. For Peplau, the "relationship core" of nursing practice was the "master-craftsman part—the art rather than the science."[149] But master craftsmen were often replaced, just as shoemakers had been replaced by shoe factories. If nurses viewed patients as objects like shoes—in need of repair—they would have limited usefulness. If nurses perceived themselves as necessary to increase patients' interpersonal competence, their usefulness would be clear and unlimited.

By the 1970s nurses were increasingly concerned with what they perceived as the erosion and possible "extinction" of nursing by technological advances.[150] In view of the "revitalized shedding propensity of physicians" whereby they continued to delegate tasks to nurses in order to extend themselves, nurses found that they were "perilously close to being radically altered without either [their] consent or knowledge." Yet they also worried that they would become obsolete if they did not master the skills of advancing technology, and they were alarmed about the increasingly "blurred" distinction between technical and professional nursing.[151] Advancing technology had widened the gray area between doctoring and true nursing, a space that was increasingly being filled with nonnurse and, perhaps even more ominously, nurse technicians.

While nurses such as Peplau stressed the humanity of the nurse as an antidote to automation, others emphasized her gender. Gertrud Ujhely, who was also in psychiatric nursing, juxtaposed the "masculine consciousness" she saw epitomized by technological innovation with the "feminine consciousness" epitomized by nursing. Ujhely cautioned nurses that although "caring," "trained intuition," and "personal skills" were being replaced with "tests, machines, drugs, and surgical procedures" and "mechanical know-how," nurses were not to become entangled in the technological matrix that valued the overpowering of nature. Nurses had to operate complex machinery for the good of patients, but they also had to "redeem and uphold the human factor in today's technological age." By acknowledging nature as the source of humanity, nurses had to take a "feminine stand" against an increasingly dominant and controlling masculine consciousness that subjugated nature to human will. Nurses had to remember that they were not just "surveiller[s] of the machine" but also "advocate[s] of the human being who is dependent on the machine." As exemplars of feminine consciousness, nurses were obligated to "translate the idea of human care into reality within an age of technology." Ujhely was resigned to the fact that "operating machines [was] par for the course in our age of technology" and that nurses were likely the only ones who even thought of making "the machine more palatable for the patient." But she called on nurses to show "courage" in reinstating true nursing. Although often lying in the shadow of "the mighty machine," nursing care still entailed, among other things, "sponging the patient's face [and] straightening his sheets." [152]

To Embrace or to Flee Technology?

By the mid-1960s nurses were seriously struggling with whether and the extent to which true nursing was technical, with nurses in practice often prizing the technical and nurse educators tending to disparage it. For the frontline nurse the core of nursing still lay in the material world: in doing things. For nurse educators the core lay beyond the corporeal and material in the ethereal and theoretical. The true nurse, to the frontline nurse, was a doer; the true nurse, according to nurse educators, was a thinker. The Nursing Theory Movement, which began in the early 1950s and reached its peak in the 1960s and 1970s, was, in part, an effort to "flee [the] technique and technology" nursing leaders perceived as preventing the advancement of nursing. A result of this movement to theorize the essence of nursing was a hardening of the "imperious distinction" between knowledge and technique, between knowing that and knowing how. [153] The position of the American Nurses' Association that technical nursing was distinguishable from professional nursing had separated nurses from one another. The Nursing Theory Movement, in turn, reinforced a polarized view of nurses as either doers who did not think or thinkers who did not do. Although nurses active in this movement invited nurses in practice to think of themselves as theorists, practicing nurses typically found nurse theorists' theories of nursing far removed from the realities of practice.

By the end of the 1970s nurses were also chiding one another for being too ready to succumb to new technology and not ready enough to learn its complexities.[154] On one hand, nurses were betraying nursing and, to a lesser extent, their feminine consciousness if they allowed themselves to "bath[e] in the reflection of [the] glory" of machines, but on the other hand, they were like "'ostrich[es]'" if they failed to take advantage of the new equipment.[155] On one hand, new technology was the "twentieth century slave" of the nurse, but on the other hand, nurses were also becoming enslaved by it.[156] As Leland Bennett, a nurse stationed in Vietnam, warned, nurses were in danger of extinction. Like the horse, whose prominent place in society was usurped by machines, nurses were, in Bennett's view, in danger of being replaced by new technologies. The electronic sensors and recording devices that had monitored the vital signs of Gemini and Apollo astronauts were already taking patients' vital signs faster and more accurately than nurses. Pneumatic and hydraulic equipment was already being used to preserve the integrity of patients' skin and to reposition patients and otherwise provide them comfort in bed. Automated pharmacies were already preparing medications for patients and reducing the likelihood of nurse error, and experiments were being conducted to create devices to dispense medications to patients automatically. Although traditional modes of care had once compelled nurses to maintain intimate body contact with patients, the new machinery required no such contact. In fact, too many nurses were not using the time these new devices saved them to maintain and deepen that intimacy.[157]

In the age of the new machinery, and in the context of the growing bureaucratization of health care, nurses were even more unsure about the nature of true nursing. One nurse described herself as an "artificial nurse."[158] Was true nursing what the nurse did to counter technology or to assimilate it into patient care? Was it primarily handwork or brain work? Was it technical or theoretical? Was the object of true nursing the "troubled body," which nurses treated with their hands and with things, or the "troubled psyche," which nurses treated by talking and listening to patients?[159] The advent of the new machinery in the post–World War II period had not created but instead had complicated the usual distinctions between manual and mental work, and between technical and true nursing. To what extent did nurses employ their brains to use their hands? To what extent did nurses' employ their hands to use their brains? Efforts to distinguish between the technical and the theoretical, and between handwork and brain work, continued to trouble nursing and to deepen the divisions among nurses.

6 Spectacular Nursing

Ever since Florence Nightingale established observation as the habit and faculty that legitimated the need for trained nurses, nursing has become synonymous with watchful care—that is, with looking for signs of improvement or decline in patient health and with looking out for patients' safety, comfort, and well-being.[1] Arguably the most enduring and evocative image of nursing remains the Lady with the Lamp, a quintessentially nurturing woman who, with only the illumination from a candle, watches out for her patients against the flickering shadows of sickness and the permanent darkness of death.

Beginning in the 1950s nurses began to use devices that radically changed the nature of this watchful care. With the advent of machine monitoring in clinical nursing practice, nursing observation was transformed from a largely embodied relation with patients and devices to an increasingly hermeneutic relation with devices.[2] Nursing became less "corporeal" and more "hyperreal."[3] Whereas nurses had once observed their patients in the "world of the tool," they were now monitoring their patients in the "world of the screen."[4] Nurses were increasingly engaged in reading, or interpreting, instrumentally mediated texts, such as rhythm strips and digital displays, as opposed merely to gathering information directly from the senses (for example, palpating the pulse with the naked finger to ascertain its rhythm and vitality) or from sense-extending devices (such as the stethoscope). Knowing the patient increasingly meant reading and then acting on the conclusions drawn from machine-generated texts. Knowing patients increasingly meant keeping them under technological surveillance.[5] This kind of knowing introduced a new kind of "hands-off" care, which contrasted sharply with traditional hands-on contact with the physical body.[6]

In the world of the tool, nurses had typically been preoccupied with the physical labor and complexities of manipulating often cumbersome, unyielding, fragile, and/or hard-to-clean items, including devices as diverse as the enema can and the iron lung.[7] Moreover, these items were oriented largely to treatment and comfort, as opposed to observation. Because of the nature of these devices and the practical difficulties nurses encountered in bending sometimes unpliable objects to their will, nurses maintained a necessarily close and hands-on relationship with both the tools of their trade and their patients. While they assisted physicians in implementing new diagnostic techniques, which tended to increase the physical and social distance between physician and patient and to alter the way physicians conceived of their patients and their diseases, nurses used these techniques in ways that altered neither the way they saw nor the way they related to their patients.[8]

In contrast, after 1950, when the first critical care nurses began to practice in the world of the screen, they also began to see their patients in terms of the traces of their bodies the new screen(ing) technology produced. This technology was oriented largely to surveillance, not treatment or comfort. Moreover, nurses became more preoccupied with the hermeneutic complexity of interpreting these machine-generated texts. Instead of the problems of handwork that characterized practice in the world of the tool, nurses now began to encounter the largely interpretive problems of distinguishing true representations from artifactual misrepresentations of patient conditions and the operational problems of minimizing false readings. In contrast to the characteristic problem of too much physical manipulation in the tool world, screen technology created the new difficulty of inadequate and insufficient physical contact. Screen technology "displaced" patients from their beds to the "cyberspace of monitors."[9] Screen technology thus seemed less to incorporate the touch of the nurse than to oppose or even replace it. In the world of the tool, devices were often physically heavy or hard to handle. In the world of the screen, devices appeared heavy because of the epistemological and even moral freight they carried. The screen technology that entered nursing practice after 1950 reshaped the aesthetics, politics, and ethics of nursing, giving nurse/patient relations a different look and feel, offering nurses the power to look, but forcing them to confront all of the practical and ethical "dilemmas of display."[10]

Surveillance as Intervention

The turn to screen(ing) technology was part of a larger shift in the orientation of medicine from treatment and diagnosis to monitoring and recording. As William Ray Arney described the change, monitoring constituted a "a new order of social control."[11] This new order was simultaneously technological and ecological, and it was oriented both inward and outward. Physicians widened their clinical gaze from the individual alone to the individual in the context of multiple (for example, physical, social, and cultural) environments, and with the aid of new visual technologies, they deepened their gaze into the interior of patients' bodies. Although new devices such as the electronic monitor did not by themselves determine this new order of social control, they "technologically amplified" and enabled it.[12] Moreover, these implements became emblematic of it. The cardiac monitor symbolized critical care just as the fetal monitor symbolized fetal intensive care.

With the advent of machine monitoring, nursing became deeply implicated in technological surveillance. Before it was imported into clinical (medical and nursing) language and practice, the term "surveillance" was used largely in connection with deviant behavior and espionage. As Arney described it (drawing from the work of French philosopher and historian Michel Foucault), surveillance in these contexts is an intervention of social control, as opposed to purely benign clinical assessment. According to Foucault, surveillance disciplines, such as the criminal justice system and medicine, acquire and maintain power by virtue of their authority to look. Foucault used the image of the panopticon (as envisioned by Jeremy Bentham) to show the relationship between seeing and power. The panopticon is a prison constructed so that all inmates are in view of a single guard who, in turn, is in view of the prison warden. Since neither prisoners nor guard know when they are being watched, the effect is to make them compliant. That is, the mere possibility of being watched created "docile bodies" ready to conform to prevailing standards of normality. Foucault conceived of the hospital as a kind of panopticon, and of medicine as a disciplinary and normalizing practice, both wielding power by means of surveillance techniques directed toward detecting deviations from normality. According to Foucault, contemporary methods of power are ensured not by right, law, or punishment but, rather, by normalization, control, and technique. In Foucault's scheme everyone watches and is being watched.[13]

One consequence of this efficient exercise of power has been the creation of a culture of risk in which the normal is problematized and in which diagnostic and surveillance techniques are construed as

benign "invitations" to receive the "gift of knowing"; another consequence is the creation of an "epidemic of risk" that ensures that individuals will constantly be on guard and thus police themselves.[14] The
at-risk status ensures that all individuals are located in a taxonomy of
health risks, thereby legitimating their being under medical supervision. As David Armstrong observed, the "cardinal feature of Surveillance Medicine is its targeting of everyone." Surveillance Medicine "requires the dissolution of the distinct clinical categories of healthy and
ill as it attempts to bring everyone within its network of visibility."[15]
The construction of surveillance technology as a gift of knowledge
(about their at-risk status) ensures that people will want to, and even
feel compelled to, receive that gift.[16] The cultural apparatus of medical
surveillance is thus reinforced by a technological apparatus designed
to make people "comply and live cleanly." Samples from and traces of
the body (such as cholesterol levels and exercise tolerance test reports)
can at any moment betray a lack of compliance and the failure to live
cleanly.[17]

In Foucauldian terms, nurses were already "bodies [made] docile"
by gender socialization and expectations to operationalize the monitoring concept and to deploy the surveillance technologies that enabled
it. As Arney observed, although "monitoring is a structure of control
that has a significant technological component . . . monitoring can be
deployed through personnel as well as machines."[18] Indeed, machine
monitoring of patients requires a cadre of highly trained and disciplined workers to exercise the "disciplinary power" of the new medical
gaze.[19] The "nursing gaze" extended the "medical gaze," as it was increasingly organized around scientific abstractions that functioned to
normalize, control, and contain.[20] Nurses began to "survey and probe
the body for physiologic and behavioral transgressions . . . beyond
the normal."[21] Nurses began actively to participate in a visual culture,
deploying technologies that "constitute privileged medical knowledge
and power."[22] Nowhere was this transformation more evident than in
obstetric nursing.

On Guard

For most of the history of childbirth in the United States,
most women and their caregivers associated maternity with pain, illness, injury, and death.[23] Maternity for women was likened to war
for men because of the fatalities and anguish it caused and the "battle

against invalidism and death" it required.[24] Well into the twentieth century, maternity-related deaths were commonplace, with maternity second only to tuberculosis as the cause of death for women fifteen to forty years old. After rising dramatically in 1918, the year of the disastrous influenza epidemic, maternal mortality rates fluctuated between 65 and 70 deaths per 10,000 live births throughout the 1920s. Maternal death rates began to decline in the mid-1930s, with the greatest improvement in maternal survival occurring between 1937 and 1945.[25]

Childbirth was the most dangerous period in the maternity cycle. If a woman carrying a fetus to term was fated to die as a result of maternity, she was most likely to die in childbirth from complications in the process itself, some preexisting condition exacerbated by childbirth, or from hospitalization. The findings of the highly influential and well-publicized New York Academy of Medicine study of maternal mortality in the early 1930s indicated that the increased use of pharmacological and surgical interventions in childbirth—which was supposed to prevent childbirth injury and death—often caused such unfortunate outcomes.[26]

Accordingly, before World War II, nursing observation during labor was directed primarily toward ensuring the physical safety and survival of laboring women, that is, toward preventing injury and death from complications in the labor process and iatrogenic injury and death from hospital practices, intervention excesses, and lapses in aseptic technique.[27] The obstetric nurse was considered the physician's "lieutenant" or, more generously, his "general" on the front lines of the battle against injury and death in childbirth.[28] Since physicians were typically absent for most of a woman's labor, obstetric observation actually meant nursing observation.

Nurses were especially "on guard" for any preventable lapses in aseptic technique that might contribute to infection, the major cause of maternal death.[29] Exercising "constant surgical watchfulness," nurses cleansed and shaved women's perineums, evacuated their bowels, and prevented women from touching their cleaned areas, an event especially likely to occur as laboring women were increasingly placed under the influence of pain-relieving drugs.[30] Inducing "twilight sleep," these drugs distorted consciousness and caused restlessness, confusion, and even frenzy.[31] Nurses ensured that physicians and nurses themselves were properly cleansed, gowned, gloved, and groomed and that instruments were properly sterilized. Didactic literature and photographs of the period of heavily masked, gowned, and gloved nurses and physicians show the great concern over infection and cleanliness and the greater burden nurses were to carry for ensuring that laboring women, their attendants, and everything that touched them were clean or sterile. Until the late 1930s, when most births were still taking place in the home, nurses were obliged to "imitate hospital conditions in the home."[32]

Nursing observation was directed not only toward the physical environment of the laboring woman—primarily to reduce the chance for infection—but also toward her body and behavior, to assess the progress of her labor and her need for comfort. Nurses observed women for the changes in demeanor, vocalizations, condition of the skin, and physical activity that indicated advancing labor. As one nurse summarized it, an experienced nurse could tell by the "sweat on her [patient's] brow, the look on her face, and the tone of her voice" how dilated a woman's cervix was and thus the stage of labor she was in.[33] Because of the great fear of infection prior to World War II and the advent of antibiotics, clinicians sought to limit the number of rectal and, especially, vaginal examinations performed to determine cervical effacement and dilatation, the physical signs of labor progress. Such examinations heightened the possibility for the introduction of bacteria into the uterus and, therefore, of puerperal infection and death for the childbearing woman. Until well into the 1970s nurses were typically not permitted to perform vaginal examinations, which were conducted under sterile conditions. If they were allowed to perform any internal examinations at all, it was the rectal exam, which did not require sterile technique. Yet rectal examinations posed the same threat as vaginal examinations to laboring women, since, if improperly conducted, fecal organisms could also be introduced into the vagina.

Largely barred from doing internal examinations, nurses had to keep their "obstetrical eyes and obstetrical ears open."[34] Nurses observed that by using their eyes and ears, they were likely to learn more about a labor than the average physician performing a rectal examination. As some nurses described them, such examinations were often misleading and could lead to unpleasant encounters between nurses and physicians when the findings of the rectal exam conflicted with findings from the nurse's observation.[35] As one nurse noted, while physicians might need to perform internal examinations to evaluate a woman's progress in labor, nurses needed only to look at women to obtain accurate information. Internal exams only confirmed what nurses already knew from studying the details and subtleties of laboring women's behavior and how these external manifestations correlated with labor progress.[36]

The most unpleasant encounter a nurse might have with a physician, however, was likely to occur over not calling him at the right time. Viewing the care of laboring women as tedious, dull, and overly time consuming, physicians had long limited their appearance in labor mainly to the delivery event. Indeed, as one pair of physician and nurse authors of an obstetric nursing text observed, in no other field of practice was so much responsibility delegated to the nurse, including even delivery itself.[37] Yet nurses were obliged to be especially accurate in determining the probable time of delivery in order to prevent precipitate deliveries, or what physicians defined as deliveries where physicians failed to be present. Instructional literature for obstetric nurses strongly emphasized the topic of "when to summon the doctor" in order to caution nurses about the importance of calling him neither too soon nor too late. Physicians thereby sought to maintain control of what they viewed as the most hazardous (for mother and infant) as well as the most dramatic (for the physician) period in the maternity cycle and thus preserve their medical control of maternity care itself. As physicians were seeking to separate themselves from midwives and other competitors for childbearing women's patronage, there was no event in childbearing that seemed to legitimate the need for physicians and to showcase their powers as well as delivery.[38]

The Technology of Nursing Observation before the 1960s

From the late nineteenth century through the 1960s nurses used relatively few instruments beyond their trained senses to observe in labor. These included the thermometer to detect maternal fever, watches and clocks with second hands to count the pulse and time contractions, the stethoscope (if permitted)[39] in combination with the sphygmomanometer to detect toxemic elevations in blood pressure, chemical strips to detect high levels of ketones and albumin in the urine (signs indicating diabetes or preeclampsia), and one of three kinds of stethoscopes to detect aberrations in rhythm and rate of the fetal heart. As shown in fig. 6-1, these devices included the traditional binaural bell-type stethoscope with a rubber band added to eliminate extraneous sounds, and two stethoscopes designed explicitly for aus-

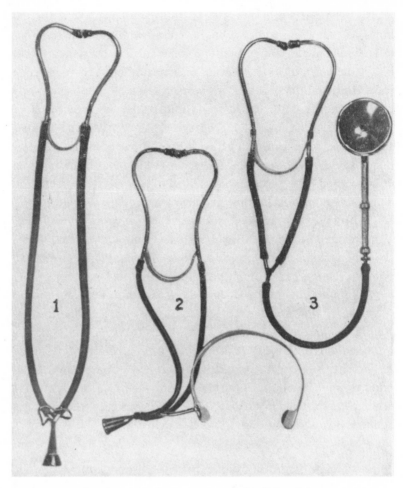

Figure 6-1. Fetal stethoscopes. (From Mae M. Bookmiller and George L. Bowen, *Textbook of Obstetrics and Obstetric Nursing*, 4th ed. [Philadelphia: Saunders, 1963], 247; by permission of Harcourt Publishers Limited)

cultation of the fetal heart: the De Lee-Hillis fetoscope and the heavier Leffscope.[40]

The technology of nursing observation included not only these instruments and the trained senses of the nurse but also the procedures for using them. Nurses auscultated the fetal heart to note whether its rhythm was regular or irregular and whether its rate was above 160 or below 120 beats per minute. The duration and the frequency with which nurses evaluated the fetal heart varied widely. Duration varied from ten seconds (multiplied by six) or fifteen seconds (multiplied by four) to one full minute; frequency ranged from one measurement every hour in the early phase of the first stage of labor, and from every hour to every five minutes as labor advanced to delivery. Nurses also listened around special events, such as before and after giving medications and after spontaneous or artificial rupture of amniotic membranes, rectal and vaginal examinations, enemas, or other treatments. Nurses used their hands to appraise uterine contractions for their frequency, duration, and intensity, but the duration and frequency of this appraisal also varied widely. Nurses looked for specific signs of fetal distress, such as heightened fetal activity and the presence of meconium in amniotic fluid discharge.

With the advent of natural childbirth and family-centered maternity care in the 1950s, nurses acquired new burdens of observation. Once obliged to imitate hospital conditions in the home—primarily to guard against maternal injury and death—nurses were now responsible for imitating home conditions in the hospital. In the early 1950s, by which time maternal mortality rates had declined dramatically and Grantly Dick Read's Natural Childbirth Method had been introduced into U.S. obstetric practice, the focus of nursing observation began to shift from an exclusive emphasis on maternal safety to include maternal satisfaction.[41] Nurses now had to make sure that women derived pleasure from their labors, to the extent that the pain of labor permitted this. Nurses were increasingly concerned with creating the right emotional and physical milieu in which women could practice natural childbirth regimens, which included the breathing techniques themselves, in addition to providing a low-noise environment and pillows and other paraphernalia women used to assist them in their breathing or to achieve comfort, as well as tending to the father of the baby himself.

Accordingly, by the time the first electronic fetal monitors entered U.S. labor rooms in the mid- to late 1960s, some equipment was already there, as well as two patients: the laboring woman and the father of her baby. Since it was designed to evaluate fetal (as opposed to maternal) health, electronic fetal monitoring added not only a machine but also another patient: the fetus. Fetal monitoring was heralded as permitting access to or revealing the previously hidden fetal patient. Labor and delivery units began to be referred to as fetal intensive care units, and obstetric medicine and maternity nursing as fetal medicine and fetal nursing.[42] As one nurse put it, with the advent of machine monitoring of the fetus, she now had three patients in the labor room. Separately and together, these patients represented—and thus challenged nurses to reconcile—three historically convergent but conceptually divergent orientations to obstetric care: the traditionally gynocentric focus on the childbearing woman herself (and, more precisely, her uterine functions); the newer, more inclusive, and more "natural" (or largely non- or even antitechnological) family-centered focus; and the newest and most technological fetocentric focus. At the center of and powering the fetocentric orientation to obstetric care was the fetal monitor. The fetal monitor became the iconic representation of the new and ostensibly more scientific approach to obstetric care and, although not a patient, yet another object requiring the nurse's care.

Intrauterine Baby Watching

In the United States electronic fetal monitoring became part of the technology of nursing observation in labor in the mid- to late 1960s and a central component of it by 1980, when up to 70 percent of all labors conducted in hospitals were electronically monitored.[43] The speed with which electronic fetal monitoring became the standard for the appraisal of laboring women in the United States was related less to its efficacy in improving obstetric outcomes than to a combination of diverse factors, including the technological imperative in U.S. health care; the desire of obstetricians to maintain control of obstetric care; the unwillingness of obstetricians to believe—against research findings—that fetal monitoring was not of value in labor; savvy marketing; and the skillful deployment of nurses.[44]

Edward Hon had established the foundation for the clinical use of fetal monitoring in 1958 in an *American Journal of Obstetrics and Gynecology* article in which he reported the preliminary findings from using a fetal electrocardiograph throughout labor, or after clinical signs of intra-partal fetal distress were detected.[45] Dubbed the father of electronic fetal monitoring by Corometrics Medical Systems, the major manufacturer of fetal monitors in the early 1970s,[46] Hon is credited with "uncod[ing] the language of the fetus as expressed through its heart rate."[47] Nurses who had worked with Hon at Yale–New Haven Hospital in the late 1950s recalled a special "monitoring room" filled with his equipment and the "monstrous" size of early models of these machines.

Articles introducing nurses to the instrumentation, operations, and research use of machine monitoring of the fetus began to appear in U.S. nursing literature in the early 1960s. A laboring woman was photographed with a tocodynamometer attached to her abdomen to record uterine contractions in a 1962 edition of the long-running *De Lee's Obstetrics for Nurses*.[48] In a 1964 essay in the *American Journal of Nursing*, a research nurse in the obstetric intensive care unit at the University of Texas in Galveston described the "intra-uterine baby watching" that was the subject of a study of 130 low-income women, most of whom had "complicated" pregnancies and/or whose labors were induced or augmented with oxytocin.[49] In that same issue two Philadelphia physicians described the technology of fetal electrocardiography.[50] In 1966 nurse Mildred Grever reported her involvement in a research project on fetal monitoring at Philadelphia's Woman's Medical College Hospital.[51]

The earliest reference describing the apparently clinical use of machine monitoring of the fetus in published U.S. nursing literature is Margaret Bergin's 1966 article, "Monitoring the Fetal Heart," which appeared in a *Nursing Clinics of North America* issue titled "The Nurse and the New Machinery."[52] Bergin, a supervisor at a county hospital in New Jersey, described a "fetal heart sound monitoring system" made by Jaeger Laboratories of Columbus, Ohio, in conjunction with a Chicago anesthesiologist, Robert Branch. As described in the article, the system consisted of an amplifier, an oscilloscope, microphones, and a cardiotachometer and could be portable or installed as a console unit. Bergin's description of the use of portions of this system at her hospital and a report of the results of a survey of staff in another twelve hospitals in nine states indicate that electronic fetal monitoring was in clinical use as early as 1965.

In contrast to intermittent auscultation of the fetal heart with a fetoscope and palpation of uterine contractions, electronic fetal monitoring provided a continuous and instantaneous visual record of the fetal heart rate in temporal relation to uterine contractions, the intensity of which were measured in millimeters of mercury. In the early years of monitoring, clinicians focused primarily on detecting fetal decelerations, or heart rates that fell below 120 beats per minute. As shown in fig. 6-2, early, or type 1, decelerations—U-shaped declines in the fetal heart rate that occurred at the peak of a uterine contraction and then returned to the baseline rate by the end of the contraction—were considered generally benign and the result of a response of the vagus nerve to compression of the fetal head. Variable decelerations, or declines in the fetal heart rate that varied in shape and timing in relation to uterine contractions, were considered less reassuring and potentially ominous and the result of compression of the umbilical cord. Late, or type 2,

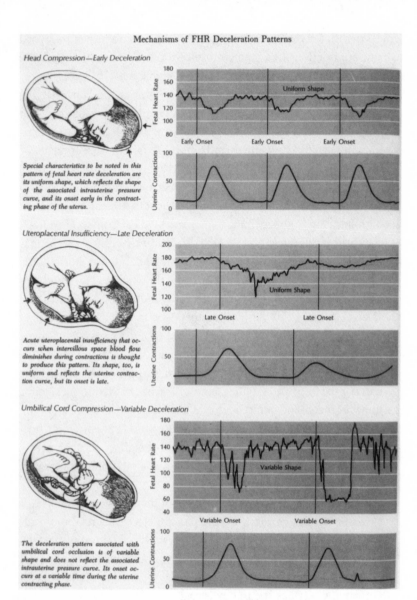

Figure 6-2. Fetal heart rate decelerations. (From *Hospital Practice* 5, no. 9 [1970]: 96; drawing by Carol Donner; reproduced by permission)

decelerations—U-shaped declines in the fetal heart rate that occurred after the beginning of a contraction, reached their lowest level after the peak, and did not return to the baseline rate until well after the contraction had ended—were considered the most ominous and the result of insufficient uteroplacental blood flow.[53] Several nurses specifically recalled hoping they would correctly discern or, even better, never see the "dreaded lates," which indicated that the fetus was not receiving enough oxygen and was "in distress."

These visual patterns were discerned from external or internal monitoring. External, or indirect, monitoring entailed the placement of sensors (phono, ultrasound, or abdominal EKG transducers and tocodynamometer) on the woman's abdomen to track the fetal heart and uterine contractions. Internal, or direct, monitoring entailed the insertion of a pressure catheter inside the woman's uterus and an electrode into the fetal scalp.[54] Since internal monitoring is invasive, requiring the rupture of amniotic membranes in order to insert the fetal heart clip or wire and uterine contraction sensors, the noninvasive external monitoring was typically used in labor before internal monitoring. But because early monitors produced poor external tracings, internal monitoring was often used to offset this problem. In teaching and research-oriented hospitals, internal monitoring was often conducted because of its greater accuracy for research purposes and to allow resident physicians to learn how to insert the sensors. Although some nurses also inserted these devices in the early 1970s, nurses initially were typically not permitted to apply them, rupture amniotic membranes, or enter the vagina at all. As one nurse recalled, physicians were concerned that the uterus might be ruptured during insertion. Another nurse recalled that nurses had to "advocate" for nurses to be permitted to insert these devices.

Continuous machine monitoring of the fetus was promoted to offset what its proponents viewed as the potentially mortal deficiencies of intermittent auscultation of the fetal heart during labor. Clinicians believed that these deficiencies were, in large part, responsible for the failure to recognize the asphyxiated "fetus destined for morbidity" and death. Although approximately 50 percent of fetal morbidity and mortality reportedly occurred in 20 percent of women appraised as high risk before labor, the other 50 percent occurred in so-called normal patients.[55] One nurse recalled hearing fluctuations in the fetal heart through her stethoscope and wondering what was then happening to babies. She described the feeling of having her "heart in her stomach" whenever the fetal heart rate dropped precipitously. She recalled also how "guilty" nurses and physicians felt, whenever a baby died, about not knowing what they might and should have known to prevent that death.

The electronic fetal monitor heralded the eradication of this guilt; electronic fetal monitoring "promised" clinicians they would know what they needed to know in time to make a difference. The monitor promised clinicians they could lower the relatively high rates of peri-natal morbidity and mortality in the United States.[56] As one nurse put it, clinicians believed naively that with electronic fetal monitoring, there would be far fewer babies with cerebral palsy or other injuries sustained during labor and delivery.[57] Clinicians hoped fetal monitoring would reduce the incidence of the neurological and mental deficits that lead to "social handicap" and the " 'poor achiever.' " [58] Indeed, reducing the incidence of such lethal or long-term injuries was the immediate motive for advocating machine monitoring.[59]

The very presence of fetal monitors caused physicians and nurses to reinterpret stethoscopic monitoring as a poor and potentially dangerous practice that yielded not only inaccurate data but also allowed important data about the fetal heart to be lost. As Edward Hon argued, evaluating the fetal heart by intermittent auscultation with a fetoscope was like "trying to decipher the plot of a movie by glimpsing two or three widely scattered frames." [60] Both nurses and physicians began to talk about early, late, and variable decelerations as if they were data that had always been there but which had hitherto been unavailable to them. That is, clinicians did not see these visual patterns as data that had no existence before and without the machine that produced them; instead, they conceived of these data as having been "missing" from fetal auscultation. Instrumental reality became clinical reality.[61]

Citing Hon's 1958 paper, early nurse and physician proponents of machine monitoring of the fetus emphasized the mistakes clinicians made in counting the fetal heart rate, especially when it was extremely high or low. Referring to findings from a key collaborative study of cerebral palsy, mental retardation, and other neurological diseases, published in 1968,[62] proponents of machine monitoring emphasized the uselessness of "stethoscopic sampling of the fetal heart rate" in predicting fetal well-being.[63] Indeed, as they repeatedly pointed out, protocols for fetal auscultation often directed clinicians to avoid listening to the fetal heart at precisely those seconds when, albeit difficult, it was most important to hear it: during or right after a contraction.[64] Even under optimal conditions, if clinicians auscultated the fetal heart every fifteen minutes for thirty seconds, they would (by some calculations) obtain only 3 percent of the information available—that is, 3 percent of the information the fetal monitor had shown them was available.[65]

In short, the proponents of electronic fetal monitoring reinforced the long-standing idea that labor was the period in the maternity cycle that most required heightened clinical vigilance, and that this heightened intrapartal vigilance would reduce fetal and neonatal morbidity and mortality. As one nurse recalled, clinicians seemed to forget that many babies were already in trouble prior to labor; machine monitoring in labor would thus not reverse the damage these babies had already sustained. Like physicians in the 1920s who had advocated the use of pharmacological and surgical interventions in labor and delivery as prophylactic measures against the dangers labor seemed to pose for every woman, physician and nurse proponents of continuous electronic fetal monitoring in labor advocated machine surveillance of the fetal heart as a prophylactic measure against the dangers labor apparently posed for every fetus.

Out of the Closet

Although some university hospitals were routinely monitoring all their patients continuously throughout labor as early as 1969, machine monitoring of the fetus was more typically used in a hit-or-miss fashion through the late 1970s.[66] One nurse recalled that the rural hospital where she worked had no monitor at all until 1979. Factors influencing whether machine monitoring was used included the type of hospital, the presence or absence of physicians on staff who had learned about machine monitoring, and the number of machines available. Richard Paul reported in 1972 that more than 50 percent of medical school teaching hospitals had fetal monitoring systems.[67] Corometrics Medical Systems, which held about 75 percent of the overall fetal monitoring market in the early 1970s, specifically directed its efforts toward "the more prestigious 'teaching hospitals' around the country."[68] These hospitals were more likely to have physicians who were oriented toward research and technological innovation and thus more likely to introduce machine monitoring on their labor units. By 1976 virtually all medical residency programs in obstetrics reportedly included electronic fetal monitoring.[69]

In the early years of machine monitoring, there were typically only one or two machines on a unit. Clinicians thus had to decide which women would undergo monitoring, but there were no uniform selection criteria for conducting machine monitoring of the fetus. The labors of women in very different circumstances were thus monitored, including both "normal" women and women deemed at higher risk for labor complications, and women across socioeconomic and racial/ethnic groups. For example, some physicians applied monitors to healthy women, primarily to teach themselves machine monitoring. One nurse jokingly recalled how she had consented to machine monitoring of her own labor as a favor to a physician wanting to learn more about it. Another nurse recalled pulling out the one monitor on her unit, which initially was rarely used, to teach women and their partners about labor and thus to heighten their enjoyment of it. Nurses saw instruments (including the new hand-held Doppler ultrasound devices) that made the fetal heart easier for couples to hear as a nice way to "share sounds" with them.[70] Some women also reportedly selected themselves for monitoring, asking for it after they learned about the procedure.

The women most likely to be selected for machine monitoring, however, had a condition or were in a circumstance indicating the need for monitoring. These patients included women who had not received prenatal care; who already had an obstetric or medical complication; who were in advanced labor or, conversely, whose labor was not progressing at all; whose fetus showed clinical signs of distress (such as a drop in fetal heart rate noted on auscultation or meconium staining of the amniotic fluid noted on visual inspection); or whose activity, size, or other circumstance made it difficult to hear the fetal heart with a fetoscope. In the 1975 issue of practice standards published by the Nurses' Association of the American College of Obstetricians and Gynecologists, the fetoscope (as opposed to the fetal monitor) was still listed among the essential equipment in labor and delivery units, and continuous machine monitoring of the fetus was only encouraged (not required) in cases of oxytocin augmentation of labor.[71]

Although the use of fetal monitors was promoted to offset what clinicians perceived as serious inaccuracies in and potentially lethal losses of important data, these machines entered many labor rooms with frequently little fanfare, little staff preparation, and even staff resistance. Monitors were initially purchased ostensibly to "modernize" labor units, but they often simply "collected dust" as nurses and/or physicians were neither trained to use them nor saw the necessity for using them.[72] Nurses recalled actually pulling monitors "out of the closet" and dusting them off, or using them to stack supplies.

Nurses and physicians initially learned about machine monitoring on-site. Nurses recalled that there was usually one physician who was knowledgeable and enthusiastic about fetal monitoring and from whom they would first learn about it. Several of the physicians that the nurses mentioned became widely known as leaders in the field of fetal monitoring, including Roger Freeman, Barry Schifrin, and Julian Parer. Afterward nurses would continue to pick up what they needed to know about machine monitoring as they used it with patients and/or from one-day professional training workshops, typically sponsored by Corometrics and Hewlett-Packard. Yet both nurses and physicians were more often than not initially forced to "fly by the seat of [their] pants." Some nurses recalled at first being told nothing more about the monitor than "here it is; use it." Or they recalled being taught only how to apply and secure the belts around women's abdomens for external monitoring.

Accordingly, the use of fetal monitors was still "not as widespread" by 1976 as proponents of monitoring had hoped, not only because of the lack of availability of monitors and institutional or other formal training and support, but also because of the presence of "apathy" and even "antipathy" toward further technological intrusions into obstetric care.[73] "Younger" physicians and nurses, or those clinicians nurses described as having no history of providing traditional labor care and as being more open to new technology, eagerly embraced machine monitoring of the fetus and wanted to pass on this exciting new development in obstetric care to others. But "older" physicians and nurses, who had practiced in obstetrics long before the advent of fetal monitors, were more likely to resist them. Nurses recalled older nurses warning that the monitor would cause them to lose their assessment and caring skills. They also described how harassed some older physicians felt when nurses advised them of a potentially ominous fetal heart rate pattern. One nurse remembered one of these physicians telling her not to call him until the woman was "complete," or her cervix was fully dilated. Another nurse described an incident in which a physician, angry that a monitor had been applied to his patient, wrote an order specifying that his patients not be monitored. For this physician and others like him, the monitor had the potential to cause trouble by producing information about which he was uncertain but which required him to act. Wary nurses and physicians hoped fetal monitoring was a "passing fad."

The variable training nurses and physicians received, and variations in openness to technological change, sometimes led to conflict between nurses and physicians, especially when better-trained nurses had to work with poorly trained and/or antagonistic physicians. Once they were introduced to electronic fetal monitoring by a physician, nurses tended to become more knowledgeable about it than many or even most of the physicians with whom they worked. Nurses were more likely than physicians to attend workshops and study groups (where monitor tracings were reviewed for teaching purposes) on fetal monitoring regularly, and they were more likely than physicians to organize and implement training programs for other nurses and physicians.[74] By the mid-1970s Corometrics had hired nurses for part-time and full-time work, specifically to travel across the country to educate clinicians about monitoring. Hewlett-Packard hired nurses on an ad hoc consultant basis, since as one nurse recalled, this company wanted nurses who were currently in practice themselves to educate other nurses about monitoring.

But physicians tended not to attend formal training sessions. Indeed, as one nurse recalled, physicians seemed not to worry about their lack of training, relying on the fact that they were physicians. That is, simply being a physician implied having knowledge. In contrast, nurses, who could never have relied on the hubris of simply being nurses (even if they had wanted to), who typically never thought they ever knew enough about anything, and who were soon left with most of the responsibility for machine monitoring, became (in the words of one nurse) almost "obsessed" with obtaining and certifying their knowledge. As one nurse put it, while the doctors she knew generally had "knowledge of the existence" of fetal monitoring, nurses generally had "knowledge of interpretation" of the data monitors produced. Observing how few physicians were schooled in fetal monitoring, physicians Roger Freeman and Thomas Garite observed that the "wise" physician turned to nurses as educational resources.[75]

When working with an untrained and resistant physician, then, the nurse who detected an ominous tracing had to convince him first to come in and then to act. One nurse described having to "go over the heads" of individual physicians—at considerable risk to herself—to advise the chief of the obstetric service that some doctors were not taking machine tracings seriously enough. After she had called one physician to report an ominous tracing, he had plaintively asked, "Why are you calling me with this information?" This nurse also suggested the extent of some physicians' ignorance of machine monitoring by describing a "classic thing" whereby one physician responded to the virtually complete loss of fetal heart rate variability (indicating impending fetal death) by saying happily, "Look. It's a perfect straight line."[76]

In addition to contending with physicians who "underreacted," nurses had to deal with physicians who "overreacted." Such physicians were too quick to respond to ominous fetal heart rate patterns or looked only at the monitor to appraise labor instead of looking at the laboring woman herself. As one nurse recalled, there were physicians who could describe in detail what a tracing looked like but could not describe what the patient looked like. Some nurses were concerned that physicians were overly relying on the fetal monitor and, thereby, losing their clinical assessment skills and subjecting laboring women to needless intervention and anxiety.

Nurses were initially less troubled, however, by physicians who overreacted, or rushed to intervene, than by physicians who underreacted. Although nurses were aware of the climbing Caesarean section rates in the 1970s, which appeared to be the direct result of increased machine monitoring of the fetus, they believed that, overall, babies were healthier and "better" as a consequence.[77] One nurse specifically recalled believing that the increased rates of Caesarean section improved fetal outcomes, even though she allowed that the "statistics" (or studies evaluating electronic fetal monitoring) later seemed to prove her wrong. Other nurses recalled thinking that rising Caesarean section rates meant that labor problems were being detected early. For them, the rising rate of Caesarean births meant that more babies were being saved from injury and death. Only later did these nurses begin to think that the "panic" and "paranoia" induced by even one instance of a drop in fetal heart rate likely led to Caesarean deliveries that might not have been necessary. As some nurses recalled, in the early days of trying to discern what a pattern meant, there was a tendency toward more "false-positive" readings (or interpretations of a pattern as indicating a compromised fetus who was ultimately born healthy). Indeed, there was a tendency to be "paranoid" if there was an interruption in the continuity of fetal monitoring for even one minute, since nurses worried that something ominous would occur in that minute and they would miss it.

Validating Nursing

Although electronic fetal monitoring contributed to some conflict between nurses and physicians, especially when nurses were better trained than physicians in reading monitor tracings, most nurses viewed it as improving the relationship between them and as fostering nurse/physician collegiality. For these nurses, electronic fetal monitoring was a tool that enhanced communication between nurse and physician in that it offered a more precise language with which to convey events in labor. With electronic fetal monitoring, the nurse could point to something visible and give it a technical name (for example, early, variable, or late deceleration). Nurses could better convey their observations to physicians and, therefore, better watch out for the mothers and babies in their care. Several nurses described their appreciation of physicians who made special efforts to share their knowledge with nurses.

Electronic fetal monitoring also "solidified the decision-making process" nurses used to determine when they should call the doctor. When to call the physician had long been a point of tension between nurses and physicians, as doctors wanted to be notified as soon as possible of aberrant events in labor and of impending delivery but did not wish to be called for what they perceived to be no valid reason, too soon in labor, or too late to conduct the delivery. As one nurse recalled, physicians did not wish to be called until the nurse saw the fetal head at the introitus. Electronic fetal monitoring relieved some of this tension by bringing some physicians (especially residents) back to the labor room for more of the first stage of labor (if only to play with the monitor or glance periodically at the monitor tracing) and by producing visual evidence of events that had occurred while the doctor was not there.[78] As one nurse put it, physicians now "listened" to nurses because nurses could now "show them what happened."

Like the vaginal or rectal examination that confirmed what expert nurses already knew about a woman's progress in labor, electronic fetal monitoring "proved the knowledge between the ears" of the nurse and made visible the accuracy of the nurse's "intuition." Before electronic fetal monitoring, a nurse might simply intuit that "something was wrong" but have nothing to confirm her feelings until an emergency developed. As several nurses recalled, there were physicians who had learned to attend to these nurse intuitions long before machine monitoring. But with electronic fetal monitoring, an intuition was "demonstrated in a pattern change." Electronic fetal monitoring offered the proof nurses desired of their value in labor and of the validity of their observations. Machine monitoring not only validated the status of the fetus; it validated nursing knowledge.

Indeed, machine monitoring of the fetus depended not on the machine alone but, rather, on the nurse's ability to properly interpret fetal heart rate patterns, to recognize patterns requiring immediate intervention, and to act appropriately in a timely fashion. The fetal monitor engaged the obstetric nurse even more fully in the diagnostic process, even if she was not officially seen as properly involved in diagnosis.[79] The nurse was the one who was in the best position to "see" fetal distress as soon as it occurred. Indeed, as nurses recalled, physicians often looked at monitor tracings only briefly and frequently did not see the tracings until hours later or days to weeks after the labor was over—too late to harness the benefits of machine monitoring. The continuous information the fetal monitor provided had no value if no one saw it as it was being produced or did not see in that information what they were supposed to see. The nurse was the critical element in electronic fetal monitoring without which the use of machine monitors was pointless.

As nurses often observed, machine monitors required skilled human monitors—namely, nurses. Nurses had sometimes felt threatened by talk that new technologies might be used to replace them.[80] The idea that one nurse could monitor several patients at a time and, therefore, allow hospital administrators to reduce personnel costs was in increasing circulation beginning in the 1950s and was specifically linked to electronic fetal monitoring in the 1970s.[81] Although there were no indications that nurses lost jobs with the advent of fetal monitoring, and many indications of the general recognition that machine monitoring of the fetus required more vigilant nursing care, just the idea that a machine might replace them worried some nurses.[82] One nurse recalled older colleagues' fears that they would become "obsolete." Another nurse had turned to electronic fetal monitoring to show that nursing—without any technology at all—was the critical element in labor. Using "objective evidence from an impersonal machine," she had demonstrated that nursing support in labor was "as effective as 100 mg of Demerol" in effecting uterine relaxation.[83]

Machine monitoring thus affirmed the value of the obstetric nurse and of obstetric nursing. Like the Cinderella status obstetrics occupied in the rank of medical specialties, obstetric nursing had a comparably low position in the nursing hierarchy.[84] In the words of one nurse, some of her colleagues saw caring for women having babies as "wasted nursing." After World War II, when maternal mortality rates had declined sharply, childbearing women were seen as basically healthy and not requiring the nursing care sick patients needed. Moreover, in contrast to established fields such as operating room nursing and newer fields such as intensive care nursing, obstetric nursing did not involve the instrumentation and machinery that made other areas of nursing practice appear more dramatic and scientific.[85]

Accordingly, nurses saw electronic fetal monitoring as proving the value of the tacit knowledge and difficult-to-express processes they used to appraise patients. In addition electronic fetal monitoring not only moved obstetric nurses closer to obstetricians; it also moved obstetric nursing, especially nursing in labor and delivery, up the hierarchy of nursing specialties.[86] Like nurses newly engaged with cardiac monitoring, many obstetric nurses were excited that they, too, could enter the Electronic Age. One nurse repeatedly referred to machine monitoring as "fabulous." Another nurse recalled how "exciting" it was using the "machinery" and "baby" EKG electrodes. Electronic fetal monitoring tied obstetric nursing more closely to the prestige and drama of critical care nursing, represented iconically by the cardiac monitor. Electronic fetal monitoring moved the labor and delivery nurse closer to the critical care nurse, who had achieved an elite status among nurses. The fetal monitor was now fact and symbol of the new intensive care nursing that nurses were privileged and proud to offer every fetus.[87] One nurse thought that machine monitoring "elevated" nurses in the eyes of patients, as it moved them from being "just bedside nurses to professional nurses"; obstetric nursing was similarly raised from only "high-touch" to "high-technology." Although she had some reservations about high-technology care, this nurse thought that becoming more "technological" was generally a "good thing" for obstetric nursing. Like physicians, nurses generally perceived technology as the embodiment of science.

(R)evolution at a Glance

In addition to engaging nurses more fully in medical diagnosis, electronic fetal monitoring extended the traditional watchful vigilance of the nurse. Electronic fetal monitoring allowed nurses to employ more of their senses to evaluate the fetus and labor and to make better use of nursing interventions to comfort laboring women. In addition to (or instead of) merely listening to the fetal heart or merely feeling uterine contractions, nurses could now see both together "at a glance." As nurses saw it, traditional fetoscopes were "cold," and a woman in active labor could tolerate a nurse using it to listen to the fetal heart only so long; a woman could endure a hand on her exquisitely sensitive abdomen feeling for contractions for just a short time.[88] As one nurse praised it, fetal monitoring "got nurses' hands off" women's abdomens. Internal monitoring, in particular, meant that the nurse did not have to "chase the baby around" with the fetoscope or external transducer to find its heartbeat. Nurses believed that electronic fetal monitoring made the appraisal work of the nurse more comfortable for the laboring woman and less physically demanding for the nurse, especially in cases where it was difficult to hear the fetal heart or that required heightened vigilance, such as labor augmentation with oxytocin. As they described it, nurses who had to care for more than one patient in labor at a time saw the monitor as watching over their patients when they could not be with them. With the volume turned up, a nurse caring for a patient in one room could hear the fetal heart in another room and thus know if it dropped. Machine monitoring of the fetus reduced the physical labor of the nurse in placing the fetoscope on her head (if using a De Lee's fetoscope) and bending over the patient for the time it took to find and listen to the fetal heart. Electronic fetal monitoring "focused" nursing observation, thereby making it more efficient; nurses now knew exactly what to look for. As nurses saw it, because the monitor paid attention to the fetal heart rate, they could concentrate more on laboring women themselves, comforting and teaching them.[89]

Moreover, in addition to being a tool for communicating with physicians and detecting aberrant conditions in the fetus as soon as they occurred, electronic fetal monitoring was a treatment tool for nurses that allowed them better to coach women through their labors. A tracing could show both the nurse and the laboring woman when the woman was hyperventilating and when a contraction was starting, even before the woman herself sensed it.[90] Nurses used this visual information to assist women to correct their breathing and to get ahead of their contractions by beginning their special breathing as soon as they saw the pen begin to rise on the paper.[91] Indeed, some nurses observed that electronic fetal monitoring was wholly compatible with the philosophy and practice of natural childbirth.[92] Machine monitoring thus became incorporated not only into the technology of prophylactic obstetrics, which had since the 1920s emphasized the use of drugs and surgery to prevent maternal and fetal morbidity and mortality, but also into the technology of natural childbirth and patient-centered care. One nurse described fetal monitoring both as a "movement," which "correlated well" with the movement toward patient-centered (as opposed to organ- or disease-centered) care, and as a "tool" of patient-centered care.

For nurses who adhered to a view of technological innovation as constituting progressive change, the fetal monitor was at the end of an evolutionary line of practices that had begun with listening to the fetal heart with the naked ear to the woman's abdomen and had advanced to hearing the fetal heart through a stethoscope. Nurses relabeled the observation they had always performed in labor as monitoring, thereby emphasizing the continuity between traditional and modern modes of evaluating the fetus and labor. Yet, echoing physician proponents of electronic fetal monitoring, nurses emphasized the deficiencies of older methods of fetal evaluation, especially of stethoscopic appraisal, noting the benefits of continuous versus intermittent assessment of the fetus and of obtaining more, and more accurate, rather than less and inaccurate information. They were impressed with how much they had "missed" in appraising their patients that the fetal monitor now revealed to them. Although they noted cases where Caesarean sections had been unnecessarily performed, they also recalled instances in which babies had been saved with the fetal monitor, or might have been saved had it been used. As one nurse recalled wondering about some of her colleagues, how could any nurse "not like" fetal monitoring?

While nurses viewed machine monitoring of the fetus as evolutionary, they also saw it as "revolutionary"—that is, as a big, but not wholly welcome, departure from traditional nursing observation in labor. The findings of a study conducted in the late 1970s of nurses' attitudes toward machine monitoring indicated that although nurses were generally positive toward it, only slightly over 50 percent of the nurses surveyed thought all labors should be routinely monitored.[93] One nurse specifically recalled her initial naïveté in thinking the fetal monitor was just another (albeit more complex) tool like the fetoscope. Another nurse lamented that machine monitoring had transformed obstetric nurses from caregivers to "electronic brokers" and "data evaluators." In contrast to nurses who saw machine monitoring as compatible with natural childbirth were those who saw it as incompatible with women's goals to avoid excessive intervention. Nurses regretted that a new generation of nurses would no longer have the skills to look at a laboring woman—without the assistance of devices—in order to determine the progress she had made and what she needed from the nurse.

Initially, electronic fetal monitoring did not necessarily alter the parameters for nursing observation and action. That is, the standard for appraisal remained the fetoscope and the hand. Nurses were still obliged to advise the physician only when the fetal heart rate dropped below 120 beats a minute and to record their evaluations of fetal heart rate and uterine contractions in the same manner and with the same frequency as they had before machine monitoring. Nurses still referred to contractions as mild, moderate, or strong—not in terms of the millimeters of mercury pressure indicated on the monitor strip.

Although some nurses were soon expected to interpret monitor tracings and to take immediate remedial action, other nurses were initially prohibited from interpreting these tracings. They could describe what they saw but not what they knew. A nurse would thus write that a deceleration was variable or late "in shape," instead of that it was a variable or late deceleration. Or she might have to tortuously describe seeing, for example, a fetal heart rate begin to drop as a contraction began, reach its lowest level when the contraction reached its greatest intensity, and then rise within ten seconds, instead of simply documenting an early deceleration. Or she might be prohibited from writing anything other than the heart rate number itself.

Some nurses, however, thought it best only to describe what they saw, especially since any one technical term was so often used to designate different events. A problem with the ostensibly more precise language of fetal monitoring was that it was used imprecisely. One nurse recalled refraining from using terms such as "late" or "variable deceleration" so as not to embarrass physicians who might not know what these expressions meant. She viewed the lengthier description nurses gave of what they saw on-screen as a way to educate such physicians. For her, not using so-called diagnostic labels was an advantage to the nurse, not a reflection of any effort by doctors to deny nurses' participation in diagnosis. Another nurse explained that if a nurse wrote, for example, "late deceleration" on a chart when the doctor had assessed the same pattern to be a "variable deceleration," legal problems might ensue. In addition to not necessarily being allowed to interpret patterns, nurses were not necessarily permitted to take any remedial action on their own other than repositioning women. In the 1960s and 1970s many nurses were still not allowed to start intravenous therapy, nor were they permitted to initiate oxygen therapy or to terminate oxytocin infusions (common actions on detection of nonreassuring fetal heart rate patterns) without a physician's order.

In Search of the Perfect Pattern

Whether or not nurses were officially permitted to diagnose fetal heart rate patterns and to take remedial action, electronic fetal monitoring entailed more work for the nurse. From its beginnings in the 1870s, nursing practice in the United States had encompassed nursing the equipment as well as the patient.[94] Nurses had historically been charged with applying instruments and connecting machines to patients; ensuring their safe, effective, and efficient operations; and obtaining patients' cooperation with, and offsetting their fears of, new devices. With the advent of electronic fetal monitoring, this tradition was continued in a modern electronic form in the "machine-body-tending" work of the nurse.[95]

In the earliest days of electronic fetal monitoring, few engineers or maintenance personnel were readily available to assist nurses. Although several nurses recalled having a Corometrics employee on-site or having a resident physician available to help them "trouble-shoot" problems with fetal monitors, nurses were more often than not on their own to manage the machine "bugs" and "quirks" that frequently arose. Nurses contended with "bulky" machines that took up a great deal of space in rooms that were already crowded, pens that stuck to the paper or that burned their fingers as they tried to change the paper, paper that was difficult to align with sprockets, belts that slipped, acoustical interference and noise that precluded a good tracing, and in general, machines that were more often "down" than functioning well. In contrast to the company claim that electronic fetal monitoring required only that a machine be turned on and off were nurses' great efforts to keep a machine running properly once it was turned on, in order to keep it from being turned off. In contrast to the claim that loading the paper was simple were nurses' recurring complaints about problems loading paper into machines.[96] Several nurses described the nightly routine of washing the nondisposable belts that held the external sensors in place on a woman's abdomen. These belts were often permanently stained a deep orange with antiseptic solution and, if not well rinsed, could cause women to suffer soap-induced skin rashes and irritations. Two nurses reported that the fetal monitors they had worked with picked up the local radio station.

Although nurses generally found that the electronic monitor made their job of tracking contractions and the fetal heartbeat easier, faster, and less bothersome to the laboring woman, the time and effort saved was offset by the energy they expended in a constant search for the "perfect pattern." As nurses described it, a perfect pattern was a technically good (as opposed to benign) tracing. (A tracing could thus be perfect but indicate a fetus either doing well or in trouble.) As the success of machine monitoring—saving babies from injury and death—depended on obtaining accurate readings of contraction patterns and fetal heart rates, nurses felt obliged to obtain the best tracings they could. Delivering a "good baby" meant obtaining a tracing technically good enough to discern patterns that would accurately indicate a troubled baby. By the late 1970s, when monitor tracings began to be used as evidence in lawsuits against obstetricians and hospitals, the responsibility for obtaining technically good tracings and to report and act on ominous fetal heart patterns became even more urgent.[97] Perfect tracings directed clinicians toward those nonreassuring tracings that required "cure," or an intervention to transform them into benign tracings.[98]

But nurses were reluctant to cause women any more discomfort during labor than they were already feeling. Accordingly, nurses were forced to walk the fine line between fitting the machine to the patient and fitting the patient to the machine. Nurses sympathized with laboring women and sought to relieve the discomfort fetal monitoring often caused them. For example, they encouraged women to move about and especially to avoid the supine position that interfered with blood flow to the fetus (a result of the pressure of the gravid uterus on the woman's inferior vena cava). Yet the initial design of fetal monitors and the operations of external monitoring, in particular, made the supine position virtually mandatory to get a reasonable tracing. One nurse recalled that some of her colleagues were so "intimidated" by the fetal monitor and its demands that they overly restricted the mobility of their patients. According to this nurse, some physicians did not want their patients to be monitored because they wanted the women to be able to move freely. At the very least, nurses had to constantly bother women to readjust the belts holding the sensors to their abdomens. One nurse left labor and delivery after machine monitoring was adopted in her hospital because she wanted to spend her time with laboring women rubbing their backs, not adjusting monitor belts.[99]

Women themselves often expressed negative feelings about these belts; they were too tight, added to their feelings of confinement, and interfered with effleurage, or the abdominal stroking used with natural childbirth breathing regimens.[100] Restless women created special problems for nurses, since these patients remained "poor candidates" for external monitoring unless "nursing intervention [could] quiet them."[101] In the late 1960s through the mid-1970s, many women in labor were still subjected to pain-relieving measures that included hallucinogenic drugs such as scopolamine (the key drug in "twilight sleep"), which caused restlessness and agitation.[102] One nurse recalled that such women could not be monitored, but that as more women received regional block treatments, such as epidural anesthesia, they were able to "participate" in fetal monitoring. Another nurse, however, recalled that such "scoped" patients were monitored, as they were already restrained in bed.

Although nurses wanted to comfort patients, the effort to obtain the perfect pattern led some nurses to control women's movements. Even laboring women themselves learned to restrict their movements. While women were largely reassured by watching and listening to the fetal heart, they were also frightened whenever there were changes in the pattern or interruptions in the visual display or the sound of their baby's heart. Women soon learned that such changes were often the result of their own movements, and nurses recalled women who overly confined themselves when they realized that they were causing these changes.

External fetal monitoring sometimes entailed the imposition of virtual restraints on women no different in effect from the physical restraints traditionally used to control agitated patients in hospitals. Fetal monitoring thus served to control the behaviors of both women and nurses. The fetal monitor exemplified the "new order of social control" achieved through "the creation of fields of visibility."[103] Fetal monitoring kept both women and their caregivers under visual control. Just as a fetal tracing might show an instance of medical malpractice, it could also reveal a nurse's inability to obtain a perfect pattern and/or a laboring woman's part in the failure to achieve that pattern.[104]

Internal monitoring also entailed more work for nurses and some discomfort for women. Although few nurses inserted internal monitoring devices, they were responsible for maintaining the integrity of pressure catheters placed inside the uterus and the spiral electrodes inserted into the fetal scalp. Laboring women with internal sensors were not as restrained from moving as women being externally monitored, but they often experienced discomfort during insertion of these devices and the feeling of being invaded, especially if they were also receiving intravenous fluids and epidural anesthesia.[105] Some of these women worried about damage to the fetal head from the electrode.[106]

Accordingly, there were women undergoing both internal and external monitoring who saw the fetal monitor as a "mechanical monster" that increased their physical discomfort and anxiety, limited their mobility, and produced distracting noise.[107]

Yet nurses recalled, and studies conducted in the 1970s on women's responses to machine monitoring in labor indicated, that women were generally positive about the procedure.[108] Women saw the monitor as providing information they could not give if they were anesthetized and not able to feel their contractions. Some women were relieved not to have the responsibility for providing information that could mislead their attendants. Like nurses who saw the monitor as confirming nurses' intuitions, some women saw the monitor as confirming that their contractions were real and intense to attendants who might not otherwise have believed them. As opposed to women who negatively anthropomorphized the monitor as a mechanical monster, women favorably inclined to the monitor positively anthropomorphized it as an extension of the physician, their bodies, and/or their babies. Women also viewed the monitor as something to look at to distract them from their labor and as allowing their partners also to see what was going on and thus to share the labor.

Women who responded positively to fetal monitoring were especially likely to have previously lost a baby. These women welcomed the monitor as a device that would protect or save their baby. But, more importantly, women who responded well to fetal monitoring were especially likely to have been "prepared" for it. Women who were properly prepared reportedly learned not to fear the monitor and to see it as a useful tool for themselves and their professional attendants. Nurses assumed much of the responsibility for educating women about monitors, primarily to reduce their fears, but also to have them accept monitoring. Having no knowledge of electronic fetal monitors was viewed as causing women greater anxiety than the monitors themselves. One very young woman who had never heard of the fetal monitor before coming to the labor room thought her baby had died after the physician had attached her to one.[109]

With the advent of machine monitoring, the idea of "prepared" childbirth expanded to include women "prepared" to accept monitors as normal in the labor room and even as adjuncts to natural childbirth. Nurses were instrumental in normalizing and naturalizing machine monitoring. They prepared themselves to explain to couples wanting natural childbirth why fetal monitoring was necessary and to assist these couples to relax and concentrate on their breathing and coaching regimens while being monitored.[110] As one nurse put it, educating women not only reduced their fears and enhanced their enjoyment of labor, but it also made them better members of the health care team. Indeed, women's cooperation was deemed at least as important in obtaining the perfect pattern as the instrumentation itself. Women's cooperation with monitoring was causally linked to "data quality." "Pre-conditioning" to reduce women's anxieties was, therefore, seen as essential.[111] Nurses were advised to help women understand the benefits of monitoring, not only for their own comfort but also specifically to "decrease baseline interference."[112] Obtaining the perfect pattern seemed to require that technological birth and natural birth come together in prepared birth, and nurses were the pivotal point at which these births converged. In order to harness the benefits of and minimize any harm from fetal monitoring, physicians eager to incorporate machine monitoring into obstetric practice relied on nurses' cooperation, and nurses wanting to comply, in turn, relied on and sought the compliance of women in labor.

Temptation Eyes

Electronic fetal monitoring required that nurses not only coordinate patient and machine to each other, in order to secure the best tracings from the monitor and the most comfort for laboring women, but also accommodate nurse and machine to each other, in order to preserve the essence of nursing. Nurses recurringly reminded themselves and each other that the fetal monitor was only a tool to augment nurses' observation skills, not the center of nursing care. Nurses sought to preserve the esteemed place that their trained senses had always held in obstetric nursing in watching over and comforting laboring women. Even the most ardent nurse proponents of machine monitoring of the fetus believed that the nurses' emotional and physical presence ought always to prevail over machine surveillance.

The accommodation between nursing and machine monitoring was difficult to achieve conceptually and practically, however, because machine monitoring was not the objective measure it was touted to be, and it required that the nurse divide her attention between the patient and the monitor. Although nurses thought fetal monitors provided valuable and objective information, they also did not wholly trust this information. They knew that so-called benign tracings sometimes resulted in damaged babies (a false-negative tracing) and, more often, that so-called ominous tracings resulted in healthy babies (a false-positive tracing).[113] One nurse recalled a monitor that continued to show a benign tracing when the fetus had long since died. As one nurse joked, "babies had not necessarily read the book" on monitoring. That is, their true condition was not always accurately revealed on monitor tracings.

Nurses who had practiced before the advent of machine monitoring sought to maintain their ausculatory, palpation, and behavioral observation skills by always using them to validate machine tracings, especially when their sixth sense indicated these tracings might be misleading. They viewed nurses who had not practiced in labor and delivery before machine monitoring and/or who relied solely on information obtained from machines as novice or poor practitioners. According to one nurse, machine monitoring required that clinicians have not only the technical skill to look at tracings but also a belief in what they saw. This belief could mislead the nurse, however, as tracings were often the result not of actual events in labor but, rather, of artifacts of machinery. Electronic fetal monitoring was supposed to offset clinician errors in counting the fetal heart rate, but machine errors were common, as for example, when fetal heart rates were halved or doubled.[114] Moreover, although electronic fetal monitoring seemed to promise clearly defined patterns with unequivocal courses of action, clinicians often disagreed on what a pattern meant. There was a great deal of interpretive flexibility in reading tracings, as any one tracing could be used to support more than one inference. Objective machine tracings ultimately depended on subjective human readings.[115]

As one nurse noted, she always had to "hear" the fetal heart herself by listening to it with the fetoscope and to use "the hand method" for appraising uterine contractions. She recalled an incident during an oxytocin augmentation when "my hand knew" the woman's uterus was not relaxing sufficiently, even while the monitor showed that it was. She attributed her hand-knowledge to having felt this woman's contractions before the oxytocin drip was initiated. Other nurses emphasized the importance of "never forgetting your ears" when evaluating the fetal heart. Nurses recognized that machine monitoring could easily become a "crutch factor" for nurses, especially those who had little experience using their senses in labor or who had never been "people persons" and preferred interacting with machinery over patients.[116] While one nurse observed that machine monitoring had decreased the time it had taken her to move from novice to expert, another nurse remarked that machine monitoring prevented novice nurses from ever becoming experts.[117]

Nurses were concerned early about the tendency to become overly engrossed with fetal monitors.[118] Observing that it was "human nature" to be attracted to such devices, several nurses described how difficult it was to "take [their] eyes away" from it to look at the laboring woman. The fetal monitor not only required that it be looked at, it seemed to demand it. Nurses judged this corruption of the eyes harshly. One nurse specifically recalled catching herself watching the monitor instead of the patient, and then chiding herself by saying, "bad girl, don't do that." Another nurse described the "classic image"—an image she feared, not an event she had ever witnessed—of "six nurses staring at a machine" with a laboring woman "huffing and puffing all alone." Similarly, another nurse recounted the apocryphal story of doctors and nurses staring at the monitor while the "baby precipitated in bed." Nurses worried about the "temptations" of monitoring that could move them farther from women in labor. In one textbook, nurses were even advised to turn the monitor away from view periodically so that neither the nurse nor the patient would be "tempted to become fixated" on it.[119]

In short, nurses were concerned that while they were looking at monitors, they were literally and figuratively "losing touch" with laboring women. Nurses used touch as a metaphor for true nursing: the traditional practice in which nurses used their bodies—not machines—as tools to watch over and minister to their patients. One nurse interpreted the advent of lay doulas (laywomen who attend women in labor) and birthing centers as an indicator that nurses were not meeting their patients' needs for personalized and touching care in labor. Lois Vice, a nurse and perinatal systems specialist for Roche Medical Electronics (another manufacturer of fetal monitoring systems), reminded nurses of the importance of touch to comfort patients and to obtain information that was not available from machines.[120] Some nurses saw the monitor as yet another piece of equipment that physically and figuratively "got in the way" of nursing care and "came between" nurses and their patients. Although useful as a tool in coaching laboring women to do their breathing regimens, the belts of machine monitoring interfered with abdominal effleurage and other touching nurses used to provide comfort. Moreover, machine monitoring seemed to require more "paper" than "patient" nursing. Nurses were responsible not only for maintaining the supply, flow, and proper speed of monitor paper, but they increasingly had to perform the "double charting" (recording the same information on the patient's chart and on the monitor tracings) that maintained the integrity of fetal monitor tracings as evidence in courts of law. Machine monitoring, by its very nature and demands, inclined or pulled nurses toward reading and tending to machines instead of women's bodies and emotions.

Some nurses were also disturbed by their colleagues' efforts to make patients comply with monitoring—that is, by nurses' efforts to "prepare" women to accept monitoring when its value in improving perinatal outcomes as well as all of its dangers had yet to be shown.[121] Nurses were worried that their socialization into hospital and high-risk obstetric care prejudiced them away from alternative, less interventive approaches. Such well-socialized nurses were opponents of rather than advocates for parents wanting these other approaches.[122] Margot Edwards, a strong nonnurse proponent of low-technology birth alternatives, was "saddened" that nurses were promoting the use of the fetal monitor by talking women into liking it. Conjuring up the hated image of the nurse restraining her patient, she observed that "talking a patient into liking the monitor [was] like medicating people in nursing homes to keep them quiet."[123]

In Between

Electronic fetal monitoring has continued to be a flash-point of controversy and a subject about which few people are "neutral."[124] The "paradox" of electronic fetal monitoring has more clearly and recurringly emerged. That is, more data do not always yield more knowledge or the ability to predict or prevent unwanted obstetric outcomes but, rather, often generate more ambiguity about what to do with those data.[125] The lack of standardization in definitions of fetal heart rate tracings and subjectivity in interpreting them are still matters of grave concern.[126] Nurses have continued to worry that too much and, alternatively, not enough attention was being paid to machine monitoring vis-à-vis other issues in the care of laboring women.[127] As one nurse observed, competency in fetal monitoring, instead of larger competencies in the care of laboring women, has become a "hallmark" of good nursing care. Moreover, the findings of additional clinical trials of fetal monitoring conducted in the 1980s and 1990s indicated no significant advantages of electronic fetal monitoring over intermittent fetal auscultation with a fetoscope.[128] Whereas obstetricians had denigrated intermittent auscultation as a method of fetal appraisal in the 1970s, the American College of Obstetricians and Gynecologists (and the American Academy of Pediatrics) concluded in 1988 that intermittent fetal auscultation was equivalent to continuous electronic fetal monitoring in detecting fetal distress.[129]

Although electronic fetal monitoring turned out to be "a disappointing story," it remains a "default technological intervention" and standard of care.[130] Physicians are more often in the position of having to defend not using machine monitoring, and strong advocates of machine monitoring continue to find the idea "implausible" that monitoring the fetus with a mere fetoscope could equal the "enlightened analysis of electronic monitoring tracings."[131] Protocols for intermittent auscultation have become more precise to bring them closer to continuous machine monitoring and in order to obtain more of the data available from machine monitoring. Like machine monitoring, these protocols demand expert nursing and a "1:1 nurse-fetus ratio."[132]

Although never explicitly designed by its inventors as a nursing technique, electronic fetal monitoring was as much a component of the technology of nursing as (and arguably even more than) of medicine. Electronic fetal monitoring was depicted as superior to intermittent auscultation of the fetal heart in labor. Since nurses usually practiced this form of appraisal, electronic fetal monitoring was actually positioned against a traditional and largely nursing practice. The much-maligned intermittent auscultation of the fetal heart was actually intermittent *nursing* auscultation of the fetal heart.

From its beginnings as an experimental device and a clinical tool, however, the electronic fetal monitor also depended on and was largely deployed by nurses. Nurses were important data collectors in research to develop fetal monitoring and key actors who put machine monitoring into clinical use. Since the electronic fetal monitor was designed to produce a continuous record of the fetal heartbeat, someone had to be constantly present to read and, if necessary, to act on that record. Like continuous cardiac monitoring, continuous machine monitoring of the fetus required a cadre of skilled readers and reactors to be on guard. The critical practice context for machine monitoring was never the standardization of the technique; an attendant could never simply read a self-evident result off a strip, like someone could read a number from a thermometer or a urine manometer. Fetal monitoring was and remains a technique requiring highly skilled but subjective readings of individual patient conditions. The critical practice context for machine monitoring was the historical spatiotemporal asymmetry between medicine and nursing.[133] Nurses were generally present at the bedside; physicians were virtually absent from it. Continuous monitoring required constant attendance. Moreover, as a result of this asymmetry, nurses rather than physicians were in the better position to have greater knowledge about actually monitoring patients. As one nurse recalled, she often taught attending physicians about monitoring at the bedside of their patients.

Nurses were almost immediately considered and targeted as the primary users of fetal monitors. Corometrics Medical Systems "wined and dined nurses," sponsored training sessions for them, advertised directly to them in nursing journals, and employed them as product representatives to sell monitors and to educate other nurses and physicians about them.[134] Companies such as Corometrics and Hewlett-Packard understood that nurses were the consumers to woo; if manufacturers could not sell their products to nurses, they would not be able to sell them to hospitals.[135] One nurse recalled that after a particular company hired her and a colleague to conduct seminars in several states, the sales of that company's monitors dramatically increased there.[136] Nurses often decided which product line a hospital would buy, and they also refused products they found difficult to use. Nurses advised company detailmen and engineers of design flaws and of ways to make their products more user-friendly.[137] Nurses thereby also played a significant (albeit undocumented) role in design improvements. One nurse recalled nurses' suggestions to a group of engineers to design wall-mounted units to conserve space and to mount these appliances at an angle to prevent damage to equipment caused by coffee spilling from cups often placed on top of machines. Nurses also made suggestions about the maintenance of machines and potential safety hazards, such as wires that tended to fray.

Although nurses did not invent machine monitoring or decide whether monitors would be purchased for a unit or that women in labor would be monitored, continuous electronic fetal monitoring would neither have been possible nor have made sense without them. The professional literature on and public rhetoric around electronic fetal monitoring have always depicted physicians as the detectors of early signs of fetal distress, but the person much more likely to have perceived those signs was the nurse. In actual practice, even if not in professional and public representations, electronic fetal monitoring was largely nursing work. Indeed, as one nurse summarized it, the advent of machine monitoring of the fetus altered primarily nurses'—not physicians'—work, since nurses soon carried the major responsibility for machine monitoring. Nothing really changed for physicians so far as their work in the first stage of labor was concerned. As another nurse observed, fetal monitoring did not change the "model of labor and delivery" that dictated that the "nurse does everything."[138] Except for "academically inclined" physicians, doctors were generally happy to leave the "science [that is, the understanding of the technology] and utilization of fetal monitoring to nurses." In hospitals, labor was still women's work, and attendance in labor was nurses' work. Machine monitoring simply gave women and nurses more and/or different work to do.[139]

As a technology that became routine within a decade and still maintains its hold on obstetric care—despite equivocal evidence that it improves perinatal outcomes—electronic fetal monitoring has often been used to exemplify or to dramatize the technological imperative in U.S. medicine.[140] Once the technology was introduced, few clinicians or prospective parents wanted to "take the risk" of not using monitors, no matter how uncertain their benefits were or how "slim the odds" that a baby would be injured or die as a consequence of labor. Fueling the move toward routine machine monitoring in labor and the "industry potential" of Corometrics, in particular, was the recognition that Americans "abhor preventable death and injury and will tolerate the expenses of seeing medicine become a more exact science."[141] Despite the subjectivities involved in electronic fetal monitoring, it was still viewed as more scientific than fetal auscultation, which produced no numbers to see, graphs to hold, or monitor tracings to study and to store.[142]

Electronic fetal monitoring also exemplifies and dramatizes recurring features of the nursing/technology relation, however, including the role nurses play as the soft technology that enables new hardware to be used; the penchant nurses have for, but the dilemmas they encounter in, "enrolling" technology to improve patient care and to advance nursing;[143] and the largely conservative impact on nursing of ostensibly radical technological change.

Auscultation of the fetal heart with the fetoscope and visualization of fetal heart rate patterns on monitor screens are both techniques employed to detect signs of fetal distress in labor, but they entail radically different ways to know and objects to see. Auscultation necessitates an embodied human/technology relation in that the fetoscope directly extends the sense of hearing.[144] Moreover, the fetoscope and the hand require close body relations between clinician and patient. In contrast, electronic fetal monitoring entails a largely hermeneutic human/technology relation in that clinicians do not directly sense the fetus but, rather, interpret its condition from visual traces that represent the fetus. (Although the fetal heart can be heard with machine monitoring, the parameters for the evaluation of the fetus are visual, not auditory.) Once the monitor is applied and functioning properly, machine monitoring does not require bodily contact for appraisal the fetus.

Although it was a radically different epistemic departure from fetal auscultation, electronic fetal monitoring still depended on nurses to use and to make sense of a tool that allowed the early detection of a compromised fetus. As the human interface between fetal monitor and laboring woman, nurses performed virtually all of the machine-body tending and sentimental work of fetal monitoring, ensuring the safe, effective, and comfortable use of monitors, trouble-shooting bugs, and enlisting women's cooperation. As primary caregivers to women in labor and as primary users of and product representatives for fetal monitors, nurses helped to sell fetal monitoring to women and other nurses and ensured that an expensive piece of hospital equipment did not remain in the closet collecting dust. Although nurses saw themselves as educating nurses and physicians about monitoring—not selling monitoring to them—companies manufacturing monitoring equipment used nurses' desires to educate and to be educated, to make a "difference," and to garner "respect," as vehicles to sell monitoring in general and their products in particular. One nurse employee of one of these companies recalled that, although she went out of her way to encourage her colleagues to compare for themselves the merits of different monitoring systems, the fact that her classes were held in the buildings of the company that employed her and that she herself had comparison-shopped and favored that company's product inclined the nurses she taught toward that product.[145]

Nurses also maintained the "purity" of electronic fetal monitoring as a clinical tool for physicians and, thereby, assisted physicians to sell themselves as the preeminent practitioners of scientific obstetric care at a time when feminist and natural childbirth activists were questioning obstetricians' dominance in the care of childbearing women. That is, nurses performed all of the "defiling acts" and "dangerously routine work" of machine monitoring, leaving physicians with only the work of officially interpreting monitor strips.[146] Nurses thereby preserved physicians' professional prestige and the "cultural machinery of [medical] jurisdiction" over fetal monitoring.[147] Nurses in concert with laboring women performed the hard and skilled work of producing the perfect strips physicians could read, and they increasingly performed the actions necessary to transform nonreassuring patterns into benign patterns.

To perform the machine-body tending and the sentimental and purification work of electronic fetal monitoring that allowed it to be incorporated into medical practice, however, nurses also had to do the work of accommodation and reconciliation—the "articulation work"—required to incorporate monitoring comfortably into nursing practice and childbearing. Articulation work is the invisible task that is the counterpoint to the routine that allows the routine to appear to be achieved naturally.[148] Machine monitoring of the fetus did not initially fit childbearing well, as it contrasted sharply with women's efforts to enjoy and control their own labors and the traditionally embodied relation between laboring women and their female attendants. Machine monitoring of the fetus did not initially fit nursing well either, as it interfered with nurses' efforts to preserve true nursing. Accordingly, nurses had to retrofit electronic fetal monitoring to both childbearing and nursing, but the very nature of this work often inclined nurses to subordinate the "nursing gaze" to accommodate the "medical gaze."[149]

Although nurses had always looked out for laboring women, looking had never compromised nurses' efforts to comfort them. Nurses had always looked—in order to care—but that looking had never seriously interfered with caring. Yet electronic fetal monitoring often undermined the comfort work of nurses by forcing them to care, in part, in order to look—that is, to obtain the perfect pattern. Machine monitoring often required that nurses use touch more acquisitively, to obtain information, than therapeutically, to provide comfort. Before machine monitoring, nurses placed their hands on the laboring woman's abdomen to obtain information about contractions but also to comfort and communicate caring to the woman. They "deployed . . . tactility" to see and to convey empathy and sympathy.[150] With external monitoring, nurses used their hands in the service of seeing—that is, to secure the belts and straps to obtain the perfect pattern. But this activity often impeded empathetic and sympathetic touch. Machine monitoring also required nurses to perform work they disliked. "Paper nursing"—charting and record keeping—were tasks nurses traditionally hated, yet machine monitoring obliged nurses to be the safekeepers of information.[151]

Perhaps, most unfitting and discomfitting for nursing was that machine monitoring sometimes intimidated nurses into acting as agents of compliance and control, rather than of comfort. As the proximate agents of fetal monitoring, nurses were most exposed to any "venting of anger" by women striving to have a birth free of technological intervention.[152] Obstetric nurses had already been the target of the wrath of the first generation of women delivering in hospitals (from the 1930s to the 1950s) because of their role in implementing hospital regimens. Nurses were the ones who separated laboring women from their families and their clothing, shaved them, administered enemas and injections, confined them to bed, and generally performed the frightening and painful tasks mandated by the practice of a highly interventive form of obstetrics. Many of these first-generation women thus perceived nurses as cruel and uncaring, even if only because they saw them more often than physicians during labor.[153]

Fetal monitoring again inclined and pulled nurses to be agents of compliance and, therefore, targets of criticism. Indeed, although most of their wrath was directed against physicians, childbirth activists (some of whom were nurses themselves) charged nurses with colluding with physicians to co-opt efforts to empower women in labor. As Margot Edwards observed, nurses were "the visible arm—the enforcers—in the medical power structure." The "price" nurses paid for being "inside" this structure was to "be compliant, to run machines, and to run interference." Edwards quoted prominent nursing leader Lavinia Dock, who in 1903 had cautioned nurses to avoid being used as tools by those who did not serve women.[154] Similarly, Madeleine Shearer charged both physicians and nurses with using their influence—as hired agents and targets of advertising by companies selling fetal monitors—to effectively silence criticism of these devices.[155] Although nurses saw themselves as fulfilling their true nursing function of educating and comforting patients, critics of fetal monitoring perceived nurses as gratifying physicians' desires to maintain control over and profit from childbearing women and obstetric practice.

Given the responsibility to make electronic fetal monitoring function for physicians, hospitals, and manufacturers, nurses sought to make the best of this new technique. They used the "rheto*·* re-assurance of access, competence, and culture" to re*·*

selves that electronic fetal monitoring was compatible with natural and prepared childbirth and with true nursing.[156] Nurses used machine monitoring of the fetus as a technique to improve the nursing care of laboring women and thereby demonstrated how technology could be utilized in a caring, as opposed to dehumanizing, manner.[157] They also saw electronic fetal monitoring as a way to advance obstetric nursing and employed it to advance themselves as nurses. Some nurses began, in the 1970s, to earn their living as full-time "educators" for companies manufacturing fetal monitors and as contracted or private entrepreneurs, consulting with hospitals and delivering education programs across the country. Nurses also naturalized machine monitoring by conceiving of and using it as an instrument of natural or nontechnological childbirth. By means of these acts of accommodation and reconciliation, nurses demonstrated their considerable ingenuity for making the best of the things delegated to their care and for trying to manage the conflicts machine monitoring aroused. They also demonstrated that putting a technology into use requires at least as much creativity as bringing a technology into existence.[158]

Although the articulation work that nurses performed, which allowed machine monitoring to be put into use, sometimes exposed them to rebuke, it also, ironically, reinforced the invisibility of nursing. Articulation work is generally visible only when it is not done well, when the routine shows itself not to be so routine after all. By virtue of their position as interface between monitor and patient, nurses and the work they performed were effaced. Indeed, electronic fetal monitoring exemplifies the traditional and problematic position nurses occupy "in between" patients and machines and patients and physicians.[159] While necessary, interfaces and other things and people in-between tend not to be seen.[160] Electronic fetal monitoring dramatized the irony of a spectacular technology—which had brought a new (fetal) patient and discoveries into view—obscuring nurses from view. For both better or worse for nurses, electronic fetal monitoring continues to be seen as a medical tool that physicians use to save babies.

Electronic fetal monitoring thus arguably exemplifies more continuity than change for nursing. Anja Hiddinga and Stuart Blume observed that "threads of practice" sometimes link dissimilar technologies, and Diana Forsythe proposed that technological change often maintains the cultural status quo.[161] In the case of the nursing/electronic fetal monitoring relation, the more things changed, the more they seemed also to have remained the same. Nurses used tools, and they were used as tools. With electronic fetal monitoring, nurses again turned to technology to enhance their care and the reputation of nursing. But machine monitoring of the fetus entailed a paradox; it was a surveillance technology that served both to showcase and to conceal their work.

CHAPTER 7

Troubled Borders

We are becoming increasingly familiar and even comfortable with the cyborg, the human/machine hybrid that has become an "emblem of postmodern identity."[1] Cyborgs, in the form of "hermaphrodite patients," "posthuman bodies," and "vital machines," are now part of everyday and virtual reality in the West.[2] We are used to people who have implanted pacemakers, artificial hips, and transplanted organs and who are tethered to ventilators. We depend on computers that seem to think like us. Moreover, the cyborg and cyborg imagery carry the "potential to disrupt the . . . troublesome dualisms" that have contributed to the "logics and practices of domination of women, people of color, nature, workers, [and] animals."[3] As Donna Haraway noted in her much-cited "cyborg manifesto," "couplings between organism and machine" emphasize continuity as opposed to difference by blurring the lines traditionally drawn between self and other, the natural and the artificial—between us and them, and us and it.[4]

Arguably, however, cyborgs and cyborg imagery also retain the power to legitimate logics and preserve practices of domination.[5] As manifested in the nursing/technology relation, the cyborg may be emblematic also of the problems and even contradictions women generally face in "enrolling" technology to serve their own ends and, in the case of nurses, to construct a socially valued place and distinctive identity.[6] Technological innovations promise gender equality, but while they may be disseminated in gender-neutral language, they are often "articulated with traditional and ideological narratives about gender."[7] Often indistinguishable from technology, nurses have yet to benefit fully from the promise of the cyborg to disrupt practices supporting domination.

Since the beginnings of trained nursing in the United States, nurses have attempted to construct their practice as distinctive from its technology and from other ministrations, occupations, and professions.[8] In the late nineteenth and early twentieth centuries, nurses sought to show that nursing was not like ordinary women's work. By the middle of the twentieth century, they were also seeking to differentiate nursing from medicine and, after World War II, from other newly created ancillary and technical occupational groups, some of whose members (such as practical nurses, nurse's aides, and nursing assistants) were also designated as nurses. Throughout their history, nurses have been the "undifferentiated other" among a growing list of health care providers.[9] Nursing has remained a residual domain by including work that must be done but which nurses themselves do not necessarily define as nursing work and which other providers are neither available nor inclined to do. Nursing has also remained a "hybrid practice" by virtue of its location "in between" patient and illness, patient and physician, patient and machine, and other "classificatory divides."[10] As cyborg and hybrid, the nurse is thus an "ambiguous figure."[11] The opportunity and danger for nurses is that nurses "trouble the borders . . . between a number of normatively bounded entities within health care."[12]

At the turn of the twenty-first century, and against the postmodern turn toward effacing difference, nurses confront arguably the greatest obstacle to their goal of constructing difference. There are now not only a plethora of health care providers claiming to care for patients, but there is also an increasing democratization of health care functions and access to technology. Physicians, nurses, nurse's aides, emergency medical technicians, and patients and their family caregivers use stethoscopes, sphygmomanometers, infusion pumps, dialyzers, defibrillators, and other, increasingly complex technology on the road and in the home as well as in the hospital, the clinic, and the physician's office. In the era of managed care and health care restructuring, cross-training (whereby one nurse is trained to function in more than one domain of practice) and personnel substitution (whereby one group of typically less expensive providers do work formerly done by another, more expensive group) are the orders of the day.[13] Provider roles have never been so blurred, as physicians, nurses, nutritionists, social workers, pharmacists, health technologists, and health educators all claim to be offering many of the same services. Minimally trained personnel "nurse," and nurses "doctor." Nurses diagnose, doctors promote health, and pharmacists manage chronic illness. Even anthropologists and sociologists claim or strive to "intervene" in health care arenas.[14] Since nurses have never wholly succeeded in differentiating themselves from either other lay women or other health-related professionals or workers, they are now even more challenged to distinguish themselves among all the contenders for (and, some would argue, pretenders to) caring. Not just doctors and nurses find themselves angling for space in the "narrow passageway" leading to the (bed)side of patients.[15] But primarily nurses encounter this passageway as a "gendered space"—that is, as a "literal and metaphorical space in which the concerns and interests of a certain gender are rendered invisible."[16]

The preceding exploration of the nursing/technology relation suggests another explanation for why the construction of difference continues to elude nursing. Nursing has been identified—in deed, word, and image, by others and by nurses themselves—both with and against technology and thus, in an ironic way, with and against itself. Early in their history, American nurses identified nursing with technology in order to align themselves with an entity associated with science and progress and thus highly valued in Western culture. Physicians identified nursing with technology and thereby appropriated the nurse's body and mind as instruments of medicine. Yet nurses have also positioned nursing against technology to disassociate nursing from an entity that, especially after World War II, was increasingly viewed as dehumanizing patient care. But, in order to separate themselves from technology, nurses realigned their practice with an entity traditionally denigrated in Western culture: feminine caring.

The irony of the nursing/technology relation is that nurses have turned both to and from technology to make their work more visible. Early in their history nurses believed that the tangibility of things and the visibility of procedures embracing those things would make their knowledge and work more perceptible and discrete. Nurses used things and did things to help patients and to help physicians help patients. Beginning in the late 1970s they also turned to technology as a way to redefine the "tender loving care" (TLC) that nurses had always identified as true nursing. That is, nurses began discursively to treat technology as a component of care. The caring nurse was the nurse who was technically competent and able to fit technology to care. They also began to treat activities such as touching patients,[17] talking and listening to them, and being present for them as technologies in an effort to raise their work above the level of mere TLC; that is, they sought to "scientize . . . caring."[18] In order to counter the "everydayness" and seeming "ordinariness" of true nursing and to document the traditionally "undocumented" components of nursing that remain "essential ingredients of nursing practice and patient care," nurses began to reformulate these activities as discrete interventions initiated after specific nursing diagnoses.[19] Such diagnoses and interventions could be classified, analyzed, and then, hopefully, remunerated, just as physicians' diagnoses and treatments were. More importantly, nursing considered in terms of diagnoses and interventions seemed less resistant to objective representation than nursing perceived simply as care.

Yet the devices of actually and discursively incorporating new technologies into nursing practice have yet to fulfill nurses' desires to differentiate their work from other health-related pursuits, and for professional autonomy and visibility. Indeed, these devices have often further eclipsed the knowledge, skill, and creativity required to put technology into use, and they have contributed to more confusion about what nursing is and ought to be. The turn to technology has yet to overcome the tenacious influence of gender and to translate into power and control for nurses to the extent that it has for physicians.[20] Although new technologies and the reconceptualization of nursing in technological terms have created new jurisdictions for nurses, nursing remains a "classic case" of the failure to subdivide a full professional jurisdiction.[21]

Nursing is also an anomalous case among the professions in that it, as Robert Brannon proposed, "contradicts major theories of professionalization and proletarianization."[22] That is, the post–World War II technologizing and bureaucratizing of health care (which included and, in part, depended on the "hospitalization" of the nurse) neither wholly proletarianized (or deskilled) nor wholly professionalized nursing. Professional status is said to be enhanced when an occupational group acquires what are deemed higher-level skills and more responsibility and when its members can delegate what are deemed lower-level skills to ancillary personnel. The team or functional nursing that characterized the primary mode of delivering nursing care in the 1950s and 1960s made nurses vulnerable to substitution by these personnel. Moreover, although team nursing enskilled nurses in domains delegated to them by physicians, it deskilled nurses in true nursing, the activities of which were delegated to ancillary personnel by transferring to them the knowledge and power nurses once had by virtue of their constant presence at the bedside and their unmediated relationship with patients. The nurse at the head of the team became like the physician who was dependent on nursing observation to prescribe medical care. In team nursing, nurses themselves became dependent on ancillary personnel for knowledge of the patient to prescribe nursing care. Nurses remain ambivalent about what they lost by giving up tasks such as bathing and toileting and by designating these encounters with patients as routine work and thus not in the domain of the truly professional nurse.[23] That is, they remain ambivalent about whether moving farther from true nursing actually shifted them toward professional nursing.[24]

Nurses were and remain key components of the infrastructure of medical technology, yet they continue to retain the invisibility that all infrastructures, interfaces, and connecting links have. Nurses continue to be described as the glue or cement that holds the U.S. health care delivery system together, but like all glue and cement, they are not noticed in the overall structure. The irony is that the very, often dramatic presence of devices, even those "spectacular" technologies that allowed clinicians new ways and new things to see, has not remedied the traditional cultural invisibility of nursing. New technologies have not so much resolved as dramatized the in-betweenness of the nurse. Indeed, as the quintessential boundary workers, regularly crossing the terrain between patient and physician, disease and illness, and medical and everyday practices, nurses have found and have actively positioned themselves between patient and machine.[25] The nature of the work they perform as interface between patient and machine, however, maintains their invisibility. What is in-between is typically not seen.[26] Moreover, the "equivocal location" of the nurse in-between is "precarious," both opening spaces for nursing practice and confining nurses within them.[27]

While nurses at the bedside turned to technology largely to improve their care and their status, academically oriented nurses eager to undermine the image of the nurse as merely a doer and nursing as a set of procedures began to turn away from technology after World War II. Theories of nursing that emerged in the 1950s and 1960s etherealized, disembodied, and dematerialized nursing in order to emphasize the minds, as opposed to the hands, of nurses.[28] The "discourse on caring" that emerged in the 1980s, with its explicitly antitechnology bias, was itself a "technology of gender [and] morality" that academic nurses used to revalorize the feminine in nursing.[29] These nurses used language as a technology to construct nursing as beyond or as frankly opposed to technology.[30] Yet in the process, they reinstated the cultural association between technology and masculinity and between antipathy to technology and femininity. That is, they reinstated gender—as opposed to science and technology—as the factor that legitimated nursing.

Truly and Technically Nursing

As boundary workers, nurses regularly traverse the terrain between care and cure and move between sympathy and skill and thus remain subject to the ambiguities of boundary work. These ambiguities are well illustrated in nurses' current embrace of a disease and a category of disease, namely AIDS and chronic illness; a technology, namely computerized information systems; and a role, the nurse practitioner. The disease, which emerged in the United States in the 1980s; the technology, which appeared in nursing in the late 1970s; and the role, which first arose in the 1960s and reemerged in the 1990s, together exemplify nurses' continuing desire to embrace both true and technical nursing.

AIDS, Chronic Illness, and the Revitalization of True Nursing

The increase in chronic illness (a result of both the decline in premature deaths from acute infections and advances in pharmacotherapeutics and surgery allowing individuals to survive and to live longer with potentially fatal diseases) over the course of the twentieth century has been a boon to nursing. Although attributable, in part, to some of the same advances in therapies that have undermined the traditional ministrations of the nurse, the rise in the numbers of persons with chronic illness has also reemphasized the importance of "caring" over "curing." The general public and probably most nurses associate caring with nursing and curing with medicine. Indeed, the metaphoric line between caring and curing constitutes a key "narrative and symbolic boundary" by which nurses have sought to differentiate themselves from medicine and to revalorize true nursing.[31] For many nurses, what distinguishes nurse-care from physician-care is that although physicians care about their patients, nurses care both about and for them.[32] That is, nurses emphasize the direct, intimate, and embodied caring of true nursing to differentiate it from the more spatio-temporally distant and abstract caring of the physician.

Diseases that as yet have no cure allow care to assume priority and, therefore by association, to privilege nursing care. As nurse and philosopher Sally Gadow observed, conflicts between care and cure arise only when cure is possible. Although certainly desirable, advances in medical treatment have "cast a shadow" on caring, which has increasingly come to be seen as a failure to cure (as in hospice care for persons without hope of cure).[33] They have also cast a shadow on nursing by virtue of its association with care. Gadow sought to move nursing care out of the shadow of medical cure by privileging care. For her, care is the "highest form of commitment to patients." The "frustrating situation" is not when there is "nothing but care" to offer patients but, rather, when there is "nothing but cure." Moreover, caring morally legitimates cure, as cure entails the exercise of an extreme form of power over patients and often an intense form of pain and suffering that would, in an uncaring context, be considered torture. For Gadow and for other contemporary nurses emphasizing the moral covenant between nurse and patient, "care is the moral end" of health care. In contrast, cure is the "morally problematic" means toward care that often diverts nurses and physicians from care. Nurses, the health professionals who experience the "ethical differences between care and cure" most "poignantly" and who regularly "tack back and forth" between them by virtue of their position "in the middle," are thus charged by these nurse scholars with the "arduous task" of and the greatest responsibility for "reconciling" cure and care, or more precisely, legitimating cure with care.[34]

As an as yet incurable illness, AIDS especially provides an occasion to revitalize the "culture of caring" nurses have sought to sustain.[35] Indeed, many nurses see the incurability of AIDS as an opportunity to return to the "hands-on, face-to-face forms of physical and interpersonal care that constitute the very core of nursing, and in which nurses, above all other health professionals, excel."[36] Persons with HIV/AIDS require embodied care. Moreover, there is as yet no technological cure that constitutes either a physical or a figurative impediment to this kind of care. As one nurse put it, AIDS is a quintessentially "nursing disease" that allows nurses to recommit themselves to true nursing.[37]

Nursing Informatics and the Renewed Turn to Technical Nursing

While AIDS is a disease that positions nursing against and privileges nursing over medical/technical cure, nursing informatics is a field of nursing that positions technology as a tool of nursing care. Indeed, nursing informatics is depicted as a site where "caring and technology meet."[38] Like HIV/AIDS nursing, nursing informatics is a newly defined specialty in nursing.[39] But whereas the HIV/AIDS nurse revitalizes the traditional role of the nurse as carer, the "informatics nurse" formalizes and expands the traditional role of the nurse as primary information handler, and as boundary spanner.[40] Trained to "integrate . . . computer science, information science, and nursing science," the informatics nurse promises to produce computerized information systems that both "reflect and support nursing practice" and thereby improve the quality and cost effectiveness of health care.[41]

Most significantly, the nursing informatics field includes an array of initiatives aimed at making the quintessentially invisible and undifferentiated practice of nursing visible as a scientific field different from other health care practices, and nurses visible as key players in the health care arena. These initiatives include efforts to redefine nursing as comprising diagnoses unique to nursing and interventions that can be classified, computerized, and linked to measurable outcomes. As Stefan Timmermans and his colleagues noted, " 'Difference' is the prime negotiated entity in the construction of a classification system."[42] Nursing informatics is aimed largely at establishing visible differences for nursing. Accordingly, efforts to classify nursing work such as the North American Nursing Diagnosis Association Taxonomy of Nursing Diagnoses, the University of Iowa Nursing Interventions Classification (NIC) system, and the University of Iowa Nursing Outcomes Classification system are means to "make visible what is wrongly invisible," to re-present work that had always existed but that required taxonomic representation to "create" it.[43] These systems are "manifestos" of a group eager to make their work manifest.[44]

The taxonomy of nursing diagnoses re-presents nursing observation and appraisal as diagnostic work like the physicians' and yet uniquely nursing. Seeking "professionalization through visibility," the claim to diagnosis is a claim to professional status.[45] The NIC system, in turn, depicts the wide range of everyday nursing activities and thereby documents the discrete practices (433 interventions are listed) comprising nursing. The NIC system thus counters the "lack of objectivity" of nursing work. Although "opinions, impressions, and hunches may form the keystone of expert practice," they "resist clinical documentation."[46] The NIC system also offsets the common practice of documentation by exception, whereby nurses deliberately do not document on the patient record any activity that is considered ordinary and routine. As much of nursing care entails the routine that is usually denigrated and the "making ordinary" of extraordinary events (such as illness, hospitalization, birth, and death), documentation by exception leaves most nursing care unrecorded.[47]

Like skill, the routine and the ordinary here are not objective entities but, rather, ideological devices used to maintain existing social hierarchies that are then re-inscribed in patient records. Kathryn Hunter noted that the "hierarchy of disciplines obtains in the chart as elsewhere in medicine."[48] Marc Berg and Geoffrey Bowker observed that the typical patient record "centralize[s] the physician's agency as core decision maker and reduce[s] the nurse's role to the provision of primary data and execution of the doctor's plan." Even though nurses spend far more time with patients than physicians, and nurses often advise physicians on what to do, the patient record elides the spatio-temporal asymmetry between nursing and doctoring and reproduces the "preferred account" of the physician as ordering nursing actions.[49] The ultimate goal of the NIC and other classification systems is thus to put the nurse back into the record by re-presenting the everyday, often tacit, but essential practices of nurses in forms that will be recognized as scientific and as conforming to current imperatives of managed health care. The nurse creators of these systems use the language of science and economics as a tool to show the contribution of nursing to quality care, cost containment, and "evidence-based" practice.[50]

Yet the discursive construction of nursing in these classification systems in terms of diagnoses, interventions, measurable outcomes, and cost effectiveness has been roundly criticized by nurses who view this "new nursing language" as moving nursing even farther from true nursing.[51] Australian nursing scholar Jocalyn Lawler argued against the characteristic tendency of nursing in the United States to use a scientific or economic discourse to get into the contemporary health care "game" that is not only alien to true nursing but also silences its voice. Although these discourses might be familiar to physicians, hospital administrators, insurance companies, and policy makers, they remain foreign to most nurses. As Lawler observed, not all nursing knowledge or activity can be expressed in language, yet those "forms which can be encased in language are the most pervasive and . . . the most powerful." Although nurses might "borrow" the language of science and economics to "try [them] out in nursing" or to "respond pragmatically to a prevailing economic climate," they needed to be aware of the extent to which nursing was being "subjected to the imposition" of these languages and thus distorted.[52]

Indeed, as Lawler contended, these languages threaten nursing, as they remain incapable of capturing (that is, classifying, measuring, and determining the cost of) true nursing activities. How, for example, could any classification scheme based on scientific or economic language account for the time and skill it took to be physically, personally, and existentially available to patients?[53] Yet "limitless [availability]" of all kinds remains exactly what patients and physicians want from nurses.[54] Indeed, as Lawler asked, how could any such rational language scheme even capture the nature of this critical component of true nursing?[55] Nurses thus remain caught in a double bind, as activities failing such capture do not exist so far as an information system is concerned, but expressing those activities in scientific and economic terms fails to make sense or even to make non-sense of them. For example, humor is listed as a nursing "intervention," but how does it get reimbursed? As Stefan Timmermans and his colleagues asked, how does it get defined or measured? Humor is "by its very nature a situated and subjective action" and thus not amenable to standardization and technique.[56] On either side of the double bind, nursing appears eternally subject to the "epistemological silence" arising from efforts to verbalize the "unspeakable."[57] Other U.S. and Canadian nurses have also voiced their concern with remaking the watchful vigilance of the nurse into nursing diagnosis and the TLC of the nurse into nursing interventions.[58] Like Lawler, they have lamented the mismatch between true nursing and the language used to describe and thereby to re-create it. Scholars in and out of nursing have also observed how current patient and clinical information systems tend to assume medical and economic orientations to health care while failing to inscribe nursing orientations.[59]

There is thus concern that nursing classification systems may actually thwart rather than advance the goal of difference and visibility for nursing, not only by inscribing a way of speaking about nursing that fails to capture it, but also by reinforcing the idea that nursing is only what nurses visibly and measurably do. Although nurses value the hands-on tradition of nursing, the focus on the hands has not always served nursing well. What nurses visibly do may not sufficiently differentiate nursing hands from other hands, and it is always less than what nurses know.[60] What nurses know and how they come to know their patients may, in turn, resist representation in these systems. As nurses have argued, "knowing the patient" entails an expenditure of time, a relationship of intimacy, and a kind of knowing different from the analytic models of clinical decision making inscribed in these systems.[61]

Moreover, there is the possibility that seeking professionalization through visibility will make nursing, ironically, too visible. As Susan Leigh Star observed, the "more visible and differentiated tasks are made, the more vulnerable they become to Tayloristic intervention, and the more likely it is that discretionary power may be taken away."[62] Modern classification systems promise to be no more liberating for nursing than the time-and-motion studies conducted in the first half of the twentieth-century, which conceptualized nursing as a series of discrete tasks completed in discrete intervals of time. Not only did these studies fail to capture the processual (as opposed to episodic) nature of nursing work, but they also subjected nurses to time and task management. Professionalization achieved through the visibility provided by information systems puts nursing at risk again by placing it under surveillance and, thereby, making it a target for management by others. The attraction of itemizing nursing activities is that they become discernible as "'billable categories.'" Nursing would no longer be an imperceptible part of the patient's hospital bill but, rather, a set of revenue-generating activities. The danger of billable categories, however, is that they can also serve to regulate the nurse's work; nurses would have to "comply with regulators' and employers' definitions of 'billable categories.'" If "back rubs and talking to patients are billed at a lower rate than giving injections and starting IVs, will nurses be 'free' to decide how to care for their patients?"[63] Moreover, how long should a back rub take? And is there ever a clear beginning and ending to the activity of talking to patients?

In summary, there is a concern that nurses will again be subject to the alien "'politics' of voice and values" already embedded in a technology they are embracing to advance their own politics.[64] There is a concern that information technology will simply reinforce the link between invisible work, gender, and status and thereby constitute a "technology of silence" for nursing.[65] There is a concern that information technology will turn nurses' desire for visibility against them by acting as a technology of panoptic surveillance and control—that is, as an "informatics of domination."[66] There is a concern that nursing will again be used as a "site where technology can be deployed" to further nonnursing ends.[67] There is a concern that the burden for working out the contradictory demands of systematizing and personalizing health care will again be placed on the shoulders of the nurse.[68] In short, there is the concern that nurses will have again turned to a device that will not fulfill and perhaps will even thwart their desires.

If there is any role that dramatizes the dilemma nurses confront by virtue of their desire to embrace both true and technical nursing, it is that of the nurse practitioner. Invented in the 1960s to deliver largely primary care to medically underserved populations (or populations that physicians typically did not wish to serve, such as lower-income patients and patients in rural settings) and revitalized in the 1990s as a tool for managed (or more cost-efficient) primary and acute health care, the function of the nurse practitioner "straddle[s] the classificatory divide" between true and technical nursing and between nursing and doctoring.[69]

Although an important constituency of physicians and nurses have variously opposed the position of nurse practitioner since it emerged in the 1960s,[70] in the 1990s it appears to have become "just what the doctored ordered." Not only do nurse practitioners offset physician shortages in medically underserved areas; they also make up for the decline in numbers of resident physicians in hospitals (deliberately engineered in response to an anticipated oversupply of specialist physicians) and relieve physicians of tasks they found mundane, routine, and thus eminently delegable to nurses.[71] The nurse practitioner of the 1990s is just what health care administrators, financers, and insurers ordered to provide quality care at lower cost. And the nurse practitioner is just what nurses ordered to return professional nurses with advanced education and clinical skills to the bedside as well as to gain more autonomy and visibility there.[72]

The key factor differentiating nurse practitioners from other nurses and from other advanced, enhanced, and/or expanded nursing practice roles, such as the clinical nurse specialist, is both the use of medical instruments and the use of instruments in ways previously denied nurses.[73] For example, whereas nurses have routinely used stethoscopes since the 1930s, primarily to ascertain blood pressure and auscultate the fetal heart, nurse practitioners use stethoscopes to detect heart and respiratory ailments. Whereas nurses used to hand the vaginal speculum to physicians during the pelvic examination, nurse practitioners conduct these examinations themselves. Whereas nurses' association with x-ray and laboratory testing used to be confined largely to collecting and transporting specimens, nurse practitioners order and interpret the results of these tests. Moreover, nurse practitioners perform diagnostic procedures (including ultrasound examinations, lumbar punctures, sigmoidoscopies, colposcopies, bone marrow biopsies, and thoracenteses) and prescribe drugs and other treatments that were once wholly in the physicians' domain. In short, since their emergence in the 1960s, nurse practitioners have been differentiated from other nurses, in large part, by having gained deeper and cleaner entry into the bodies of patients and, more importantly, into the domains of medical diagnosis and treatment.

Yet the very instrumental entries characterizing the role of the nurse practitioner have also made it controversial. From the time of its emergence to the present day, the nurse practitioner role has been for nurses a contested portal of entry to professional advancement and autonomy and to cultural authority and visibility. Although the role was invented from and supported by the collaboration of many individual physicians and nurses, the idea of the nurse practitioner has inspired continued efforts by organized medicine to limit practitioners' prescriptive authority and ability to be reimbursed for their services.[74] Although individual physicians have fully collaborated with individual nurses to deliver enhanced health care services, organized medicine has typically viewed any physician/nonphysician collaboration as preserving the existing hierarchical structure of health care. The American College of Physicians 1994 position paper on "non-physician providers" makes it clear that at the level of organized medicine and health policy, even if not at the level of individual physicians, collaboration with nurses is neither the egalitarian view of it nurses hold nor an outcome of nurses' increasing abilities to work with physicians as equal partners.[75] Indeed, this position reveals the reluctance of organized medicine to accept research evidence that nurse practitioners are as good as or better than physicians at providing the same services. As the college argued, independent nursing practice would have to be compared to physician practice (which is already independent) for this research finding to be accepted as valid. But since organized medicine has also worked to maintain barriers to independent practice for nurses, the college's position was, in effect, to make its support of the nurse practitioner contingent on studies of a kind of nursing practice organized medicine had sought to prevent.

When the role first emerged, many academic nurses also opposed it because it too uncomfortably reprised for them nurses' tendencies to abandon nursing imperatives in favor of medical tasks. As noted nurse educator and theorist Martha Rogers observed, nurses were too easily "gull[ed]" to abandon true nursing "to play handmaiden to medical

mythology and machines." They naively "fall victim to a mythologi-
cal 'status rainbow.'"[76] Viewing the clinical nurse specialist as the true
advanced nurse—that is, as the mind and spirit of nursing—and the
nurse practitioner as little more than the hand of the doctor, many academic nurses initially considered nurse practitioners "traitors to nursing" and, therefore, resisted programs to educate them in schools of
nursing. As nurse practitioners were a new type of elite nurse, they also
engendered the kind of enmity or envy from nonpractitioner nurses
that the critical care nurse had aroused.[77]

Nurse practitioners have confronted obstacles not only from physicians and other nurses but also from the instrumental nature of the
role itself. The ability of nurse practitioners to nurse is constrained
whenever, in the words of one neonatal nurse practitioner, their day
is spent "perform[ing] medical procedures, such as intubation, lumbar puncture, umbilical line placement, and circumcision."[78] Indeed,
because of the time required to perform such activities in acute care
settings and the time limits imposed on the encounter between nurse
practitioners and their patients in primary care settings, nurse practitioners too often have had to delegate many of the bodily ministering, teaching, and interpersonal relationship functions comprising the traditional core of true nursing to nonpractitioner nurses or
to members of other established and emerging disciplines, such as
psychologists, social workers, grief counselors, and lay patient advocates. Since nurse practitioners have often been sought to perform one
highly skilled function repeatedly, the role has reprised the one-nurse-
to-one-technique, as opposed to one-nurse-to-one-patient, model of
nursing care. Furthermore, by performing the physical examination
as a separate and discrete procedure (as opposed to as an integral or
disguised part of the traditional embodied encounter between nurse
and patient) and by performing tasks such as colposcopies and bone
marrow biopsies, nurse practitioners have made their encounters with
patients more like the experiences physicians have with their patients:
deeply penetrating and instrumental. Nurse practitioners have often
exchanged the embodied intimacies of true nursing for the instrumentally mediated intimacies of medicine.

Although nurse advocates always envisioned the nurse practitioner
as returning nurses to nursing—that is, to the bedside after years of
abandoning it for the desk and the classroom—the public demand for
nurse practitioners derived not from a desire for expanded nursing services but, rather, from a need to "cover the [health care] house" and to

render health care more inexpensively. Nurse advocates construe the nurse practitioner as fulfilling the nursing imperative for comprehensive, holistic, personalized, and otherwise improved health care and as an equal partner with the physician in offering that care. The use of instruments is considered only one means to achieve that end. Indeed, the nurse practitioner's deeper entry into the domains of medical diagnosis and treatment is seen not as a departure from nursing but as an affirmation of the "heritage and philosophy" of nursing.[79]

In the prevailing discourse around the nurse practitioner, however, the role emerges as a largely economically and "medically-driven model of practice" for nurses.[80] In this discourse the traditional image is maintained of nurses as the extra hands and eyes of physicians willingly and cheaply filling voids and bridging gaps in health care.[81] Indeed, as Barbara Daly noted with reference to the acute care nurse practitioner, the "best recognized function" of the nurse practitioner is to "substitute for physicians [and] to deliver cost-effective bedside care."[82] The primary point of reference for the nurse practitioner is arguably not truly nursing (no matter how much nurses insist it is) but, instead, medicine and economics. Nurse practitioners have recurringly been promoted and have presented themselves as a cheap albeit excellent alternative to physicians.[83] Medicine and economics, not nursing ideals, remain the "gold standard" against which the nurse practitioner is promoted and judged.[84]

So powerful is this standard that even nurse proponents of the nurse practitioner recurringly caution nurses not to forget the *nurse* in nurse practitioner. Advocates continue to worry that identification with medicine will simply reinforce medical dominance in health care.[85] Nurse practitioner pioneer Loretta Ford noted the problem of nurses retaining their "nursing identities." Concerned by the expressed desire of one nurse practitioner to be recognized as "more than just a nurse," Ford observed that nurse practitioners had to "resolve their identity crisis by joining the family of nursing."[86] Educator and nurse practitioner Mary Kohnke recalled when the "height of prestige" for the nurse was to "wear narcotic keys around [her] neck." Nurses were now increasingly finding prestige in wearing "a stethoscope or carry-[ing] an otoscope . . . in an expanded role." Kohnke worried that nurses were "expanding right out of nursing."[87] Barbara Daly reminded nurses that they had a "moral commitment to do more than imitate medicine." She advised nurses that what would "save" them from "giving in to the temptation to take the easier road, to simply prepare physician extenders," was their special "mission" as nurses. By becoming a nurse practitioner, a nurse was not simply fulfilling the need for a warm body "to write fluid orders and insert arterial lines" but, rather, using these added responsibilities and skills to realize the goal of nursing: to "restore patients to a state of health."[88] In response to the concern that the nurse practitioner role precluded nurses from nursing, advocates asserted that the position enabled nurses finally to nurse.[89]

Although patients and individual nurses have undeniably benefited from the nurse practitioner role, nursing—as a discrete and differentiated domain of practice—continues to be also undermined by it. Nurses are again being recruited to offset personnel shortages in and the high costs of health care. They are again in danger of "selling themselves short" by (over)producing nurse practitioners to the virtual exclusion of other advanced practice roles and by marketing themselves as the cheap alternative to physicians.[90] Moreover, in a manner reminiscent of the early-twentieth-century promotion of x-ray and laboratory work for nurses, they are again being advised that they will find performing procedures such as endoscopies more fulfilling than just doing ostensibly ordinary nursing.[91]

The role of nurse practitioner has returned the professional nurse to the bedside but, arguably, not always as a nurse. In medical and public policy discourse, the identity of the nurse practitioner as a nurse is elided. The nurse practitioner is a "mid-level" provider in a vertical hierarchy still dominated by the physician. The nurse practitioner is a "physician extender": the Hamburger Helper of health care. Most ominously, though, the nurse practitioner is a nonentity most often referred to as a "non-physician."[92] Despite the sustained contributions of individual nurse practitioners to improved health care, especially for persons who have traditionally been denied it, the nurse practitioner role continues to serve as "ideological cover for continued inequality."[93] Built primarily around the technologies of medical diagnosis and prescription, the nurse practitioner role constitutes arguably yet another effort to create a full jurisdiction for nurses that has yet to be fully realized. For all of the nurse practitioner's autonomy in actual practice, and despite the considerable gains made in removing restrictive barriers to practice, the role still constitutes a significant but limited incursion into the larger domain of medical diagnosis and treatment. Nurse practitioners actually care for patients far removed from any medical supervision, but they remain nominally under the supervision of physicians and legally as border-crossers into medicine.

The incursion of nurses and others into the domain of medical practice is likely to continue as the lines separating health professionals become increasingly blurred, as health care restructuring and reengineering increasingly follow market forces, and as specific tasks are no longer tied to specific kinds of providers. The best person for a job is more often considered to be the person who can be quickly trained to do the job competently and efficiently. Accordingly, the transfer of the "dangerously routine work" of diagnosis and prescription to nurses and others is likely the most hazardous act of delegation for physicians, whose claims to dominance have historically rested on their exclusive possession of the special and "secret" knowledge required to diagnose and prescribe.[94] Such knowledge legitimates professional jurisdictions.[95] Physicians have learned from their experience in trying to reclaim contested fields such as anesthesia and midwifery that it is difficult to take back what has been delegated, and it is hard to reconstruct what was once dismissed as easy enough for a nurse to do as once again too complex for anyone but a physician[96] One physician, for example, worried about a colleague's advocacy of the transfer of endoscopic examinations from residents to nurses, argued for keeping this activity in the medical domain by teaching medical students to do them.[97]

Although physicians now face the greatest challenge to their dominance in health care and nurses now have their best chance of promoting nursing as an independent and reimbursable venture, cultural norms and the gender narratives purveying them continue to reinforce existing arrangements.[98] The general public expects physicians—whether male or female—to be at the top of the health care hierarchy, assumes that physicians know more about all matters of health and disease than any other provider, and is thus highly responsive to "professional discourses" that reinforce these gendered expectations.[99] Even the most ardent advocates of nursing and of the nurse practitioner role in particular propagate the notion that primary care, health promotion, and psychosocial support are inherently less complicated services than those deemed "medically complex." Indeed, nurses and other nonphysician providers are typically represented as saving physicians for these more complex services. Physicians, in turn, are never represented as saving nursing for complex nursing services.

The nurse practitioner role again illustrates how insufficient technology is by itself to assert professional supremacy and to overcome gender. The nurse practitioner role exemplifies how language and gender can operate as technologies to limit nurses' use of medical technologies to advance nursing. The nurse practitioner role illuminates the possibilities and problems of hybrid nursing, of nurses' efforts to cross the entrenched divides between care and cure and between true and technical nursing.

The Equivocal Nursing/Technology Relation

Technology has provided a portal of entry for nurses, but one that nurses have entered at some risk to nursing. As physical object and activity, technological innovations have undeniably enskilled nurses and enlarged the scope of nursing practice. In nurses' hands, the benefits of new technologies have been harnessed and their liabilities minimized. Yet although new technologies have enskilled nurses in practice, the discursive practices around these technologies have also deskilled nurses in law and custom. Indeed, these practices themselves have constituted devices that have both advanced and thwarted the fulfillment of nurses' desires.

Chapter 1

1. Alexandra Chasin, "Class and Its Close Relations: Identities among Women, Servants, and Machines," in *Posthuman Bodies*, ed. Judith Halberstam and Ira Livingston (Bloomington: Indiana University Press, 1995), 73–96 (quote on p. 73).

2. Janet K. Schultz, "Nursing and Technology," *Medical Instrumentation* 14, no. 4 (1980): 211–14 (quote on p. 211).

3. Burton J. Bledstein, *The Culture of Professionalism: The Middle Class and the Development of Higher Education in America* (New York: Norton, 1976), 95.

4. Shizuko Y. Fagerhaugh, Anselm Strauss, Barbara Suczek, and Carolyn L. Wiener, *Hazards in Hospital Care: Ensuring Patient Safety* (San Francisco: Jossey-Bass, 1987) (quote on pp. 81–82).

5. Anselm Strauss, Shizuko Y. Fagerhaugh, Barbara Suczek, and Carolyn L. Wiener, "Sentimental Work in the Technologized Hospital," *Sociology of Health and Illness* 4, no. 3 (1982): 254–78.

6. Richard Willens, "A Nurse Equipment Specialist: Innovative Addition to the Perioperative Team," *Perioperative Nursing Quarterly* 2, no. 3 (1986): 1–7.

7. See, for example, *Pathway Evaluation Program for Nursing Professionals: Specialty Profiles* (Research Triangle Park, N.C.: Glaxo Wellcome, 1995).

8. See, for example, Lynda P. Nauright, Linda Moneyham, and Julianna Williamson, "Telephone Triage and Consultation: An Emerging Role for Nurses," *Nursing Outlook* 47, no. 5 (1999): 219–26.

9. Pamela A. DeVisser, "The Effects of Technology on Critical Care Nursing Practice," *Focus on Critical Care* 8 (July–August 1981): 26–29 (quote on p. 27).

10. Rosemary Stevens, *In Sickness and in Wealth: American Hospitals in the Twentieth Century* (New York: Basic Books, 1989) (quote on p. 18).

11. "Suggestions for National Hospital Day Publicity," *Bulletin of the American Hospital Association* 1, no. 1 (1927): 3–23. Rosemary Stevens observed that incubators, x-rays, and laboratory services "tempted" paying patients; see her *In Sickness and in Wealth*, 108.

12. Jeffrey P. Baker demonstrated the link between technology and spectacle in his description of the "incubator show movement" in the early twentieth

century, which put premature infants, the new incubators developed to house them, and nurses and physicians on display for the education and entertainment of the public; see chap. 5 in his *The Machine in the Nursery: Incubator Technology and the Origins of Newborn Intensive Care* (Baltimore: Johns Hopkins University Press, 1996). Rosemary Stevens observed that the American hospital has been a focus for "community pride, conspicuous waste, and cultural display" (*In Sickness and in Wealth*, 203). See Rosemary Stevens, "Times Past, Times Present," in *The American General Hospital: Communities and Social Contexts*, ed. Diana Elizabeth Long and Janet Golden (Ithaca, N.Y.: Cornell University Press, 1990), 191–206.

13. G. H. M. Rowe, "The Training of Nurses," *Boston Medical and Surgical Journal* 109, no. 1 (1883): 1–4 (quote on p. 2).

14. Temple Burling, Edith M. Lentz, and Robert N. Wilson, eds., *The Give and Take in Hospitals: A Study of Human Organization in Hospitals* (New York: Putnam's, 1956), 266.

15. Anselm Strauss, "The Structure and Ideology of American Nursing: An Interpretation," in *The Nursing Profession: Five Sociological Essays*, ed. Fred Davis (New York: John Wiley, 1966), 60–108 (quote on p. 99).

16. Agnes B. Meade, *Manual of Clinical Charting*, 2nd ed. (Philadelphia: Lippincott, 1938), vii; David C. Figge, "The Tyranny of Technology," *American Journal of Obstetrics and Gynecology* 162, no. 6 (1990): 1365–69 (quote on p. 1365); Caroline Rogers, "Phoenix Seminar: Keynote Speech," *AORN Journal* 16, no. 4 (1972): 165–70 (quote on p. 166).

17. See, for example, Daniel M. Fox and Christopher Lawrence, *Photographing Medicine: Images and Power in Britain and America since 1840* (New York: Greenwood Press, 1988).

18. Baker, *Machine in the Nursery*, 74, 78.

19. John D. Thompson and Grace Goldin, *The Hospital: A Social and Architectural History* (New Haven: Yale University Press, 1975), 215.

20. Adeline C. Jenkins, "Successful Cardiac Monitoring," *Nursing Clinics of North America* 1, no. 4 (1966): 537–47 (quotes on p. 538).

21. Isabel A. Hampton, *Nursing: Its Principles and Practice* (Philadelphia: Saunders, 1893), 93; Ruby M. Harris, "Symposium on the Nurse and the New Machinery," *Nursing Clinics of North America* 1, no. 4 (1966): 535–36; Barbara B. Minckley, "The Multiphasic Human-to-Human Monitor (ICU Model): Nursing Observation in the Intensive Care Unit," *Nursing Clinics of North America* 3, no. 1 (1968): 29–39; Edwina A. McConnell, "The Nature of Human-Machine Interface: An Exploratory Study" (Ph.D. diss., University of Illinois, Chicago, 1987).

22. Evelyn M. Heath, "How the Rural Hospital Can Best Serve Its Community," *Minutes of the Tri-State Hospital Conference*, Columbia, S.C., April 14–16, 1938, North Carolina Collection, University of North Carolina, Chapel Hill, 104–6 (quote on p. 105).

23. Kim Walker, "Confronting 'Reality': Nursing, Science, and the Micro-Politics of Representation," *Nursing Inquiry* 1, no. 1 (1994): 46–56 (quotes on p. 52).

24. Ibid., 51–52.

25. See Robbie E. Davis-Floyd, *Birth as an American Rite of Passage* (Berkeley: University of California Press, 1992), 47.

26. I intend to convey a semiotic link. Semiotics is a diverse and complex domain of cultural study concerned with signs and how they come to have meaning. A sign is anything and everything (e.g., words, objects, visual images, events) that can be taken as signifying something else or that has meaning to particular groups of people. A sign is always experienced as the thing, or signifier, plus its meaning, or what is signified. See, for example, Martha S. Feldman, *Strategies for Interpreting Qualitative Data* (Thousand Oaks, Calif.: Sage, 1995), 21–41, and Peter K. Manning, *Semiotics and Fieldwork* (Newbury Park, Calif.: Sage, 1987).

27. Leonard Riessman and John H. Rohrer, "The Changing Role of the Professional Nurse," in *Change and Dilemma in the Nursing Profession: Studies of Nursing Services in a Large General Hospital*, ed. Leonard Riessman and John H. Rohrer (New York: Putnam's, 1957), 3–17 (quote on p. 14).

28. Bruce Mazlish, "The Fourth Discontinuity," *Technology and Culture* 8, no. 1 (1967): 1–15.

29. Ruth Schwartz Cowan, "Technology Is to Science as Female Is to Male: Musings on the History and Character of Our Discipline," *Technology and Culture* 37, no. 3 (1996): 572–82.

30. See, for example, Carolyn Merchant, *The Death of Nature: Women, Ecology, and the Scientific Revolution* (San Francisco: Harper and Row, 1980). In the study of signs, referent systems constitute the knowledge that we already have and that we bring to a sign that endows it with meaning. These systems are ideological in that ideas already exist in societies that are continually and imperceptibly being reproduced (by virtue of being continually referred to by other sign systems), thereby giving them the qualities of timelessness and inevitability. Because they are there and seem always to have been there, such ideological or knowledge systems take on the appearance of eternal truths—that is, as being outside history or culture. See, for example, Stephen R. Barley, "The Codes of the Dead: The Semiotics of Funeral Work," *Urban Life* 12, no. 1 (1983): 3–31, and Judith Williamson, *Decoding Advertisements: Ideology and Meaning in Advertising* (Boston: Marion Boyars, 1978).

31. See, for example, Pat Ashworth, "Technology and Machines: Bad Masters but Good Servants," *Intensive Care Nursing* 3 (1987): 1–2, and Alan Barnard, "A Critical Review of the Belief That Technology Is a Neutral Object and Nurses Are Its Master," *Journal of Advanced Nursing* 26, no. 1 (1997): 126–31.

32. Chasin, "Class and Its Close Relations," 78; Marie Francoise Colliere, "In-

visible Care and Invisible Women as Health Care Providers," *International Journal of Nursing Studies* 23, no. 2 (1986): 95–112.

33. Susan M. Reverby, *Ordered to Care: The Dilemma of American Nursing, 1850–1945* (Cambridge: Cambridge University Press, 1987).

34. See, for example, Cheryl Bland Jones and Judith W. Alexander, "The Technology of Caring: A Synthesis of Technology and Caring for Nursing Administration," *Nursing Administration Quarterly* 17, no. 2 (1993): 11–20, and Marilyn Anne Ray, "Technological Caring: A New Model in Critical Care," *Dimensions of Critical Care Nursing* 6, no. 3 (1987): 166–73.

35. See, for example, Sally Gadow, "Touch and Technology: Two Paradigms of Patient Care," *Journal of Religion and Health* 23, no. 1 (1984): 63–69, and Margarete Sandelowski, "A Case of Conflicting Paradigms: Nursing and Reproductive Technology," *Advances in Nursing Science* 10, no. 3 (1988): 35–45.

36. Marianne C. Lovell, "The Politics of Medical Deception: Challenging the Trajectory of History," *Advances in Nursing Science* 2, no. 3 (1980): 73–86; Gertrud B. Ujhely, "Current Technological Advances and the Nurse-Patient Relationship," *Journal of New York State Nurses Association* 5, no. 3 (1974): 25–28.

37. Barnard, "Critical Review," 126.

38. Jocalyn Lawler, *Behind the Screens: Nursing, Somology, and the Problem of the Body* (Melbourne: Churchill Livingstone, 1991).

39. Cortney Davis, "Poetry about Patients: Hearing the Nurse's Voice," *Journal of Medical Humanities* 18, no. 2 (1997): 111–25 (quotes on p. 114).

40. Lawler, *Behind the Screens*.

41. Zane Robinson Wolf, "Nurses' Work: The Sacred and the Profane," *Holistic Nursing Practice* 1, no. 1 (1986): 29–35, and *Nurses' Work: The Sacred and the Profane* (Philadelphia: University of Pennsylvania Press, 1988).

42. Everett C. Hughes, *Men and Their Work* (Glencoe, Ill.: Free Press, 1958), 49–53.

43. Peter Short, "Picturing the Body in Nursing," in *The Body in Nursing*, ed. Jocalyn Lawler (Melbourne: Churchill Livingstone, 1997), 7–9 (quote on p. 9).

44. Cortney Davis, "Poetry about Patients," 120; Lawler, *Behind the Screens*, 216.

45. Christopher William Crenner, "Professional Measurement: Quantifying Health and Disease in American Medical Practice, 1880–1920" (Ph.D. diss., Harvard University, Cambridge, Mass., 1993), 24, 38. Crenner used these terms to describe the kind of interaction between physicians and patients that the use of such devices as the thermometer and the stethoscope allowed.

46. Colliere, "Invisible Care."

47. Susan Leigh Star, "The Sociology of the Invisible: The Primacy of Work in the Writings of Anselm Strauss," in *Social Organization and Social Process: Essays in Honor of Anselm Strauss*, ed. David R. Maines (New York: Aldine De Gruyten, 1991), 265–83 (quotes on p. 266). Star cited "technology of silence" from Adrienne Rich, "Cartographies of Silence," in *The Dream of a Common Language* (New York: Norton, 1978), 17.

48. Susan Leigh Star, "Epilogue: Work and Practice in Social Studies of Science, Medicine, and Technology," *Science, Technology, and Human Values* 20, no. 4 (1995): 501–7 (quote on p. 503).

49. Faye G. Abdellah, "Method of Identifying Covert Aspects of Nursing Problems: A Key to Improving Clinical Teaching," *Nursing Research* 6, no. 1 (1957): 4–23.

50. Deborah Heath, "Bodies, Antibodies, and Modest Interventions," in *Cyborgs and Citadels: Anthropological Interventions in Emerging Sciences and Technologies*, ed. Gary Lee Downey and Joseph Dumit (Santa Fe, N.M.: School of American Research Press, 1997), 66–82. Heath described how Western scientists cling to mind/body distinctions between scientists and technicians, relegating technicians and the "embodied materiality . . . [and] corporeality of technoscientific knowledge" (69, 71) to an inferior place in the "hierarchical order" (68) of science.

51. James Dickoff and Patricia James, "Highly Technical but Yet Not Impure: Varieties of Basic Knowledge," in *Perspectives on Nursing Theory*, 2nd ed., ed. Leslie H. Nicoll (Philadelphia: Lippincott, 1992), 572–75 (quote on p. 573).

52. Sharon Traweek, "An Introduction to Cultural and Social Studies of Sciences and Technologies," *Culture, Medicine, and Psychiatry* 17, no. 1 (1993): 3–25.

53. See, for example, Keith Grint and Rosalind Gill, eds., *The Gender-Technology Relation: Contemporary Theory and Research* (London: Taylor and Francis, 1995); Gill Kirkup and Laurie Smith Keller, eds., *Inventing Women: Science, Technology, and Gender* (Cambridge: Polity Press, 1992); Steve Woolgar, ed., "Feminist and Constructivist Perspectives on New Technology," *Science, Technology, and Human Values* 20, no. 3 (1995), special issue; and Judy Wajcman, *Feminism Confronts Technology* (University Park: Pennsylvania State University Press, 1991).

54. On the gender/technology relation, see, for example, Cynthia Cockburn, *Brothers: Male Dominance and Technological Change* (London: Pluto Press, 1983) and *Machinery of Dominance: Women, Men, and Technical Know-How* (London: Pluto Press, 1985); Ruth Schwartz Cowan, *More Work for Mother: The Ironies of Household Technology from the Open Hearth to the Microwave* (New York: Basic Books, 1983); Wendy Faulkner and Erik Arnold, eds., *Smothered by Invention: Technology in Women's Lives* (London: Pluto Press, 1985); Eileen Green, Jenny Owen, and Den Pain, eds., *Gendered by Design? Information Technology and Office Systems* (London: Taylor and Francis, 1993); Maurita Harney, "Computation and Gender," *Research in Philosophy and Technology* 13 (1993): 57–71; H. Patricia Hynes, ed., *Reconstructing Babylon: Essays on Women and Technology* (Bloomington: Indiana University Press, 1991); Judith A. McGaw, "Women and the History of American Technology," *Signs: Journal of Women in Culture and Society* 7, no. 4 (1982): 798–828; Ruth Perry, ed., "From Hard Drive to Software: Gender, Computers, and Difference," *Signs: Journal of Women in Culture and Society* 16, no. 1 (1990), special issue; Kathryn S. Ratcliff, ed., *Healing Technology: Feminist Perspectives* (Ann Arbor: University of Michigan Press, 1989); Joan Rothschild, ed., *Machina ex Dea: Feminist Perspectives on Technology* (New York:

Pergamon Press, 1983); Patricia Spallone and Deborah Lynn Steinberg, eds., *Made to Order: The Myth of Reproductive and Genetic Progress* (Oxford: Pergamon Press, 1987); Autumn Stanley, *Mothers and Daughters of Invention: Notes for a Revised History of Technology* (New Brunswick, N.J.: Rutgers University Press, 1995); Michelle Stanworth, ed., *Reproductive Technologies: Gender, Motherhood, and Medicine* (Minneapolis: University of Minnesota Press, 1987); and Martha M. Trescott, ed., *Dynamos and Virgins Revisited: Women and Technological Change in History* (Metuchen, N.J.: Scarecrow Press, 1979).

55. Nina Lerman, Arwen Mohun, and Ruth Oldenziel, "Versatile Tools: Gender Analysis and the History of Technology," *Technology and Culture* 38, no. 1 (1997): 1–8.

56. Anne Balsamo, *Technologies of the Gendered Body: Reading Cyborg Women* (Durham, N.C.: Duke University Press, 1997), 9. The virtual lack of attention to nursing as a site for gender/technology study is due to a tendency, even among feminists themselves who argue against such stereotypes, to see nursing as a quintessentially woman's occupation and, therefore, not as a science and technology field. Moreover, there is a heritage of mistrust between nursing and feminism around what Ellen Baer has described as "the feminist disdain for nursing" (see "The Feminist Disdain for Nursing," *New York Times*, February 19, 1991.) Whereas feminists have often been insufficiently pro-female for many nurses, nurses have apparently been too uncomfortably female for many feminists.

57. Judy Wajcman, "Feminist Theories of Technology," in *Handbook of Science and Technology Studies*, ed. Sheila Jasanoff, Gerald E. Markle, James C. Petersen, and Trevor Pinch (Thousand Oaks, Calif.: Sage, 1995), 189–204 (quote on p. 200).

58. See, for example, Julie Fairman and Joan Lynaugh, *Critical Care Nursing: A History* (Philadelphia: University of Pennsylvania Press, 1998), and Barbara Melosh, *"The Physician's Hand": Work Culture and Conflict in American Nursing* (Philadelphia: Temple University Press, 1982) and "Doctors, Patients, and 'Big Nurse': Work and Gender in the Postwar Hospital," in *Nursing History: New Perspectives, New Possibilities*, ed. Ellen Condliffe Lagemann (New York: Teachers College Press, 1983), 157–79 (quote on p. 158).

59. Barbara A. Koenig, "The Technological Imperative in Nursing Practice: The Social Creation of a 'Routine' Treatment," in *Biomedicine Examined*, ed. Margaret Lock and Deborah Gordon (Dordrecht: Kluwer Academic, 1988), 465–96.

60. Strauss, "Structure and Ideology."

61. David Wagner, "The Proletarianization of Nursing in the United States, 1932–1946," *International Journal of Health Services* 10, no. 2 (1980): 271–90.

62. Lovell, "Politics of Medical Deception," 85.

63. Candace West and Don H. Zimmerman, "Doing Gender," *Gender and Society* 1, no. 2 (1987): 125–51 (quote on p. 129).

64. See, for example, Carolyn Huffman and Margarete Sandelowski, "The Nurse-Technology Relationship: The Case of Ultrasonography," *Journal of Obstetric, Gynecologic, and Neonatal Nursing* 26, no. 6 (1997): 673–81.

65. See, for example, Susan M. Reverby, "A Legitimate Relationship: Nursing, Hospitals, and Science in the Twentieth Century," in Long and Golden, *American General Hospital*, 135–56.

66. See, for example, Hurdis M. Griffith, Nancy Thomas, and Laura Griffith, "MDs Bill for These Routine Nursing Tasks," *American Journal of Nursing* 91, no. 1 (1991): 22–27, and Hurdis M. Griffith and Karen R. Robinson, "Current Procedural Terminology (CPT) Coded Services Provided by Nurse Specialists," *Image: Journal of Nursing Scholarship* 25, no. 3 (1993): 178–86.

67. Marc Berg, "Of Forms, Containers, and the Electronic Medical Record: Some Tools for a Sociology of the Formal," *Science, Technology, and Human Values* 22, no. 4 (1997): 403–33 (quote on p. 424).

68. See, for example, Linda S. Williams, "The Overlooked Role of Women Professionals in the Provision of In Vitro Fertilization," *Resources for Feminist Research* 18, no. 3 (1989): 80–82.

69. Pam Linn, "Gender Stereotypes, Technology Stereotypes," in *Gender and Expertise*, ed. Maureen McNeil (London: Free Association Books, 1987), 127–51; Flis Henwood, "Establishing Gender Perspectives on Information Technology: Problems, Issues, and Opportunities," in Green, Owen, and Pain, *Gendered by Design?*, 31–49 (quote on p. 43).

70. See, for example, Barbara Keddy, Kelly Acker, Dianne Hemeon, Donna MacDonald, Anne MacIntyre, Thayne Smith, and Brenda Vokey, "Nurses' Work World: Scientific or 'Womanly Ministering'?," *Resources for Feminist Research* 16, no. 4 (1987): 37–39, and Celine Marsden and Anna Omery, "Women, Science, and a Women's Science," *Women's Studies* 21, no. 4 (1992): 479–89.

71. Lerman, Mohun, and Oldenziel, "Versatile Tools," 6.

72. See, for example, Don Ihde, *Technology and the Lifeworld: From Garden to Earth* (Bloomington: Indiana University Press, 1990), and Chapter 2 of this book.

73. Star, "Sociology of the Invisible."

74. Judith Parker and Glenn Gardner, "The Silence and the Silencing of the Nurse's Voice: A Reading of Patient Progress Notes," *Australian Journal of Advanced Nursing* 9, no. 2 (1992): 3–9 (quote on p. 8).

75. In his thoughtful review of a draft of this book, Christopher Crenner observed that the "traces [nurses] leave behind, at best, are anonymous [and] at worst, seem not to be a product of human effort at all," as, for example, a "direct transcription of a measurement/machine reading." Geoffrey C. Bowker observed that nursing has been viewed as an "intermediary profession that does not need to leave a trace." Often having no "official trace" of their own in the medical record, nurses act to ensure that the work of others is preserved; "nursing . . . acts as a distributed memory system for doctors and hospital ad-

ministrators." See Bowker "Lest We Remember: Organizational Forgetting and the Production of Knowledge," available on-line at http://weber.ucsd.edu/~gbowker/forget.html.

76. Alberto Manguel, *A History of Reading* (Toronto: Knopf, 1996), 233. I thank Joy Johnson and Pamela Ratner for the gift of this book.

77. H. Tristram Engelhardt, "Physicians, Patients, Health Care Institutions — and the People in Between: Nurses," in *Caring, Curing, Coping: Nurse, Physician, Patient Relationships*, ed. Anne H. Bishop and John R. Scudder (University: University of Alabama Press, 1983), 62–79; Jenny Littlewood, "Care and Ambiguity: Towards a Concept of Nursing," in *Anthropology in Nursing*, ed. Pat Holden and Jenny Littlewood (London: Routledge, 1986), 170–89 (quote on p. 185); Arthur Kleinman, *Writing at the Margin: Discourse between Anthropology and Medicine* (Berkeley: University of California Press, 1995).

78. Indeed, academic nurses have often talked of borrowing concepts from other fields, as if they eventually had to give them back, and as if only nurses borrowed from others.

79. See, for example, Monica J. Casper and Marc Berg, "Constructivist Perspectives on Medical Work: Medical Practices and Science and Technology Studies," *Science, Technology, and Human Values* 20, no. 4 (1995): 395–407, and Monica J. Casper and Barbara A. Koenig, "Reconfiguring Nature and Culture: Intersections of Medical Anthropology and Technoscience Studies," *Medical Anthropology Quarterly* 10, no. 4 (1996): 523–36.

80. See, for example, Guenter B. Risse and John Harley Warner, "Reconstructing Clinical Activities: Patient Records in Medical History," *Social History of Medicine* 5 (1992): 183–205.

81. See, for example, Joel D. Howell, *Technology in the Hospital: Transforming Patient Care in the Early Twentieth Century* (Baltimore: Johns Hopkins University Press, 1995).

82. See, for example, C. A. Hale, L. H. Thomas, S. Bond, and C. Todd, "The Nursing Record as a Research Tool to Identify Nursing Interventions," *Journal of Clinical Nursing* 6, no. 3 (1997): 207–14, and Parker and Gardner, "Silence and the Silencing." I learned this myself through my own futile efforts to locate patient records that would yield readable information about early-twentieth-century nursing practice and from a set of patient records spanning the 1970s, which contained hardly any information about nursing practice. My research assistant, Donna Bailey, systematically reviewed a random sample of more than 2,000 hospital records in the 1970s for information about nursing practice around electronic fetal monitoring. We found that the records allowed few inferences about nursing activities. Indeed, if these records were the only evidence of nursing procedures, a researcher would wrongly infer that nurses hardly practiced at all.

83. According to Agnes B. Meade, a key writer in the area of nursing records, the topic of charting had become "absorbing" by the early 1930s. See her

"Charting Manual Tool in Ward Teaching," *Hospital Management* 38, no. 1 (1934): 53, 55 (quote on p. 53). See also her "Clinical Recording," *Trained Nurse and Hospital Review* 98, no. 4 (1937): 401–4; "Clinical Charting, Part II," *Trained Nurse and Hospital Review* 98, no. 5 (1937): 495–99; and *Manual of Clinical Charting*.

84. See, for example, Lester Adams, "A Rubber Stamp for Hospital Charts," *Modern Hospital* 3 (1914): 131–32, and Margaret Busche, "Concerning Charting," *American Journal of Nursing* 28, no. 1 (1928): 17–20.

85. See, for example, T. R. Ponton, "Medical Records Bring Obligations," *Hospital Management* 21, no. 2 (1926): 52–54.

86. See, for example, Malcolm T. MacEachern, "Nurses' Clinical Records," *Trained Nurse and Hospital Review* 86, no. 6 (1931): 760–63.

87. Mary A. Merrill, "The Role of the Student Nurse in the 'Clinical Record,' " *Trained Nurse and Hospital Review* 86, no. 1 (1931): 84–86.

88. Gladys M. Bayne, "Patients or Charts?," *Hospital Management* 31, no. 10 (1931): 34–38 (quotes on p. 35).

89. LaVerna L. Balzar, "Improved Clinical Recording Aid to Better Charts," *Hospital Management* 41, no. 3 (1936): 50–51 (quote on p. 50).

90. It is a common contemporary legalistic notion that if an event is not in the record, it never happened. Although the primary purpose of the record is to serve clinical work, it has increasingly become subject to secondary purposes: for example, as a repository of billable categories, as evidence in court cases, and as a time-, task-, and labor-management tool.

91. See, for example, Marc Berg, "Medical Work and the Computer-Based Patient Record: A Sociological Perspective," *Methods of Information in Medicine* 37 (1998): 294–301, and "Practices of Reading and Writing: The Constitutive Role of the Patient Record in Medical Work," *Sociology of Health and Illness* 18, no. 4 (1996): 499–524.

92. Berg, "Practices of Reading and Writing," 512.

93. See, for example, Berg, "Of Forms, Containers, and the Electronic Medical Record," and David Hughes, "When Nurse Knows Best: Some Aspects of Nurse-Doctor Interaction in a Casualty Department," *Sociology of Health and Illness* 10, no. 1 (1988): 1–22.

94. See, for example, Tony Hak, "Psychiatric Records as Transformations of Other Texts," in *Text in Context: Contributions to Ethnomethodology*, ed. Graham Watson and Robert M. Seiler (Newbury Park, Calif.: Sage, 1992), 138–55. On the history of the patient record, see also Stanley J. Reiser, "The Clinical Record in Medicine," pt. 1, "Learning from Cases," and pt. 2, "Reforming Content and Purpose," *Annals of Internal Medicine* 114, nos. 10, 11 (1991): 902–7, 980–85, and "Creating Form out of Mass: The Development of the Medical Record," in *Transformation and Tradition in the Sciences: Essays in Honor of I. Bernard Cohen*, ed. Everett Mendelsohn (Cambridge: Cambridge University Press, 1984), 303–16.

95. I came to Christopher Crenner's work long after I had written Chapter 4, in which I—like he—explore nurses' use of diagnostic instruments. He

used medical records in addition to the sources I used, including nursing and medical texts and advertisements. We both reached similar conclusions.

96. Mary Jo Arndt, "Caring as Everydayness," *Journal of Holistic Nursing* 10, no. 4 (1992): 285–93; Charles E. Rosenberg, "Clio and Caring: An Agenda for American Historians and Nursing," *Nursing Research* 36, no. 1 (1987): 67–68.

97. Ruth Schwartz Cowan, *A Social History of American Technology* (New York: Oxford University Press, 1997), 3. See also Carroll Pursell, *The Machine in America: A Social History of Technology* (Baltimore: Johns Hopkins University Press, 1995), xi–xii.

98. Sandra J. Tanenbaum, *Engineering Disability: Public Policy and Compensatory Technology* (Philadelphia: Temple University Press, 1986), vii.

99. See, for example, Balsamo, *Technologies of the Gendered Body*.

100. Cowan, *Social History*, 204.

101. As Lawler described it in *Behind the Screens*.

Chapter 2

1. Carl Mitcham, *Thinking through Technology: The Path between Engineering and Philosophy* (Chicago: University of Chicago Press, 1994), 152.

2. See, for example, Joseph J. Corn, "Object Lessons/Object Myths? What Historians of Technology Learn from Things," in *Learning from Things: Method and Theory of Material Culture Studies*, ed. W. David Kingery (Washington, D.C.: Smithsonian Institution Press, 1996), 35–54; Sandra Harding, "Knowledge, Technology, and Social Relations" (review of *Medicine and the Reign of Technology*), *Journal of Medicine and Philosophy* 3, no. 4 (1978): 346–58; Hughie Mackay and Gareth Gillespie, "Extending the Social Shaping of Technology Approach: Ideology and Appropriation," *Social Studies of Science* 22, no. 4 (1992): 685–716; and Ruth Oldenziel, "Object/ions: Technology, Culture, and Gender," in Kingery, *Learning from Things*, 55–69. I chose the title for this chapter, *Object Lessons*, several years before I discovered Corn's paper with the same title.

3. See, for example, John Pickstone, "Objects and Objectives: Notes on the Material Cultures of Medicine," in *Technologies of Modern Medicine*, ed. Ghislaine Lawrence (London: Science Museum, 1994), 13–24 (quote on p. 15).

4. See, for example, Audrey B. Davis, "Historical Studies of Medical Instruments," *History of Science* 16 (1978): 107–33, and *Medicine and Its Technology: An Introduction to the History of Medical Instrumentation* (Westport, Conn.: Greenwood Press, 1981); James M. Edmonson, "Learning from the Artifact: Surgical Instruments as Resources in the History of Medicine and Medical Technology," *Caduceus* 9, no. 2 (1993): 87–95; Ghislaine Lawrence, "The Ambiguous Artifact: Surgical Instruments and the Surgical Past," in *Medical Theory, Surgical Practice: Studies in the History of Surgery*, ed. Christopher Lawrence (London: Routledge, 1992), 295–314; and Gretchen Worden, "Steel Knives and Iron Lungs: Medical Instruments as Medical History," *Caduceus* 9, no. 2 (1993): 111–18.

5. Mitcham, *Thinking through Technology*, 267.

6. Technology scholars often differentiate among tools, machines, utilities, and other objects, but these differences are not emphasized here.

7. See, for example, Barbara Duden, *Disembodying Women: Perspectives on Pregnancy and the Unborn* (Cambridge, Mass.: Harvard University Press, 1993), and Daniel J. Boorstin, *The Americans: The Democratic Experience* (New York: Vintage Books, 1974), chap. 39.

8. Alexandra Chasin, "Class and Its Close Relations: Identities among Women, Servants, and Machines," in *Posthuman Bodies*, ed. Judith Halberstam and Ira Livingston (Bloomington: Indiana University Press, 1995), 73–96 (quote on p. 75).

9. See, for example, David F. Channell, *The Vital Machine: A Study of Technology and Organic Life* (New York: Oxford University Press, 1991), and Donna J. Haraway, *Simians, Cyborgs, and Women: The Reinvention of Nature* (New York: Routledge, 1991).

10. Simon J. Williams, "Modern Medicine and the 'Uncertain Body': From Corporeality to Hyperreality?," *Social Science and Medicine* 45, no. 7 (1997): 1041–49.

11. See Ruth Oldenziel's review of Bernice L. Hausman's *Changing Sex: Transsexualism, Technology, and the Idea of Gender*, in *Technology and Culture* 39, no. 1 (1998): 179–81 (quote on p. 181).

12. See, for example, Monica J. Casper, "At the Margins of Humanity: Fetal Positions in Science and Medicine," *Science, Technology, and Human Values* 19, no. 3 (1994): 307–23; Emiko Ohnuki-Tierney, "Brain Death and Organ Transplantation: Cultural Bases of Medical Technology," *Current Anthropology* 35, no. 3 (1994): 233–54 (with comments); and Pickstone, "Objects and Objectives," 14.

13. Casper, "At the Margins of Humanity," 307–8.

14. See, for example, Alice E. Adams, *Reproducing the Womb: Images of Childbirth in Science, Feminist Theory, and Literature* (Ithaca, N.Y.: Cornell University Press, 1994); Dion Farquhar, *The Other Machine: Discourse and Reproductive Technologies* (New York: Routledge, 1996); and Karen Newman, *Fetal Positions: Individualism, Science, Visuality* (Stanford, Calif.: Stanford University Press, 1996).

15. See Lennart Nilsson, *A Child Is Born* (New York: Delacorte Press, 1990) and "Drama of Life before Birth," *Life*, April 30, 1965, 54–72A.

16. Bruce Mazlish, "The Fourth Discontinuity," *Technology and Culture* 8, no. 1 (1967): 1–15.

17. Keith Grint and Steve Woolgar, "On Some Failures of Nerve in Constructivist and Feminist Analyses of Technology," *Science, Technology, and Human Values* 20, no. 3 (1995): 286–310. Another version of this paper appears in *The Gender-Technology Relation: Contemporary Theory and Research*, ed. Keith Grint and Rosalind Gill (New York: Taylor and Francis, 1995), 48–75.

18. J. David Bolter, *Turing's Man: Western Culture in the Computer Age* (Chapel Hill: University of North Carolina Press, 1984), chap. 2, and David Rothenberg,

Hand's End: Technology and the Limits of Nature (Berkeley, Calif.: University of California Press, 1993), xiv.

19. Judy Wajcman, "The Masculine Mystique: A Feminist Analysis of Science and Technology," in *Pink Collar Blues: Work, Gender, and Technology*, ed. Belinda Probert and Bruce W. Wilson (Melbourne: Melbourne University Press, 1993), 20–40 (specific information on p. 30).

20. See, for example, Anne Balsamo, *Technologies of the Gendered Body: Reading Cyborg Women* (Durham, N.C.: Duke University Press, 1997).

21. Ruth Oldenziel, *Making Technology Masculine: Men, Women, and Modern Machines in America, 1870–1945* (Amsterdam: Amsterdam University Press, 1999), 190.

22. Ibid., 14–15, 18. She referred to "technology" as a "neologism" (14) emerging in the 1930s. Technology, as term and domain of knowledge and practice, is frequently tied to narrative. See, for example, Jose Van Dyck, *Manufacturing Babies and Public Consent: Debating the New Reproductive Technologies* (New York: New York University Press, 1995), 11, and John M. Staudenmaier, *Technology's Storytellers: Reweaving the Human Fabric* (Cambridge, Mass.: MIT Press, 1985).

23. Werner Rammert, "New Rules of Sociological Method: Rethinking Technology Studies," *British Journal of Sociology* 48, no. 2 (1997): 171–91 (quote on p. 173).

24. Mitcham, *Thinking through Technology*, 152; Jens F. Jensen, "Computer Culture: The Meaning of Technology and the Technology of Meaning: A Triadic Essay on the Semiotics of Technology," in *The Computer as Medium*, ed. Peter Bogh Andersen, Berit Holmqvist, and Jens F. Jensen (New York: Cambridge University Press, 1993), 292–336.

25. Bryan Pfaffenberger, "Fetishized Objects and Humanized Nature: Towards an Anthropology of Technology," *Man* 23 (June 1988): 236–52 (quote on p. 250).

26. Alan Trachtenberg, *Brooklyn Bridge: Fact and Symbol*, 2nd ed. (Chicago: University of Chicago Press, 1979).

27. Mitcham, *Thinking through Technology*, 160–61. See also Jennifer Clark, "The American Image of Technology from the Revolution to 1840," *American Quarterly* 39, no. 3 (1987): 431–49; Brooke Hindle, "The Exhilaration of Early American Technology: An Essay," in *Early American Technology: Making and Doing Things from the Colonial Era to 1850*, ed. Judith A. McGaw (Chapel Hill: University of North Carolina Press, 1994), 40–48; and Merritt Roe Smith and Leo Marx, eds., *Does Technology Drive History? The Dilemma of Technological Determinism* (Cambridge, Mass.: MIT Press, 1994).

28. Claudia Springer, *Electronic Eros: Bodies and Desire in the Postindustrial Age* (Austin: University of Texas Press, 1996), 4.

29. Professor of English N. Katherine Hayles cautioned that we not forget the "materiality of informatics . . . that makes the information age possible," even as we are increasingly confronted with the "immateriality of information." To counter the "postmodern orthodoxy" that disembodies and

dematerializes the body (or the view that the body is largely a "discursive and informational construction"), she reminded us of the ways that our engagement with information technology is reconfiguring our bodies: altering habits of posture, eye and hand movement, and neural connections. See her "The Materiality of Informatics," *Configurations: A Journal of Literature, Science, and Technology* 1, no. 1 (1993): 147–70 (quotes on pp. 147, 149).

30. Alan Barnard, "A Critical Review of the Belief That Technology Is a Neutral Object and Nurses Are Its Master," *Journal of Advanced Nursing* 26, no. 1 (1997): 126–31 (quote on p. 126); Leo Marx and Merritt Roe Smith, introduction to Smith and Marx, *Does Technology Drive History?*, ix–xv (quote on p. xiv).

31. See, for example, Balsamo, *Technologies of the Gendered Body*; Haraway, *Simians, Cyborgs, and Women*; and Paula Treichler and Lisa Cartwright, eds., "Imaging Technologies, Inscribing Science," *Camera Obscura* 28, 29 (1992). Moreover, in Judy Wajcman's view, "many protagonists of postmodernism" are technological determinists in a more "fashionable" guise, as they depict new information and communication technologies as "causing a new form of society and consciousness to emerge" ("Masculine Mystique," 21).

32. Don Ihde, *Technology and the Lifeworld: From Garden to Earth* (Bloomington: Indiana University Press, 1990), 70.

33. Loucine M. D. Huckabay and Asdghig D. Daderian, "Effect of Choices on Breathing Exercises Post–Open Heart Surgery," *Dimensions of Critical Care Nursing* 9, no. 4 (1990): 190–201.

34. Leelamma Thomas, Helen Ptak, Lynne S. Giddings, Lucille Moore, and Corrine Opperman, "The Effects of Rocking, Diet Modifications, and Anti-flatulent Medication on Post–Cesarean Section Gas Pain," *Journal of Perinatal and Neonatal Nursing* 4, no. 3 (1990): 12–24.

35. For a recent discussion of how women and minority groups have been excluded from the domain of technology, see, for example, Oldenziel's "Object/ions" and *Making Technology Masculine*.

36. On the significance but invisibility of "female" technologies, see, for example, Martha M. Prescott, ed., *Dynamos and Virgins Revisited: Women and Technological Change in History* (Metuchen, N.J.: Scarecrow Press, 1979), and Autumn Stanley, *Mothers and Daughters of Invention: Notes for a Revised History of Technology* (New Brunswick, N.J.: Rutgers University Press, 1995).

37. Ruth Schwartz Cowan, *A Social History of American Technology* (New York: Oxford University Press, 1997), 2. Yet, alternatively, Mitcham proposed that it is not merely the presence or absence of artifacts in a human activity that determines whether it is a technology but, rather, the prominence of artifacts in relation to human users. Accordingly, it is possible to argue that the nurse using a stuffed animal to relieve a patient's pain is not engaged in a technology but in a technique, as she and, specifically, her hands are more central to the activity than the toy. In contrast, when a nurse uses an electronic fetal monitor to appraise the fetus, she is engaged in a technology, as the ma-

chine predominates in the activity of appraisal. See Mitcham, *Thinking through Technology*, 235–36. See also Tim Ingold, "Tools, Minds, and Machines: An Excursion in the Philosophy of Technology," *Techniques et Culture* 12 (1988): 151–76. Rammert, in "New Rules of Sociological Method," 176–78, differentiated among three kinds of "technicization": "habitualization," where human actions become drill- or machine-like; "mechanization," where human labor is delegated to physical artifacts; and "algorithmization," where "technological schemata" are separated from the material and human action and constructed as "sign systems," as in the case of computer programs. According to Rammert's typology, any practice of the nurse in the service of an end is included in the social process of technicization.

38. Stanley, *Mothers and Daughters of Invention*, xvii.

39. Ihde, *Technology and the Lifeworld*, 128; Wiebe E. Bijker, Thomas P. Hughes, and Trevor J. Pinch, eds., *The Social Construction of Technological Systems: New Directions in the Sociology and History of Technology* (Cambridge, Mass.: MIT Press, 1987); Donald MacKenzie and Judy Wajcman, eds., *The Social Shaping of Technology: How the Refrigerator Got Its Hum* (Philadelphia: Open University Press, 1985); Trevor J. Pinch and Wiebe E. Bijker, "The Social Construction of Facts and Artefacts: Or How the Sociology of Science and the Sociology of Technology Might Benefit Each Other," *Social Studies of Science* 14, no. 3 (1984): 399–441.

40. Stefan Timmermans, "Resuscitation Technology in the Emergency Department: Towards a Dignified Death," *Sociology of Health and Illness* 20, no. 2 (1998): 144–67 (quote on p. 148). See also his "High Touch in High Tech: The Presence of Relatives and Friends during Resuscitation Efforts," *Scholarly Inquiry for Nursing Practice* 11, no. 2 (1997): 153–68, and "Saving Lives or Saving Multiple Identities? The Double Dynamic of Resuscitation Scripts," *Social Studies of Science* 26, no. 4 (1996): 767–97.

41. Timmermans, "Resuscitation Technology," 155.

42. Margarete Sandelowski, "Channel of Desire: Fetal Ultrasonography in Two Use-Contexts," *Qualitative Health Research* 4, no. 3 (1994): 262–80.

43. Janelle S. Taylor, "The Public Fetus and the Family Car: From Abortion Politics to a Volvo Advertisement," *Public Culture* 4, no. 2 (1992): 67–80.

44. See, for example, Marveen Craig, "The Other Side of the Story," *Journal of Diagnostic Medical Sonography* 12, no. 3 (1996): 142–47; M. E. Furness, "Fetal Ultrasound for Entertainment?," *Medical Journal of Australia* 153, no. 7 (1990): 371; and Wayne H. Persutte, "Videotaping of Obstetrical Examinations for Patients," *Journal of Diagnostic Medical Sonography* 11, no. 1 (1995): 1–2.

45. See, for example, Rosalind P. Petchesky, "Fetal Images: The Power of Visual Culture in the Politics of Reproduction," in *Reproductive Technologies: Gender, Motherhood, and Medicine*, ed. Michelle Stanworth (Minneapolis: University of Minnesota Press, 1987), 57–80.

46. Jeffrey P. Baker, *The Machine in the Nursery: Incubator Technology and the Origins of Newborn Intensive Care* (Baltimore: Johns Hopkins University Press, 1996).

47. Diane M. Douglas, "The Machine in the Parlor: A Dialectical Analysis of the Sewing Machine," *Journal of American Culture* 5, no. 1 (1982): 20–29 (quotes on p. 26).

48. Sandra J. Tanenbaum, *Engineering Disability: Public Policy and Compensatory Technology* (Philadelphia: Temple University Press, 1986), 19.

49. Nina Lerman, Arwen Mohun, and Ruth Oldenziel, "Versatile Tools: Gender Analysis and the History of Technology," *Technology and Culture* 38, no. 1 (1997): 1–8.

50. The feminist confrontation with technology began in the 1970s and now encompasses a range of widely divergent positions. For example, liberal feminists view technology as a largely gender-neutral entity helping women to overcome the biological and social constraints of gender. Fundamentalist feminists view technology largely as a purveyor of masculine norms that exposes women to mortal danger and furthers women's subordination to men. Feminist social constructionists and cultural theorists view technology as neither absolutely liberating nor enslaving and emphasize the mutually shaping interactions between technology and gender. There are several points of view within each of these larger positions. There is now a vast literature on the women/gender/technology relation. To capture quickly the content and debates in this field since its beginnings, see, for example, Grint and Gill, *Gender-Technology Relation*; Judith A. McGaw, "Women and the History of American Technology," *Signs: Journal of Women in Culture and Society* 7, no. 4 (1982): 798–828; Martha M. Trescott, ed., *Dynamos and Virgins Revisited: Women and Technological Change in History* (Metuchen, N.J.: Scarecrow Press, 1979); and Judy Wajcman, *Feminism Confronts Technology* (University Park: Pennsylvania State University Press, 1991). Dion Farquhar used the terms "liberal" and "fundamentalist" to describe feminist and other "discourses" on reproductive technology. See her *Other Machine*, chaps. 3 and 4.

51. Candace West and Don H. Zimmerman, "Doing Gender," *Gender and Society* 1, no. 2 (1987): 125–51 (quote on p. 126).

52. Cowan, *Social History*, 204.

53. Balsamo, *Technologies of the Gendered Body*, 9, 11.

54. See, for example, Cynthia Cockburn, *Machinery of Dominance: Women, Men, and Technical Know-How* (London: Pluto Press, 1985), and Oldenziel, *Making Technology Masculine*.

55. Richard Butsch, "Crystal Sets and Scarf-Pin Radios: Gender, Technology, and the Construction of American Radio Listening in the 1920s," *Media, Culture, and Society* 20, no. 4 (1998): 557–72 (quotes on pp. 558, 557, and 562, respectively).

56. Sherrie A. Inness, "On the Road and in the Air: Gender and Technology in Girls' Automobile and Airplane Serials, 1909–1932," *Journal of Popular Culture* 30, no. 2 (1996): 47–60 (quotes on p. 48).

57. See Chapter 4 of this book.

58. See, for example, Marianne Bankert, *Watchful Care: A History of America's Nurse Anesthetists* (New York: Continuum, 1989); Audrey B. Davis, "Anesthetist and Anesthesiologist: Technology in the Social Context of a Medical and Nursing Specialty," *Transactions and Studies of the College of Physicians of Philadelphia*, 5th ser., 11, no. 2 (1989): 123–34; and Virginia S. Thatcher, *History of Anesthesia, with Emphasis on the Nurse Specialist* (Philadelphia: Lippincott, 1953). Quote from Bankert, *Watchful Care*, 52.

59. See, for example, Margery W. Davies, *Woman's Place Is at the Typewriter: Office Work and Office Workers, 1870–1930* (Philadelphia: Temple University Press, 1982); Ruth Perry, ed., "From Hard Drive to Software: Gender, Computers, and Difference," *Signs: Journal of Women in Culture and Society*, 16, no. 1 (1990), special issue; and Charis Cussins, "Producing Reproduction: Techniques of Normalization and Naturalization in Infertility Clinics," in *Reproducing Reproduction: Kinship, Power, and Technological Innovation*, ed. Sarah Franklin and Helena Ragone (Philadelphia: University of Pennsylvania Press, 1998), 66–101.

60. Butsch, "Crystal Sets," 569.

61. Ibid., 570 n. 1. See also, for example, Ruth Schwartz Cowan, *More Work for Mother: The Ironies of Household Technology from the Open Hearth to the Microwave* (New York: Basic Books, 1983).

62. Inness, "On the Road," 56.

63. Langdon Winner, "Do Artifacts Have Politics?," in MacKenzie and Wajcman, *Social Shaping of Technology*, 26–37; Judith Lorber, "In Vitro Fertilization and Gender Politics," *Women and Health* 13, no. 1/2 (1988): 117–33. See also Anne-Jorunn Berg and Merete Lie, "Feminism and Constructivism: Do Artifacts Have Gender?," *Science, Technology, and Human Values* 20, no. 3 (1995): 332–51.

64. Anne Phillips and Barbara Taylor, "Sex and Skill: Notes towards a Feminist Economics," *Feminist Review* 6 (1980): 78–88 (quote on p. 85).

65. Judy Wajcman proposed that technology may "represent 'frozen gender relations.'" See her "Patriarchy, Technology, and Conceptions of Skill," *Work and Occupations* 18, no. 1 (1991): 29–45 (quote, in quotes in the original, on p. 30).

66. Cowan, *More Work for Mother*, 10.

67. Oldenziel, "Object/ions," 63, and Corn, "Object Lessons," 47, noted the irony that being "objective," even in an "object-centered" field like the history of technology, usually entails "suppressing experience with actual objects." Corn lamented the cultural and, specifically, academic tendency to privilege talking about technology, as opposed to learning directly from it, or to favor the abstract and cognitive over the "experiential" and "personally particularized" (46).

68. Alan Prout, "Actor-Network Theory, Technology, and Medical Sociology: An Illustrative Analysis of the Metered Dose Inhaler," *Sociology of Health and Illness* 18, no. 2 (1996): 198–219 (quote on p. 199). Recently the term "actor" is increasingly being replaced by the term "actant" to refer to "any entity endowed with the ability to act." See, for example, Michael Callon, "Four

Models for the Dynamics of Science," and Wiebe E. Bijker, "Sociohistorical Technology Studies," in *Handbook of Science and Technology Studies*, ed. Sheila Jasanoff, Gerald E. Markle, James C. Petersen, and Trevor Pinch (Thousand Oaks, Calif.: Sage, 1995), 29–63 (quote on p. 53) and 229–56, and John Law and John Hassard, eds., *Actor Network Theory and After* (Malden, Mass.: Blackwell, 1999).

69. Julian E. Orr, *Talking about Machines: An Ethnography of a Modern Job* (Ithaca, N.Y.: Cornell University Press, 1996), 3.

70. Ibid., chap. 6.

71. Cowan, *More Work for Mother*, 9.

72. Corlann Gee Bush, "Women and the Assessment of Technology: To Think, to Be; to Unthink, to Free," in *Machina ex Dea: Feminist Perspectives on Technology*, ed. Joan Rothschild (New York: Pergamon Press, 1983), 151–70 (quote on p. 155); Rothenberg, *Hand's End*, xv; Don Ihde, *Technics and Praxis* (Boston: Dordrecht, 1979), 42–43.

73. Bush, "Women and the Assessment of Technology," 155.

74. Ibid.

75. Barron H. Lerner, "The Perils of 'X-Ray Vision': How Radiographic Images Have Historically Influenced Perception," *Perspectives in Biology and Medicine* 35, no. 3 (1992): 382–97.

76. Lisa Cartwright, "'Experiments of Destruction': Cinematic Inscriptions of Physiology," *Representations* 40 (fall 1992): 129–52.

77. Newman, *Fetal Positions*, 107–8.

78. Edward Yoxen, "Seeing with Sound: A Study of the Development of Medical Images," in Bijker, Hughes, and Pinch, *Social Construction of Technological Systems*, 281–303.

79. Kathleen Biddick, "Stranded Histories: Feminist Allegories of Artificial Life," *Research in Philosophy and Technology* 13 (1993): 165–82 (quote on p. 170).

80. Roger C. Sanders, *Clinical Sonography: A Practical Guide* (Boston: Little, Brown, 1984), 29.

81. J. F. Dyro, *Impact of Technology on Biomedical Engineering and Nursing* (Arlington, Va.: Association for Advancement of Medical Instrumentation, 1983), 14; Ihde, *Technics and Praxis*, 21.

82. Adeline C. Jenkins, "Successful Cardiac Monitoring," *Nursing Clinics of North America* 1, no. 4 (1966): 537–47 (quote on p. 539).

83. Bush, "Women and the Assessment of Technology," 155.

84. Philip Phenix, *Realms of Meaning* (New York: McGraw-Hill, 1964), 144.

85. Ibid.

86. Natalie Goldberg, *Writing Down the Bones: Freeing the Writer Within* (Boston: Shambhala, 1986), 7.

87. On the displacement of the self and diffusion of identity in the world of the screen, see, for example, Debra Grodin and Thomas R. Lindlof, eds., *Constructing the Self in a Mediated World* (Thousand Oaks, Calif.: Sage, 1996), and Albert B. Robillard, "Communication Problems in the Intensive Care Unit,"

in *Reflexivity and Voice*, ed. Rosanna Hertz (Thousand Oaks, Calif.: Sage, 1997), 252–64.

88. June C. Abbey and Marvin D. Shepherd, "Responding to the Challenge of Education of Nurses and Allied Health Personnel on Safe Use of Medical Devices," in *The Medical Device Industry: Science, Technology, and Regulation in a Competitive Environment*, ed. Norman F. Estrin (New York: Marcel Dekker, 1990), 587–622.

89. Mitcham, *Thinking through Technology*, 164.

90. Ihde, *Technics and Praxis*, 44.

91. Ibid., 43.

92. Micki L. Cabaniss, *Fetal Monitoring Interpretation* (Philadelphia: Lippincott, 1993), 536, 521 (emphasis is mine).

93. Edwin T. Layton, "Technology as Knowledge," *Technology and Culture* 15, no. 1 (1974): 31–41.

94. See, for example, H. David Banta and Clyde J. Behney, "Policy Formulation and Technology Assessment," *Milbank Quarterly* 59, no. 3 (1981): 445–79; Ada Jacox, "Health Care Technology and Its Assessment: Where Nursing Fits In," in *Charting Nursing's Future: Agenda for the 1990s*, ed. Linda H. Aiken and Claire M. Fagin (Philadelphia: Lippincott, 1992), 70–84; and Diane W. Wardell and Joan Engebretson, "Technology Assessment for Nursing Innovations," *Applied Nursing Research* 6, no. 4 (1993): 172–83.

95. Eugene S. Ferguson, "The Mind's Eye: Nonverbal Thought in Technology," *Science* 197, no. 4306 (1977): 827–36 (quotes on p. 827).

96. See, for example, Ingold, "Tools, Minds, and Machines," 152–53, and Oldenziel, *Making Technology Masculine*, chap. 1.

97. Otto Mayr argued that the very effort to understand the science/technology (or technology/science) relationship is, in part, self-interested. That is, engineers (and nurses) might find it in their self-interest to argue for the priority of technology over science. As Mayr summarized it, any effort (and there have been too many, in his view) to arrive at one answer to the "problem" of the science/technology relationship is bound to fail, as all such attempts are based on different assumptions and refer to different things. What would be more fruitful for those attempting to clarify the relationship is to understand how different people in different times comprehended it. See his "The Science-Technology Relationship as a Historiographic Problem," *Technology and Culture* 17, no. 4 (1976): 663–73. Accordingly, my choice of a conceptualization that privileges technology over science can be seen, in part, as a reflection of my interest in privileging nursing, with which technology is often identified. See Chapter 1 of this book.

98. See, for example, Ihde, *Technics and Praxis* and *Technology and the Lifeworld*, and Bruno Latour and Steve Woolgar, *Laboratory Life: The Construction of Scientific Facts* (Princeton: Princeton University Press, 1986).

99. Richard Rorty, *Philosophy and the Mirror of Nature* (Princeton: Princeton University Press, 1979).

100. Lynn White, *Medieval Technology and Social Change* (Oxford: Oxford University Press, 1962).

101. James H. Maxwell, "The Iron Lung: Halfway Technology or Necessary Step?," *Milbank Quarterly* 64, no. 1 (1986): 3–29.

102. Sandra Harding, *Whose Science? Whose Knowledge? Thinking from Women's Lives* (Ithaca, N.Y.: Cornell University Press, 1991).

103. Wendy Faulkner, "Conceptualizing Knowledge Used in Innovation: A Second Look at the Science-Technology Distinction and Industrial Innovation," *Science, Technology, and Human Values* 19, no. 4 (1994): 425–58.

104. Don Ihde, *Instrumental Realism: The Interface between Philosophy of Science and Philosophy of Technology* (Bloomington: Indiana University Press, 1991).

105. Ibid., 45.

106. Michael Lynch and Steve Woolgar, eds., *Representation in Scientific Practice* (Boston: Kluwer Academic, 1988).

107. Latour and Woolgar, *Laboratory Life*.

108. Rothenberg, *Hand's End*, xvi.

109. Ibid., 194.

110. Allucquere Rosanne Stone, preface to *Electronic Culture: Technology and Visual Representation*, ed. Timothy Druckrey (New York: Aperture, 1996), 6.

111. Ibid.

112. Sherry Turkle, *The Second Self: Computers and the Human Spirit* (New York: Simon and Schuster, 1984).

113. Stone, preface, 7.

114. Pfaffenberger, "Fetishized Objects," 244.

115. Joseph F. Fletcher, *The Ethics of Genetic Control: Ending Reproductive Roulette* (Buffalo, N.Y.: Prometheus, 1988), 44.

116. Mitcham, *Thinking through Technology*, 231.

117. Ihde, *Technics and Praxis*, 18.

118. Ihde, *Technics and Praxis* and *Technology and the Lifeworld*.

119. Ihde, *Instrumental Realism*, 118.

120. Duden, *Disembodying Women*, 4.

121. Ibid., 8.

122. Martin Buber, *I and Thou* (New York: Charles Scribner's Sons, 1958).

123. See, for example, Stephen R. Barley, "The Social Construction of a Machine: Ritual, Superstition, Magical Thinking, and Other Pragmatic Responses to Running a CT Scanner," in *Biomedicine Examined*, ed. Margaret Lock and Deborah Gordon (Boston: Kluwer Academic, 1988), 497–539 (specific information on pp. 519–20).

124. There is a large feminist literature analyzing the impact of reproductive technology on women. See, for example, Farquhar, *Other Machine*; Franklin and Ragone, *Reproducing Reproduction*; Janice G. Raymond, *Women as Wombs: Reproductive Technologies and the Battle over Women's Freedom* (San Francisco: Harper, 1993); Patricia Spallone and Deborah Lynn Steinberg, eds., *Made to Order: The Myth of*

Reproductive and Genetic Progress (Oxford: Pergamon Press, 1987); Stanworth, Reproductive Technologies; and Kathryn Strother, ed., Healing Technology: Feminist Perspectives (Ann Arbor: University of Michigan Press, 1989).

125. See, for example, Margarete Sandelowski, "Culture, Conceptive Technology, and Nursing," International Journal of Nursing Studies 36, no. 1 (1999): 13–20.

126. See, for example, Cowan, More Work for Mother.

127. Rima D. Apple, Mothers and Medicine: A Social History of Infant Feeding, 1890–1950 (Madison: University of Wisconsin Press, 1987).

128. Phillips and Taylor, "Sex and Skill," 85.

129. Diana E. Forsythe, "New Bottles, Old Wine: Hidden Cultural Assumptions in a Computerized Explanation System for Migraine Sufferers," Medical Anthropology Quarterly 10, no. 4 (1996): 551–74.

130. See, for example, Chapter 7 in this book and Gro Bjerknes and Tone Bratteteig, "Florence in Wonderland: System Development with Nurses," in Computers and Democracy: A Scandinavian Challenge, ed. Gro Bjerknes, Pelle Ehn, and Morten Kyng (Aldershot: Avebury, 1987), 279–95; Geoffrey C. Bowker, Stefan Timmermans, and Susan Leigh Star, "Infrastructure and Organizational Transformation: Classifying Nurses' Work," in Information Technology and Changes in Organizational Work, ed. Wanda Orlikowski, Geoff Walsham, Matthew R. Jones, and Janice DeGross (London: Chapman and Hall, 1995), 344–70; Suzanne Bakken Henry and Charles N. Mead, "Nursing Classification Systems: Necessary but Not Sufficient for Representing 'What Nurses Do' for Inclusion in Computer-Based Patient Record Systems," Journal of the American Medical Informatics Association 4, no. 3 (1997): 222–32; and Judith Parker and Glenn Gardner, "The Silence and the Silencing of the Nurse's Voice: A Reading of Patient Progress Notes," Australian Journal of Advanced Nursing 9, no. 2 (1992): 3–9.

131. Laura R. Woliver, "The Deflective Power of Reproductive Technologies: The Impact on Women," Women and Politics 9, no. 3 (1989): 17–47.

132. Sandelowski, "Culture, Conceptive Technology, and Nursing."

133. Heather Lechtman and Arthur Steinberg, "The History of Technology: An Anthropological Point of View," in The History and Philosophy of Technology, ed. George Bugliarello and Dean B. Doner (Urbana: University of Illinois Press, 1979), 135–60.

134. Jensen, "Computer Culture," 312.

135. Margarete Sandelowski, "'This Most Dangerous Instrument': Propriety, Power, and the Vaginal Speculum," Journal of Obstetric, Gynecologic, and Neonatal Nursing 29, no. 1 (2000): 73–82.

136. Trachtenberg, Brooklyn Bridge.

137. Bolter, Turing's Man, 11.

138. Ibid.

139. Jensen, "Computer Culture," 326–28; George Lakoff and Mark Johnson, Metaphors We Live By (Chicago: University of Chicago Press, 1980).

140. Turkle, Second Self.

141. Bolter, *Turing's Man*, 42.

142. Wanda J. Orlikowski, "The Duality of Technology: Rethinking the Concept of Technology in Organizations," *Organization Science* 3, no. 3 (1992): 398–427. See also Anthony Giddens, *Central Problems in Social Theory: Action, Structure, and Contradiction in Social Analysis* (Berkeley: University of California Press, 1979) and *The Constitution of Society: Outline of the Theory of Structure* (Berkeley: University of California Press, 1984), and Wanda J. Orlikowski and Daniel Robey, "Information Technology and the Structuring of Organizations," *Information Systems Research* 2, no. 2 (1991): 143–69. I thank my doctoral student Donna Bailey for leading me to Orlikowski's work.

143. Springer, *Electronic Eros*, 4, specifically links devices to desires by referring to electronic technology as an "object of erotic attraction." Sally L. Hacker linked pleasure to technology in *Pleasure, Power, and Technology* (Boston: Unwin Hyman, 1989). In "The Eye of the Beholder: An Essay on Technology and Eroticism," in *Doing It the Hard Way: Investigations of Gender and Technology — Sally L. Hacker,* ed. Dorothy E. Smith and Susan M. Turner (Boston: Unwin Hyman, 1990), 205–23, Hacker observed that technology, like eroticism, excites the body and mind, both emerging from common sources of pleasure learned in a cultural context (specific information on p. 208).

Chapter 3

1. Until the 1930s most graduates worked as private duty nurses. The nurses providing care in hospitals were usually students. For example, graduate nurses were not added to the staff of Watts Hospital in Durham, North Carolina, until 1932. These graduates replaced student nurses as head nurses. See Report of Trustees, Watts Hospital, *The Eightieth Year of Quality Health Care to the Community* (Durham, N.C., 1975).

2. See, for example, *A Handbook of Nursing for Family and General Use* (New Haven: Connecticut Training School for Nurses, 1878); *A Manual of Nursing Prepared for the Training School for Nurses Attached to Bellevue Hospital* (New York: Putnam's, 1878); Annual Report, January 1878, Records of Woman's Hospital of Philadelphia, Center for the Study of the History of Nursing, School of Nursing, University of Pennsylvania, Philadelphia (hereafter cited as CSHN); Carolyn C. Van Blarcom, *Obstetrical Nursing: A Textbook on the Nursing Care of the Expectant Mother, the Woman in Labor, the Young Mother and Her Baby,* 1st, 2nd, 3rd eds. (New York: Macmillan, 1922, 1928, 1933); Joseph B. De Lee, *Obstetrics for Nurses,* 5th, 10th eds. (Philadelphia: Saunders, 1917, 1933); Joseph B. De Lee and Mabel C. Carmon, *Obstetrics for Nurses,* 11th ed. (Philadelphia: Saunders, 1937); Minnie Goodnow, *The Technic of Nursing* (Philadelphia: Saunders, 1928); Isabel A. Hampton, *Nursing: Its Principles and Practice,* 2nd ed. (Cleveland: E. C. Koeckert, 1903); Bertha Harmer, *Textbook of the Principles and Practice of Nursing,* 1st, 2nd, 3rd eds. (New York: Macmillan, 1922, 1928, 1934); Bertha Harmer and Virginia Henderson, *Text-*

book of the *Principles and Practice of Nursing*, 4th ed. (New York: Macmillan, 1939); Anna C. Maxwell and Amy E. Pope, *Practical Nursing: A Textbook for Nurses*, 2nd rev. ed. (New York: Putnam's, 1910); Clara S. Weeks-Shaw, *A Textbook of Nursing: For the Use of Training Schools, Families, and Private Students*, 3rd ed. (New York: D. Appleton, 1914); and Henry L. Woodard and Bernice Gardner, *Obstetric Management and Nursing* (Philadelphia: F. A. Davis, 1936).

3. Jocalyn Lawler, *Behind the Screens: Nursing, Somology, and the Problem of the Body* (Melbourne: Churchill Livingstone, 1991), 29. Lawler distinguished between the "object body" as a material thing and the "lived body" as experienced by living people. Nurses in this period focused on the material body, providing physical care and comfort as opposed to helping people live with and through what was happening to their bodies. Nurses did not yet integrate these two bodies in their practice or in body care in this period of time. See also David Armstrong, "The Fabrication of Nurse-Patient Relationships," *Social Science and Medicine* 17, no. 8 (1983): 457–60.

4. John Wiltshire, "Medical Science, Nursing, and the Future," *Nursing Inquiry* 5, no. 3 (1998): 187–93 (quote on p. 192).

5. Peter Short, "Picturing the Body in Nursing," in *The Body in Nursing*, ed. Jocalyn Lawler (Melbourne: Churchill Livingstone, 1997), 7–9 (quote on p. 9).

6. Donald Ihde, *Technics and Praxis* (Boston: Dordrecht, 1979), 18.

7. The observation functions of the nurse are detailed in Chapter 4 of this book.

8. See, for example, Harmer, *Textbook of the Principles*, 1st ed., 7, 45; *Nursing Procedures*, 1924, 120, Philadelphia General Hospital, School of Nursing, CSHN; Lecture no. 1, 1902, Chautauqua School of Nursing Lecture Notes, CSHN, 4.

9. W. Gilman Thompson, "Efficiency in Nursing," *Journal of the American Medical Association* 61, no. 24 (1913): 2146–49 (quote on p. 2146). Nurses initially worked ten to twelve hours a day for up to seven days a week. In 1897 student nurses at Watts Hospital in Durham, North Carolina, worked seventy to eighty hours a week. In 1932 the graduate nurses who replaced them as head nurses worked a minimum of fifty-six hours a week. See Report of Trustees, *Eightieth Year*.

10. Lecture, November 17, 1887, Mary U. Clymer Papers, CSHN.

11. Maurine Ligon, "The Psychology of Anesthesia," *Trained Nurse and Hospital Review* 96, no. 3 (1936): 260–62 (quote on p. 260). As physicians sought to claim the specialty practice of anesthesia for themselves, the womanly traits once thought appropriate to what physicians saw as lowly work became disadvantages. That is, anesthesia, once considered an "effeminate procedure" (260), was masculinized. See, for example, Marianne Bankert, *Watchful Care: A History of America's Nurse Anesthetists* (New York: Continuum, 1989).

12. Marie Koeneke, *Nursing Procedures: The Lankenau Hospital*, 1927, Lankenau Hospital School of Nursing Records, CSHN. As noted in the editorial "Anybody Can Nurse!," *Trained Nurse and Hospital Review* 105, no. 6 (1940): 470–72, nursing

practice did not lend itself to definite lines of demarcation, with some tasks bordering on housework while others absorbed the latest medical techniques, such as blood transfusions.

13. Emily A. M. Stoney, *Practical Points in Nursing for Nurses in Private Practice*, 2nd ed. (Philadelphia: Saunders, 1897), 25.

14. Martin S. Pernick, *A Calculus of Suffering: Pain, Professionalism, and Anesthesia in Nineteenth-Century America* (New York: Columbia University Press, 1985), 223.

15. Viola K. Swindler, "The Care and Arrangement of Flowers," *American Journal of Nursing* 34, no. 8 (1934): 749–52.

16. Only after features were added to the traditional bed, such as siderails and cranks, did the bed visibly become a sickbed, or hospital bed, distinctive to nursing practice and patienthood.

17. Harmer, *Textbook of the Principles*, 1st ed., 33. The Harmer and Henderson textbooks were mainstays of American nursing education through the 1970s.

18. Lecture no. 13, ca. 1904, Chautauqua School of Nursing Lecture Notes, CSHN, 4. Hospital stays could last up to three months in the late nineteenth century. The average stay at Boston City Hospital in 1870 was twenty-seven days. See Morris J. Vogel, *The Invention of the Modern Hospital: Boston, 1870–1930* (Chicago: University of Chicago Press, 1980), 74.

19. Forty-three varieties of beds and bed making were listed in an unpublished study referred to in Ethel Johns and Blanche Pfefferkorn, *An Activity Analysis of Nursing* (New York: Committee on the Grading of Nursing Schools, 1934), 25.

20. See, for example, the citations listed in n. 2, above; K. L. Milligan, "Bandaging," *Trained Nurse and Hospital Review* 41, no. 5 (1908): 299–301; and E. M. Simpson, "The Bath as a Healing Agent," *American Journal of Nursing* 3, no. 5 (1903): 333–37. Effectiveness, efficiency, comfort given to the patient, and a finished appearance were criteria for judging nursing procedures. See, for example, two students' rendering of these standards in Irma M. Campbell and Corinne Crawford, "Standards for Judging Nursing Procedures," *American Journal of Nursing* 33, no. 10 (1933): 997.

21. See, for example, William R. Houston, *The Art of Treatment* (New York: Macmillan, 1937).

22. According to Edna L. Foley, "Standing Orders," *American Journal of Nursing* 13, no. 6 (1913): 452, patients often objected to baths in cold weather but accepted them "philosophically when told that 'the doctor ordered it.'" Baths were also mainstays of the nurse/patient encounter throughout this period, as they served as a major opportunity for nurses to observe patients closely, to provide comfort, and to forge intimacy. Baths epitomized the nurse at work. Physician R. G. Schroth, in *Instructions for Nurses* (Chicago: Illinois Post Graduate and Training School for Nurses, 1913), 11, observed that "bathing gives the nurse a chance to show that she is earning money and it makes the patient feel better. Also makes it pleasant to visitors." Esther Lucille Brown, in the

landmark *Nursing for the Future: A Report Prepared for the National Nursing Council* (New York: Russell Sage Foundation, 1948), 90–91, noted that there were still head nurses who believed that any staff nurse not in motion was not working. "In the past, the giving of the bed-bath to the patient afforded opportunity for the establishment of an intimate although brief nurse/patient relationship, and yet satisfied the head nurse that work was going on. Now the bath is coming to be given by a nongraduate nurse, before much provision has been made for other ways in which this important relationship can be established." After the 1940s, nurses continued to express ambivalence about relinquishing bathing and other kinds of "bodily care" to ancillary personnel. See, for example, Marion Lesser and Vera Keane, "Nursing and Bodily Care," *American Journal of Nursing* 55, no. 7 (1955): 804–6, and Chapter 5 in this book.

23. Nurses do "dirty work" in the literal and sociological sense, as introduced in Everett C. Hughes, *Men and Their Work* (Glencoe, Ill.: Free Press, 1958), 49–53. See also Lawler, *Behind the Screens*, 45–49, and Zane Robinson Wolf, "Nurses' Work: The Sacred and the Profane," *Holistic Nursing Practice* 1, no. 1 (1986): 29–35.

24. Judith A. McGaw described the experience of early American technology as "redolent with aromas . . . offer[ing] all of the uncomfortable sensuous and visceral experiences we have worked for decades to eradicate." Nursing technology in the late nineteenth and early twentieth centuries also kept nurses in "continuous, relatively unmediated interaction with nature," or the human body. See McGaw, "The Experience of Early American Technology," in *Early American Technology: Making and Doing Things from the Colonial Era to 1850*, ed. Judith A. McGaw (Chapel Hill: University of North Carolina Press, 1994), 1–15 (quotes on pp. 5–6).

25. See, for example, Harmer, *Textbook of the Principles*, 2nd ed., 448–68, and Harmer and Henderson, *Textbook of the Principles*, 4th ed., 565–97, and 5th ed. (New York: Macmillan, 1955), 712–65.

26. See, for example, Janice R. Anderzon, "Emerging Nursing Techniques: Venipuncture," *Nursing Clinics of North America* 3, no. 1 (1968): 165–78; Jules K. Joseph, "Should We Permit Qualified Nurses to Administer Intravenous Therapy?," *Hospital Management* 64, no. 1 (1947): 65–68; "Nursing Practice and Intravenous Therapy," *American Journal of Nursing* 56, no. 5 (1956): 572–73; "Should Nurses Do Venipunctures?," *American Journal of Nursing* 51, no. 10 (1951): 603–4; and James A. Willan, "How the States Stand on IV Administration by Nurses," *Hospital Topics* 40, no. 7 (1962): 41–45. Intravenous nursing is discussed in Chapter 5 of this book.

27. See the Harmer and the Harmer and Henderson series of textbooks cited in n. 2, above. The Philadelphia General Hospital School of Nursing included this technique for the first time in their 1948 procedure book. See *Nursing Procedures*, 1948, Philadelphia General Hospital, School of Nursing, CSHN, 40. See also Chapter 4 of this book.

28. Don Ihde, *Technology and the Lifeworld: From Garden to Earth* (Bloomington: Indiana University Press, 1990), 80–97. See also Chapter 2 of this book.

29. S. Weir Mitchell, *The Early History of Instrumental Precision in Medicine*, an address before the Second Congress of the American College of Physicians and Surgeons, September 23, 1891 (New Haven, Conn.: Tuttle, Morehouse, and Taylor, 1892).

30. The practice of having one nurse take all the temperatures also worked against nurses interpreting temperature in the context of any one case. Temperatures became something the nurse obtained and recorded as efficiently as possible for the doctor's use. The nurse's use of the thermometer is discussed in detail in Chapter 4 of this book.

31. Harmer, *Textbook of the Principles*, 1st ed., 59.

32. "A Practical Point," *Trained Nurse and Hospital Review* 40, no. 1 (1908): 17.

33. Ihde, *Technology and the Lifeworld*, 70.

34. See, for example, Lyla M. Olson, *Improvised Equipment: In the Home Care of the Sick*, 1st, 2nd, 3rd eds. (Philadelphia: Saunders, 1928, 1933, 1939); Anna H. Ross, "Ingenuity and Private Nursing," *American Journal of Nursing* 5, no. 12 (1905): 873–75; Emma V. Skillman, "Improvisations in Private Duty Nursing," *American Journal of Nursing* 26, no. 4 (1926): 269–70; and Stoney, *Practical Points*.

35. Lecture, November 17, 1887, Clymer Papers, CSHN.

36. Stoney, *Practical Points*, 17; Lyla M. Olson, *Improvised Equipment*, 3rd ed., 8.

37. Log, November 4, 1930, Charlotte Tyson Rath Papers, CSHN.

38. The hospital became the technological standard against which the home was compared. Yet to offset patients' fears of hospitals, there were also efforts to make the hospital look like home, with comfortable room decor. The nurse was to be the hostess away from home. See, for example, the Simmons ad in the *Bulletin of the American Hospital Association* 1, no. 2 (1927): 121.

39. Louise Zabriskie, *Mother and Baby Care in Pictures* (Philadelphia: Lippincott, 1935), 62, 64–65; De Lee and Carmon, *Obstetrics for Nurses*, 19.

40. Louise B. Nichols, "For the Limited Budget," *Public Health Nurse* 20, no. 8 (1928): 416–18.

41. E. M. Rice, "Making the Best of Things," *Trained Nurse and Hospital Review* 41, no. 1 (1908): 22–24.

42. Ibid., 24.

43. Lyla M. Olson, *Improvised Equipment*, 3rd ed., 100; Pauline Carlson, "The Evolution of a Stupe Kettle," *American Journal of Nursing* 37, no. 6 (1937): 584–85.

44. As shown in the *American Journal of Nursing* 26, no. 11 (1926): 846.

45. Stoney, *Practical Points*, 25.

46. Ross, "Ingenuity," 874.

47. Carolyn C. Van Blarcom, "Appliances Exhibited at the Meeting of the American Society of Superintendents of Training Schools for Nurses in Pittsburgh," *American Journal of Nursing* 4, nos. 6, 9 (1904): 436–37, 681–84; Nancy E. Cadmus, "Some Hospital Devices and Procedures," *American Journal of Nursing* 16,

no. 7 (1916): 589–605; "Instruments New and Useful in Patient Care," *Trained Nurse and Hospital Review* 102, no. 15 (1939): 414–15; "Technical Exhibits," *Bulletin of the American Hospital Association* 1, no. 3 (1927): 136–62. The De Puy Manufacturing Company of Warsaw, Indiana, invited the "careful inspection of all surgeons and nurses" of their wares ("Technical Exhibits," 141).

48. Mary L. Duchesne, "A Labor-Saving Device," *American Journal of Nursing* 23, no. 3 (1923): 470–72 (quote on p. 472).

49. See, for example, Simpson, "The Bath," and "Typhoid Baths," *American Journal of Nursing* 3, no. 5 (1903): 338–43.

50. Ross, "Ingenuity," 875.

51. See, for example, Cadmus, "Some Hospital Devices"; the picture of a practical croup tent in *American Journal of Nursing* 26, no. 6 (1926): 472; and Elizabeth Berends, "An Improvised Funnel," *Trained Nurse and Hospital Review* 96, no. 3 (1936): 223.

52. See the ad in *Trained Nurse and Hospital Review* 32, no. 1 (1904): 69.

53. "An Interesting Device," *American Journal of Nursing* 26, no. 4 (1926): 280.

54. M. Theodore, "The Good Samaritan Infusion Radiator," *American Journal of Nursing* 31, no. 11 (1931): 1267–68.

55. Martha M. Russell, "Hospital Furnishings," *American Journal of Nursing* 26, no. 11 (1926): 841–46 (quote on p. 841). Nurses viewed furnishings as components of the equipment of nursing practice and important objects in the physical environment of the patient.

56. Nancy P. Ellicott, "Opportunities for Original Work in the Improvement of Hospital Appliances," *American Journal of Nursing* 14, no. 10 (1914): 843–45.

57. Amy M. Hilliard, "Equipment for Nursing Procedures," *American Journal of Nursing* 21, no. 7 (1921): 728–31.

58. Ellicott, "Opportunities for Original Work," 843–45.

59. For information on medical trade literature, see, for example, Audrey B. Davis and Mark S. Dreyfus, *The Finest Instruments Ever Made: A Bibliography of Medical, Dental, Optical, and Pharmaceutical Company Trade Literature, 1700–1939* (Arlington, Mass.: Medical History Publishing Associates I, 1986), and John Parker, "The Adventures of Dr. C. B. Hustler, or Cataloging the Library's Medical Trade Ephemera Collection," *Fugitive Leaves: From the Historical Collections, Library of the College of Physicians of Philadelphia*, 3rd ser., 9, no. 1 (1994): 1–4.

60. "Ethics of Nursing, No. IV: The Doctor," *Trained Nurse* 3, no. 1 (1889): 80–85 (quote on p. 85). At this time the "ethics of nursing" connoted the nurse's comportment and relationship with the physician, not moral dilemmas in practice.

61. P. C. Remondino, "The Trained Nurse in Private Practice," *Trained Nurse* 32, no. 2 (1904): 77–82.

62. See, for example, "Bag Equipment for Rural Nursing," *Public Health Nurse* 21, no. 7 (1929): 352; Jane Elizabeth Hitchcock, "The Story of Our Bag," *Public*

Health Nursing 27, no. 1 (1935): 29–31; and Ruth W. Hubbard, "Bag Technic and the Hourly Nurse," *American Journal of Nursing* 28, no. 6 (1928): 557–59.

63. Frank S. Betz Company, *Surgical Instruments and Supplies*, 1918, Medical Trade Ephemera Collection, College of Physicians of Philadelphia (hereafter cited as MTEC), 37.

64. See the ad for a nurse's outfit on the back of the table of contents in the *American Journal of Nursing* 29, nos. 1–6 (1929).

65. See, for example, the Christmas gift suggestions featured in RN 3, no. 2 (1939): 29–32.

66. Weeks-Shaw, *Textbook of Nursing*, 58.

67. See the ad for B-D Clinical Thermometers in *Trained Nurse and Hospital Review* 66, no. 1 (1921).

68. See the ad for Capsheaf Safety Pin in *Trained Nurse and Hospital Review* 35, no. 6 (1905).

69. See the ad for the Ideal Douche Pan in *Trained Nurse and Hospital Review* 32 (1904).

70. See the ad for Lister's Towels in *Trained Nurse and Hospital Review* 33, no. 6 (1904).

71. "Publisher's Desk," *Trained Nurse and Hospital Review* 32, no. 2 (1904): 152. Fifty years later a physician employee of a New York advertising agency advised his nurse readers that advertising in professional journals was a virtually effortless way for them to keep up with the latest medical products, especially pharmaceuticals. See Philip Reichert, "The Modern Nurse and Medical Advertising," *American Journal of Nursing* 54, no. 9 (1954): 1092–93.

72. By the early 1930s concerns were expressed about the use of the nurse and her image to sell products of all kinds, from cigarettes to toilet paper to razor blades. See, for example, Meta Pennock, "New Ethics in Publicity," *Trained Nurse and Hospital Review* 87, no. 6 (1931): 753–57, 800.

73. See the ad preceding the table of contents in *American Journal of Nursing* 27, no. 3 (1927), and Richard Young, *Illustrated Catalogue of Surgical Instruments, Hospital Furniture, Physicians' Equipment, Sick Room Supplies, Electrotherapeutic and Orthopedic Apparatus* (Philadelphia, 1925), Medical Trade Catalogue Collection, Medical Sciences Division, National Library of Medicine, Washington, D.C., 310, 318, 27.

74. See the ad in *Trained Nurse and Hospital Review* 35, no. 4 (1905): 251, and Denver Chemical Manufacturing Company, *Physician Testimonials* (for Antiphlogistine), 1900–1929, MTEC. A physician writing a testimonial for the use of the product in cases of inflammation observed, "It is conceded by all physicians that outside of the trained nurses, few people are capable of making and applying [poultices] properly, and a lesser number willing to assume the responsibility of changing them at least every hour, night and day" (*Physician Testimonials*, 17).

75. See the ad in *Trained Nurse and Hospital Review* 32, no. 1 (1904): 65.

76. See the ad in *RN*, 3, no. 7 (1940): 43.

77. See the ad for Tycos Fever Thermometer in *Trained Nurse and Hospital Review* (1915).

78. Capsheaf Safety Pin ad.

79. Lister's Towels ad.

80. Ideal Douche Pan ad.

81. Becton, Dickinson, and Company, *Physician Catalog*, 1918, MTEC, 14.

82. Greeley Laboratories, *Greeley Hypodermic Unit*, ca. 1906, MTEC, 8.

83. Hospital Supply Company of New York, *Catalogue of Sterilizers*, 1913, MTEC, 41, 10.

84. See, for example, Harmer and Henderson, *Textbook of the Principles*, 4th ed., 603, and Margaret J. Hawthorne, Virginia Henderson, Mildred Montag, and Marguerite D. Warfield, "Oxygen Therapy: A Study in Some Nursing Aspects of the Operation of an Oxygen Tent," *American Journal of Nursing* 38, no. 11 (1938): 1203–16.

85. Mary E. Benton, "Buck's Extension," *American Journal of Nursing* 34, no. 6 (1934): 539–41.

86. Harmer, *Textbook of the Principles*, 2nd ed., vi.

87. The jury absolved the nurse of criminal liability but cited the hospital for gross carelessness, as the nurse, used to hot water bottles, had not been trained in the use of the electric heating pad. See "Is Investigating Death of Infant," "Jury to Probe Infant's Death," "Nurse's Illness Prevents Action," and "Blame Hospital for Baby's Death," *Raleigh News and Observer*, October 21–24, 1925.

88. See, for example, Garnet W. Ault, "Perforation of the Rectum with Enema Tips," *Transactions: American Proctologic Society*, September 1, 1939, 203–13, and H. H. Rayner, "Injury of the Rectum Caused by the Faulty Administration of an Enema," *British Medical Journal*, March 5, 1932, 419–21.

89. "Urinary Drainage Bottle for Ambulatory Patients," *American Journal of Nursing* 30, no. 9 (1930): 1157–58 (quote on p. 1157). A nurse at Presbyterian Hospital in Chicago, after "experimenting a little," invented a muslin pocket to hold the urine flask against the leg and inside the pants of the patient. One man using it had even been able to go to the theater with his leg bag undetected.

90. See, for example, Edward T. Morman, ed., *Efficiency, Scientific Management, and Hospital Standardization: An Anthology of Sources* (New York: Garland, 1989), and Susan Reverby, "The Search for the Hospital Yardstick: Nursing and the Rationalization of Hospital Work," in *Sickness and Health in America: Readings in the History of Medicine and Public Health*, 2nd ed., ed. Judith Walzer Leavitt and Ronald L. Numbers (Madison: University of Wisconsin Press, 1985), 206–16.

91. Sr. M. Therese, "Why the Nurse Needs a Sound Education: Analysis of Elementary Nursing Procedures," *Trained Nurse and Hospital Review* 95, no. 6 (1935): 557–62. For more time and activity studies of nursing, see, for example, Martha E. Erdmann and Margaret Welsh, "Studies in Thermometer

Technique," *Nursing Education Bulletin* 2, no. 1 (1929): 8–33; Amy Owens, Elizabeth Ruppert, and Gladys Sellew, "Some Time Studies," *American Journal of Nursing* 27, no. 2 (1927): 99–101; and Chelly Wasserberg and Ethel Northam, "Some Time Studies in Obstetrical Nursing," *American Journal of Nursing* 27, no. 7 (1927): 543–44. These studies continued through the 1950s.

92. Blanche Pfefferkorn and Marion Rottman, *Clinical Education in Nursing* (New York: Macmillan, 1932), 20–21.

93. Clare Dennison, "Maintaining the Quality of Nursing Service in the Emergency," *American Journal of Nursing* 42, no. 7 (1942): 774–84.

94. See, for example, Catherine A. Bindel, "From Muslin to Metal," *American Journal of Nursing* 48, no. 11 (1948): 699, and Josephine Hughes, "Hypodermic Injection," *American Journal of Nursing* 16, no. 2 (1916): 198–200.

95. Ruth Sleeper, "The Two Inseparables: Nursing Service and Nursing Education," *American Journal of Nursing* 48, no. 11 (1948): 678–81.

96. Dennison, "Nursing Service in the Emergency," 777.

97. Martha Ruth Smith, "What Are We Doing to Improve Nursing Practice: II. Through Improvement of Nursing Methods," *American Journal of Nursing* 32, no. 6 (1932): 685–88 (quote on p. 687).

98. See, for example, the Harmer and the Harmer and Henderson textbooks cited in n. 2, above; "Comparative Nursing Methods: Lumbar Puncture, Hypodermoclysis, and Intravenous Infusion Trays," *American Journal of Nursing* 30, no. 3 (1930): 253–60; photo collection of equipment trays and *Procedure Books*, 1924–54, Philadelphia General Hospital, School of Nursing, CSHN; and "Student Experience Record of Central Surgical Service," 1935, Albert Einstein Medical Center (formerly Jewish Hospital) School of Nursing Records, CSHN.

99. See, for example, Bindel, "From Muslin to Metal," 699.

100. Weeks-Shaw, *Textbook of Nursing*, 16.

101. Evelyn Mercer, "Nursing Care in Lobar Pneumonia," *American Journal of Nursing* 37, no. 11 (1937): 1211–18.

102. See, for example, "Bulletin," 1936, Albert Einstein Medical Center School of Nursing Records, CSHN; the note on "noisiness" in *Trained Nurse* 2, no. 1 (1888): 27; and Mildred E. Newton, "The Noiseless Perineal Dressing Cart," *American Journal of Nursing* 28, no. 7 (1928): 667–68.

103. "Evaluation of Nursing Care," 1935, Albert Einstein Medical Center School of Nursing Records, CSHN.

104. Harriet M. Gillette, "A Practical Thermometer Tray," *American Journal of Nursing* 26, no. 11 (1926): 840.

105. Charlotte J. Garrison, "Teaching Care of Hospital Equipment," *American Journal of Nursing* 27, no. 10 (1927): 823–26.

106. See, for example, Hulda Helling, "The Patient in the Respirator," *American Journal of Nursing* 41, no. 11 (1941): 1322–24.

107. Thomas Craig Olson, "Laying Claim to Caring: Nursing and the Language of Training, 1915–1937," *Nursing Outlook* 41, no. 2 (1993): 68–72.

108. See, for example, Charles E. Rosenberg, *The Care of Strangers: The Rise of America's Hospital System* (Baltimore: Johns Hopkins University Press, 1987), 212–36.

109. David Rothenberg, *Hand's End: Technology and the Limits of Nature* (Berkeley: University of California Press, 1993), and Barbara Melosh, *"The Physician's Hand": Work Culture and Conflict in American Nursing* (Philadelphia: Temple University Press, 1982).

110. Rosemary Stevens, *In Sickness and in Wealth: American Hospitals in the Twentieth Century* (New York: Basic Books, 1989), 12.

111. Margaret Levi, "Functional Redundancy and the Process of Professionalization: The Case of Registered Nurses in the United States," *Journal of Health Politics, Policy, and Law* 5, no. 2 (1980): 333–53 (quote on p. 336). On p. 347 Levi also used the word "handicapped" to describe the plight of nursing.

112. See, for example, Jo Ann Ashley, *Hospitals, Paternalism, and the Role of the Nurse* (New York: Teachers College, 1976), and Susan M. Reverby, *Ordered to Care: The Dilemma of American Nursing, 1850–1945* (Cambridge: Cambridge University Press, 1987).

113. For discussions differentiating kinds of knowledge needed for practice, see, for example, Joan L. Bottorff, "Nursing: A Practical Science of Caring," *Advances in Nursing Science* 14, no. 1 (1991): 26–39, and Joy L. Johnson, "Nursing Science: Basic, Applied, or Practical? Implications for the Art of Nursing," *Advances in Nursing Science* 14, no. 1 (1991): 7–16.

114. The debate in nursing beginning in the 1960s and continuing today concerning "practice theories" and "practical knowledge" may be seen, in part, as an effort to feature a special domain of knowledge nurses could celebrate and claim exclusively for themselves and to valorize the carrying-out functions of the nurse. As good members of Western culture, nurses also tended to laud basic knowledge, to denigrate applied and practice knowledge, and, thereby, to denigrate much of the knowledge they had and that could have served as a focal point of nursing science. For key essays in this debate, most notably by James Dickoff and Patricia James, see the articles in unit 5 in Leslie H. Nicoll, ed., *Perspectives on Nursing Theory*, 2nd ed. (Philadelphia: Lippincott, 1992). See also Hesook Suzie Kim, "Practice Theories in Nursing and a Science of Nursing Practice," *Scholarly Inquiry for Nursing Practice* 8, no. 2 (1994): 144–58. Kim further dimensionalized the knowledge of application and showed it to be a highly complex domain.

115. Nurses' equivocal relation to science is discussed in Susan M. Reverby, "A Legitimate Relationship: Nursing, Hospitals, and Science in the Twentieth Century," in *The American General Hospital: Communities and Social Contexts*, ed. Diana Elizabeth Long and Janet Golden (Ithaca, N.Y.: Cornell University Press, 1990), 135–56. For a discussion of science in Canadian nursing with relevance to U.S. nursing, see Kathryn McPherson, "Science and Technique: Nurses' Work in a Canadian Hospital, 1920–1939," in *Caring and Curing: Historical Perspectives on Women*

and *Healing in Canada*, ed. Dianne Dodd and Deborah Gorham (Ottawa: University of Ottowa Press, 1994), 71–101. A later version of this paper appears in chapter 4 of McPherson, *Bedside Matters: The Transformation of Canadian Nursing, 1900–1990* (Toronto: Oxford University Press, 1996).

116. See, for example, J. Banett, "Simplifying Nursing Procedures," *American Journal of Nursing* 43, no. 8 (1943): 713–16.

117. Judith Parker and Glenn Gardner, in "The Silence and the Silencing of the Nurse's Voice: A Reading of Patient Progress Notes," *Australian Journal of Advanced Nursing* 9, no. 2 (1992): 3–9, observed that nurses still insist on "making ordinary" the extraordinary work they do in order to help patients with the "extraordinary" events happening to them, but are then "seduced by their own rhetoric" (8).

118. Barbara Melosh and Tom Olson differentiated between the rank-and-file nurse who held a craft-based image of her occupation and the nursing elite who held a professional image. See Melosh, *"Physician's Hand"*, and Tom Olson, "Apprenticeship and Exploitation: An Analysis of the Work Pattern of Nurses in Training, 1897–1937," *Social Science History* 17, no. 4 (1993): 559–76, and "Competing Paradigms and the St. Luke's Alumnae Association Minutes, 1895–1916," *Advances in Nursing Science* 12, no. 4 (1990): 53–62.

119. Diane Hamilton, "Constructing the Mind of Nursing," *Nursing History Review* 2 (1994): 3–28.

120. Mary M. Roberts, "Modification of Nursing Procedures as Demanded by Progress in Medicine," *Hospital Progress* 12, no. 9 (1931): 390–93.

121. Isabel M. Stewart, "The Science and Art of Nursing," *Nursing Education Bulletin* 2, no. 1 (1929): 1–4 (quotes on p. 1).

122. Martha Ruth Smith, "The Variability in Existing Nursing Procedures and Methods of Determining Their Validity," *Nursing Education Bulletin*, n.s., 1 (1930): 10–17.

123. Stewart, "Science and Art," 4.

124. Isabel M. Stewart, *The Education of Nurses: Historical Foundations and Modern Trends* (New York: Macmillan, 1943), 150–51.

125. Clara D. Noyes, "Response and President's Address," *American Journal of Nursing* 20, no. 10 (1920): 780–84 (quote on p. 783).

Chapter 4

1. Bertha Harmer, *Textbook of the Principles and Practice of Nursing* (New York: Macmillan, 1922), 45.

2. T. R. Ponton, "Medical Records Bring Obligations," *Hospital Management* 21, no. 2 (1926): 52–54 (quotes on p. 54).

3. See, for example, Christine A. Tanner, Patricia Benner, Catherine Chesla, and Deborah R. Gordon, "The Phenomenology of Knowing the Patient," *Image: Journal of Nursing Scholarship* 25, no. 4 (1993): 273–80; Donald A. Laird, *Applied*

Psychology for Nurses (Philadelphia: Lippincott, 1923); Hildegard E. Peplau, *Interpersonal Relations in Nursing* (New York: Putnam's, 1952); and Patricia Benner, ed., *Interpretive Phenomenology: Embodiment, Caring, and Ethics in Health and Illness* (Thousand Oaks, Calif.: Sage, 1994).

4. David Armstrong, "The Fabrication of Nurse-Patient Relationships," *Social Science and Medicine* 17, no. 8 (1983): 457–60.

5. Florence Nightingale, *Notes on Nursing: What It Is and What It Is Not* (1859; reprint, New York: Dover, 1969). Nightingale noted that "really ill," as opposed to hypochondriacal, patients did "not want to talk about themselves" (98). Armstrong, in "Fabrication of Nurse-Patient Relationships," 459, concluded that "whereas the essence of the modern [nurse/patient] relationship is communication, that of Nightingale's is silence."

6. Nightingale, *Notes on Nursing*, 105.

7. Ibid., 106, 109.

8. See, for example, Charles E. Rosenberg, *The Care of Strangers: The Rise of America's Hospital System* (Baltimore: Johns Hopkins University Press, 1987), and John H. Warner, *The Therapeutic Perspective: Medical Practice, Knowledge, and Identity in America, 1820–1885* (Cambridge, Mass.: Harvard University Press, 1986).

9. Nightingale, *Notes on Nursing*, 133.

10. Ibid., 110, 111.

11. Ibid., 116, 124.

12. See, for example, *A Manual of Nursing Prepared for the Training School for Nurses Attached to Bellevue Hospital* (New York: Putnam's, 1878), 23–35; Harmer, *Textbook of the Principles*, 45–49; and Isabel Hampton Robb, *Nursing: Its Principles and Practice for Hospital and Private Use*, 3rd ed. (Cleveland: E. C. Koeckert, 1906), 253–69.

13. *Nursing Procedures*, 1924, 120, Philadelphia General Hospital, School of Nursing, Center for the Study of the History of Nursing, School of Nursing, University of Pennsylvania, Philadelphia (hereafter cited as CSHN).

14. Clara S. Weeks, *A Textbook of Nursing* (New York: D. Appleton, 1890), 80.

15. Ibid.

16. Robb, *Nursing*, 41.

17. See, for example, the series written by physician Robert A. Kilduffe, "The Nurse and Her Relation to Symptomatology," *Trained Nurse and Hospital Review*: pt. 1, "The Pulse," vol. 65, no. 6 (1920): 498–501; pt. 2, "The Temperature," vol. 66, no. 1 (1921): 13–16; and pt. 3, "The Respiration," vol. 66, no. 2 (1921): 109–12.

18. See, for example, the series by Myer Solis-Cohen, "How to Observe Symptoms," *Trained Nurse and Hospital Review* 35 (July 1905): 8–11, (August 1905): 83–85, and (September 1905): 140–42, and Eugene A. Smith, "The Observation of Symptoms," *Trained Nurse* 1, no. 1 (1888): 52–55.

19. At one time entering the body could only be accomplished postmortem. See, for example, Stanley Joel Reiser, *Medicine and the Reign of Technology* (Cambridge: Cambridge University Press, 1978).

20. See, for example, Weeks, *Textbook of Nursing*, 80.

21. Christopher William Crenner suggested this dramatic element in "Professional Measurement: Quantifying Health and Disease in American Medical Practice, 1880–1920" (Ph.D. diss., Harvard University, Cambridge, Mass., 1993), 54.

22. This pedagogy also likely contributed to both nurses and patients not seeing nurses as performing physical assessments, thereby preserving this work as a special province of physicians until well into the 1960s and the advent of the nurse practitioner and the physician's assistant. The nurse practitioner is considered in Chapter 7 of this book.

23. Log 26 August ca. 1888, Mary U. Clymer Papers, CSHN.

24. Charting and maintaining records were critical components of nursing observation that nurses did not necessarily enjoy. See, for example, Margaret Busche, "Concerning Charting," *American Journal of Nursing* 28, no. 1 (1928): 17–20.

25. Agnes B. Meade, "Training the Senses in Clinical Observation," *Trained Nurse and Hospital Review* 97, no. 6 (1936): 540–44 (quote on p. 540), and John D. Thompson and Grace Goldin, *The Hospital: A Social and Architectural History* (New Haven: Yale University Press, 1975), 232. According to Thompson and Goldin, *The Hospital*, "Supervision/observability" (231) competed with "privacy" (207) in the history of hospital design. That is, as more patients were housed in private rooms, nurses found it harder to maintain visual control of patients and the environment surrounding them. With the increasing replacement of the ward with the private room, a nurse could no longer stand in one place and see everything she needed to see.

26. In *Reminiscences of Linda Richards: America's First Trained Nurse* (Boston: Whitcomb and Barrows, 1911), 18–19, Richards suggested an important early environmental impediment to nursing observation. Concerning night duty at Bellevue Hospital, she recalled, "No sooner had the day nurses left the wards than the gas was turned so low that the faces of the patients could not be distinguished. One could only see the dim outlines of figures wrapped in gray blankets lying upon the beds. If any work was to be done, a candle must be lighted, and only two candles a week were allowed each ward. If more were used, the nurse had to provide them. . . . The captain of the watch . . . at 5 A.M. . . . turned off all the gas, leaving us in total darkness." Richards had this practice reversed by promising that nurses would use no more gas than they required to fulfill their duties.

27. Warner, *Therapeutic Perspective*.

28. See, for example, Merriley Borell, "Training the Senses, Training the Mind," in *Medicine and the Five Senses*, ed. W. F. Bynum and Roy Porter (Cambridge: Cambridge University Press, 1993), 244–61; Malcolm Nicolson, "The Art of Diagnosis: Medicine and the Five Senses," in *Companion Encyclopedia of the History of Medicine*, vol. 2, ed. W. F. Bynum and Roy Porter (London: Routledge, 1993), 801–25; Reiser, *Medicine and the Reign of Technology*; and also by Reiser,

"Technology and the Eclipse of Individualism in Medicine," *Pharos* 45, no. 1 (1982): 10–15; "The Science of Diagnosis: Diagnostic Technology," in Bynum and Porter, *Companion Encyclopedia of the History of Medicine*, 2:826–51; and "Technology and the Use of the Senses in Twentieth-Century Medicine," in Bynum and Porter, *Medicine and the Five Senses*, 262–73.

29. S. Weir Mitchell, *The Early History of Instrumental Precision in Medicine*, an address before the Second Congress of the American College of Physicians and Surgeons, September 23, 1891 (New Haven, Conn.: Tuttle, Morehouse, and Taylor, 1892).

30. Martha E. Erdmann and Margaret Welsh, "Studies in Thermometer Technique," *Nursing Education Bulletin* 2, no. 1 (1929): 8–33 (quote on p. 11). See also, on the history of clinical thermometry, Logan Clendening, "The History of Certain Medical Instruments," *Annals of Internal Medicine* 4, no. 2 (1930): 176–89; J. Gershon-Cohen, "A Short History of Medical Thermometry," *Annals of the New York Academy of Sciences* 121, art. 1 (1964): 4–11; Hugh A. McGuigan, "Medical Thermometry," *Annals of Medical History* 9, no. 2 (1937): 148–54; and Reiser, *Medicine and the Reign of Technology*, 91–121.

31. Carl A. Wunderlich, *On the Temperature in Diseases: A Manual of Medical Thermometry*, trans. from the 2nd German ed. by W. Bathurst Woodman (London: New Sydenham Society, 1871); Edouard Seguin, *Family Thermometry: A Manual of Thermometry for Mothers, Nurses, Hospitalers, Etc., and All Those Who Have Charge of the Sick and the Young* (New York: Putnam's, 1873), and *Medical Thermometry and Human Temperature*, 2nd ed. (New York: William Wood, 1876). Excerpts of *Family Thermometry* are reprinted in *Temperature*, pt. 1, *Arts and Concepts*, ed. Theodore H. Benzinger (Stroudsburg, Pa.: Dowden, Hutchinson and Ross, 1977), 316–35.

32. Seguin, *Medical Thermometry*, 253.

33. Kathleen Lockhart Latta, "The Clinical Thermometer," *Trained Nurse and Hospital Review* 16 (1896): 584–85 (quote on p. 584).

34. See, for example, Amanda Beck, *A Reference Handbook for Nurses* (Philadelphia: Saunders, 1905), 50; Harmer, *Textbook of the Principles*, 134–51; and lecture, November 21, 1887, Clymer Papers, CSHN.

35. See the ads at the back of Bellevue Hospital's *Manual of Nursing* and Emily A. M. Stoney, *Bacteriology and Surgical Technique for Nurses* (Philadelphia: Saunders, 1900).

36. See, for example, Frank S. Betz Company, *Surgical Instruments and Supplies*, 1918, Medical Trade Ephemera Collection, College of Physicians of Philadelphia (hereafter cited as MTEC), 37; Anna M. Fullerton, *Surgical Nursing* (Philadelphia: P. Blakiston's Son, 1899), 255; E. Hibbard, "A Nurse's Requirements," *Trained Nurse* 2, no. 5 (1889): 188–89; Emily A. M. Stoney, *Practical Points in Nursing for Nurses in Private Practice*, 2nd ed. (Philadelphia: Saunders, 1897), 25; and H. W. Weed Company, *Illustrations of Surgical Instruments*, 1902, 2115, Medical Trade Catalog Collection, Division of Medical Sciences, National Museum of American History, Washington, D.C.

37. See, for example, the Becton, Dickinson ad before the table of contents in *American Journal of Nursing* 27, no. 3 (1927).

38. See, for example, Alice Ward Bailey, "Hospital Life," *Scribner's Magazine* 3 (1888): 698–715; Emily Bax, "Are Nurses Overpaid?," *Hygeia* 9, no. 8 (1931): 727–31 (quote on p. 727); and Katherine DeWitt, "Hospital Sketches," *American Journal of Nursing* 6, no. 7 (1906): 455–59.

39. Bax, "Are Nurses Overpaid?," 727.

40. Isabel A. Hampton, *Nursing: Its Principles and Practice* (Philadelphia: Saunders, 1893) (quote on p. 93).

41. Seguin, *Family Thermometry*, 4–5.

42. Ibid., 19–20.

43. Bellevue Hospital, *Manual of Nursing*, 143.

44. Connecticut Training School for Nurses, *A Handbook of Nursing for Family and General Use* (Philadelphia: Lippincott, 1879), 107–9.

45. Hampton, *Nursing*, 167–85.

46. J. C. Wilson, *Fever Nursing* (Philadelphia: Lippincott, 1899).

47. Harmer, *Textbook of the Principles*, 138.

48. Helen W. Faddis, Alice Auman, and Harkensia Bussey, "Making Temperature Taking Safe," *Pacific Coast Journal of Nursing* 24, no. 2 (1928): 73–74.

49. Latta, "Clinical Thermometer," 584.

50. Safety work is a contemporary concept with historical relevance described by Shizuko Y. Fagerhaugh, Anselm Strauss, Barbara Suczek, and Carolyn L. Wiener in "Chronic Illness, Medical Technology, and Clinical Safety in the Hospital," *Research in the Sociology of Health Care* 4 (1986): 237–70.

51. See, for example, the Becton, Dickinson ad in *Trained Nurse and Hospital Review* 66, no. 1 (1921): 73; the Faichney Instrument ad in *Hospital Management* 21, no. 2 (1926): 88; and Minnie Goodnow, *The Technic of Nursing* (Philadelphia: Saunders, 1928), 148.

52. Daisy Barnwell Jones, *My First Eighty Years* (Baltimore: Gateway Press, 1986), 250. A student at Johns Hopkins in the late 1920s and early 1930s, Jones described falling and, as a result, breaking thirty-two thermometers for which she did not have to pay.

53. Erdmann and Welsh, "Studies in Thermometer Technique." See also Ruth Ashburn, "A Bacteriological Study of Clinical Thermometer Technic," *American Journal of Nursing* 30, no. 3 (1930): 336–42, and A. Frances Fischer and Catherine Simonds, "A Modern Hospital Takes Its Temperatures," *American Journal of Nursing* 29, no. 1 (1929): 89–90.

54. See, for example, Minnie Goodnow, *First-Year Nursing: A Textbook for Pupils during Their First Year of Hospital Work*, 2nd ed. (Philadelphia: Saunders, 1919), 148; Harmer, *Textbook of the Principles*, 150; and Weeks, *Textbook of Nursing*, 67.

55. Hampton, *Nursing*, 50.

56. See, for example, Faddis, Auman, and Bussey, "Making Temperature Taking Safe," 74; Harriet M. Gillette, "A Practical Thermometer Tray," *American*

Journal of Nursing 26, no. 11 (1926): 840; and "A Method of Taking Temperatures," American Journal of Nursing 27, no. 10 (1927): 810.

57. Virginia H. Walker, Nursing and Ritualistic Practice (New York: Macmillan, 1967), 11–22, 169–71. Walker described the transformation of temperature-taking from a critical procedure that nurses valued to a ritualistic procedure and/or one delegated to ancillary personnel.

58. See, for example, Bailey, "Hospital Life."

59. See, for example, Goodnow, First-Year Nursing, 137, 299.

60. See, for example, Joseph B. Cooke, A Nurse's Handbook of Obstetrics, 10th ed., rev. Carolyn E. Gray and Philip F. Williams (Philadelphia: Lippincott, 1924); Joseph B. De Lee, Obstetrics for Nurses, 4th, 9th eds. (Philadelphia: Saunders, 1913, 1930); and Carolyn C. Van Blarcom, Obstetrical Nursing: A Textbook on the Nursing Care of the Expectant Mother, the Woman in Labor, the Young Mother and Her Baby, 1st, 3rd eds. (New York: Macmillan, 1922, 1933).

61. See, for example, Robert A. Kilduffe, "The Blood Pressure: A Consideration of Its Technique and Significance," Trained Nurse and Hospital Review 68 (March 1922): 228–30; Louise Gliem, "High Blood Pressure: Its Care and Treatment," American Journal of Nursing 24, no. 12 (1924): 1184–89; Veronica F. Murray, "Technic of Taking Blood Pressure," American Journal of Nursing 34, no. 11 (1934): 1057–64; Charles C. Sutter, "Blood Pressure," American Journal of Nursing 15, no. 1 (1915): 7–13; William S. Middleton, "Blood Pressure Determination: A Nursing Procedure," American Journal of Nursing 30, no. 10 (1930): 1219–25; and Irving Wilson Voorhies, "What Is Blood Pressure?," Trained Nurse and Hospital Review 61 (July 1918): 6–8. The Philadelphia General Hospital School of Nursing did not include the taking of blood pressure in its procedure books until 1948. See Nursing Procedures, 1948, Philadelphia General Hospital, School of Nursing, CSHN, 40. In the 1930 edition of De Lee's Obstetrics for Nurses a nurse is shown on p. 116 taking the blood pressure. Blood pressure technique is not described at all in, for example, Barbara A. Thompson, Procedures Used in the Teaching of the Principles and Practice of Nursing, Volume 1, at Associated Hospitals of the University of Minnesota School of Nursing, 1929, National Library of Medicine, Washington, D.C., or Mary C. Wheeler and Amalia Metzker, Nursing Technic, 3rd ed. (Philadelphia: Lippincott, 1930).

62. Hughes Evans, "Losing Touch: The Controversy over the Introduction of Blood Pressure Instruments into Medicine," Technology and Culture 34, no. 4 (1993): 784–807.

63. On the addition of the stethoscope to the procedure for taking blood pressure, and physicians' responses, see Crenner, "Professional Measurement" and "Introduction of the Blood Pressure Cuff into U.S. Medical Practice: Technology and Skilled Practice," Annals of Internal Medicine 128, no. 6 (1998): 488–93.

64. Blood pressure was ascertained this way by attaching an inflatable cuff wrapped around the patient's arm to a mercury manometer. By means of an air pump, the pressure in the cuff was increased until the pulse at the wrist

could no longer be felt by palpation. The point at which this occurred on the manometer was recorded as the pulse pressure.

65. Harvey Cushing, "On Routine Determinations of Arterial Tension in Operating Room and Clinic," *Boston Medical and Surgical Journal* 148, no. 10 (1903): 250–56.

66. For more on technology as a symbol and media images of nurses and physicians with technology, see, for example, Daniel M. Fox and Christopher Lawrence, *Photographing Medicine: Images and Power in Britain and America since 1840* (New York: Greenwood Press, 1988), and N. J. Krantzler, "Media Images of Physicians and Nurses in the United States," *Social Science and Medicine* 22, no. 9 (1986): 933–52. From advertisements directed to nurses, Crenner observed that when stethoscopes passed to nurses, they were called by names, such as assistoscope and nurse-o-scope, and designed in pastel colors to separate them from the black and substantial stethoscopes in the physicians' province ("Professional Measurement," 492). I interpret from his observation that an effect would thus be to trivialize nurses' use of the stethoscope and to make it seem as if nurses were playing at being doctors, much like a child might play with toy versions of devices used by grown-ups. But it is possible also to argue that advertisers wanted to appeal directly to nurses. In their ad for the Assistoscope (*American Journal of Nursing* 68, no. 6 (1968): 1190) that Crenner cited, Ormont Drug and Chemical Company advised nurses that their product was "designed with the nurse in mind . . . slim, dainty, light and flexible . . . yet sturdy and dependable." The ad assured nurses that, although designed for them to fit in their pocket or purse, the stethoscope had "all the acoustic perfection" of highly expensive devices. Moreover, the ad appealed to nurses' desire to ensure patients' comfort by noting that the diaphragm rings were made from "non-chilling" materials. In his review of a draft of this book, Crenner further noted that such devices and the advertisements for them reflected an effort to "distinguish nursing work from doctoring work especially when such distinctions became difficult to make."

67. G. S. C. Badger, "The Ideal Curriculum for a Training School," *Trained Nurse and Hospital Review* 36, no. 4 (1906), 198–201 (including discussion) (specific information on p. 199).

68. Eugene A. Smith, "Observation of Symptoms," 53.

69. See, for example, Joel D. Howell, *Technology in the Hospital: Transforming Patient Care in the Early Twentieth Century* (Baltimore: Johns Hopkins University Press, 1995), and Stanley J. Reiser, "The Test Tube as Oracle: The Domination of Diagnostics by Laboratory Analysis," in *History of Diagnostics: Proceedings of the Ninth International Symposium on the Comparative History of Medicine, East and West*, ed. Yosio Kawakita (Osaka, Japan: Taniguchi Foundation, 1987), 175–85.

70. Rosemary Stevens, *In Sickness and in Wealth: American Hospitals in the Twentieth Century* (New York: Basic Books, 1989), 105–31.

71. See, for example, S. Virginia Levis, "Some Practical Points for the Nurse

Who Is Interested in Urinalysis," *Trained Nurse and Hospital Review* 16 (1896): 656–58; P. C. Remondino, "The Trained Nurse in Private Practice," *Trained Nurse* 32, no. 2 (1904): 77–82; and Weeks, *Textbook of Nursing*, 173.

72. Hospital Day was May 13, Florence Nightingale's birthday. See, for example, *Annual Report of the Watts Hospital for the Year Ending 30 November 1922*, 41, Durham, N.C., North Carolina Collection, University of North Carolina, Chapel Hill (hereafter referred to as NCC), and "Suggestions for National Hospital Day Publicity," *Bulletin of the American Hospital Association* 1, no. 1 (1927): 3–23.

73. Edward F. Stevens, *The American Hospital of the Twentieth Century*, 2nd rev. ed. (New York: Architectural Record, 1921), 225.

74. For the varied duties and education of the nurse in these fields, see, for example, Charlotte A. Aikens, *Clinical Studies for Nurses*, 2nd ed. (Philadelphia: Saunders, 1912), 37; Sister Alma, *Clinical Laboratory Manual for Nurses and Technicians* (St. Louis: C. V. Mosby, 1932); Louise B. D'Arby, "The Hospital X-Ray Nurse," *American Journal of Nursing* 17, no. 6 (1917): 488–90, and "Suggestions for the X-Ray Room," pt. 2, "Fluoroscopic Work and Record Keeping," *Trained Nurse and Hospital Review* 70, no. 5 (1923): 416–17; Henry J. Goeckel, "A Plan for the Laboratory Training of Nurses," *Modern Hospital* 12 (June 1919): 422–23; A. Hazelwood, "The Nurse and the Clinical Laboratory," *American Journal of Nursing* 27, no. 4 (1927): 259–61; R. M. L. "My Experience in X-Ray Work," *American Journal of Nursing* 20, no. 8 (1920): 626–27; Rose M. Lorish, "The Development of the X-Ray Negative," *American Journal of Nursing* 21, no. 4 (1921): 234–36; Margaret Ossenback, "Training School for Nurses," in *Annual Report of the Watts Hospital*, 22–27, NCC; Olive B. Sweet, "A Hospital Nurse's Day," *U.S. Veterans' Bureau Medical Bulletin* 1, no. 4 (1925): 57–61; Catherine B. Washburn, "Assisting with Diagnostic Tests," *American Journal of Nursing* 29, no. 6 (1929): 645–48; Edith L. Weart, "The Nurse as Laboratory Technician," *American Journal of Nursing* 32, no. 12 (1932): 1251–54; and John B. Zingrone, "Mercy Hospital X-Ray Laboratory," *Hospital Progress* 1, no. 3 (1920): 104–7. See also the series by Henry J. Goeckel, "The Laboratory: Its Relation to the Nursing Service," *Trained Nurse and Hospital Review* 70, nos. 1–6 (1923): 44–45, 115–16, 226–27, 320–21, 413–15, 509–11.

75. See, for example, Nora D. Dean, "The Roentgenological Field for Nurses," *American Journal of Nursing* 21, no. 3 (1920): 159–61, and E. Blanche Seyfert, "Opportunities for the Nurse in the X-Ray Diagnostic Laboratory," *Trained Nurse and Hospital Review* 68 (February 1922): 136–37 (quote on p. 136).

76. J. M. Parrott, response to Edmundson S. Boice, "The Interne Problem of the Small Hospital," *Transactions of the North Carolina Hospital Association*, First Annual Meeting, April 16, 1919, Pinehurst, N.C., NCC, 14–19 (quote on p. 19).

77. See, for example, Seyfert, "Opportunities for the Nurse"; M. Warwick, "The Nurse as Laboratory Technician," *American Journal of Nursing* 27, no. 2 (1927): 95–97; and Weart, "Nurse as Laboratory Technician."

78. Seyfert, "Opportunities for the Nurse," 137.

79. Boice, "Interne Problem," 18.

80. I have found no means to determine exactly how many nurses assumed these roles. Clara D. Noyes, in her presidential address to the first meeting of the American Nurses' Association after World War I, lamented that nurses were leaving nursing to enter related fields, such as social service, anesthesia, oral hygiene, and x-ray and laboratory work. See Noyes, "Response and President's Address," *American Journal of Nursing* 20, no. 10 (1920): 780–84. A nurse is listed as a laboratory technician in *Annual Report of the Watts Hospital*, 7, NCC.

81. Weart, "Nurse as Laboratory Technician," 1251.

82. Seyfert, "Opportunities for the Nurse," 137.

83. D'Arby, "Hospital X-Ray Nurse," 488; Dean, "Roentgenological Field," 159; Seyfert, "Opportunities for the Nurse," 138.

84. Warwick, "Nurse as Laboratory Technician," 97.

85. Mabel McVicker, "The Importance of Understanding Medical Laboratory Tests," *American Journal of Nursing* 23, no. 1 (1922): 14–16 (quotes on p. 14).

86. Ethel Johns and Blanche Pfefferkorn, *An Activity Analysis of Nursing* (New York: Committee on the Grading of Nursing Schools, 1934), 83.

87. Harmer, *Textbook of the Principles*, xi; Bertha Harmer and Virginia Henderson, *Textbook of the Principles and Practice of Nursing*, 4th ed. (New York: Macmillan, 1939), ix.

88. See, for example, Charlotte A. Aikens, *Studies in Ethics for Nurses* (Philadelphia: Saunders, 1916), 112–13; George H. Hoxie, *Practice of Medicine for Nurses: A Textbook for Nurses and Students of Domestic Science, and a Handbook for All Those Who Care for the Sick* (Philadelphia: Saunders, 1980), preface; and Kilduffe, "Nurse and Her Relation to Symptomatology," pt. 1, 498.

89. Eugene A. Smith, "Observation of Symptoms," 54.

90. See, for example, J. M. Davis, "Teaching Bacteriology in School of Nursing," in *Official Proceedings of the 32nd Annual Convention of the North Carolina State Nurses' Association*, October 25–27, 1934, Fayetteville, N.C., NCC, 59–63; Kilduffe, "Nurse and Her Relation to Symptomatology"; Eugene A. Smith, "Observation of Symptoms"; and Solis-Cohen, "How to Observe Symptoms."

91. Dr. Billings, quoted in Ethel Johns and Blanche Pfefferkorn, *The Johns Hopkins Hospital School of Nursing, 1889–1949* (Baltimore: Johns Hopkins Press, 1954), 13.

92. See, for example, W. Gilman Thompson, "The Overtrained Nurse," *New York Medical Journal* 83, no. 17 (1906): 845–49. A physician could never be overtrained.

93. See, for example, Richard O. Beard, "The Education of the Nurse in America," *Transactions of the American Hospital Association* 12 (1910): 345–59; Richard C. Cabot, "Suggestions for the Improvement of Training Schools for Nurses," *Boston Medical and Surgical Journal* 145, no. 21 (1901): 567–69; "Nursing as a Profession," *Boston Medical and Surgical Journal* 149, no. 5 (1903): 133–34; John H. Packard, "On the Training of Nurses for the Sick," *Boston Medical and Surgical Journal* 95, no. 20 (1876): 573–79; "The Reciprocal Relations of the Nurse and the

Physician," *Boston Medical and Surgical Journal* 121, no. 17 (1889): 417–18; and G. H. M. Rowe, "The Training of Nurses," *Boston Medical and Surgical Journal* 109, no. 1 (1883): 1–4. For a history of these views, see Thelma Ingles, "The Physicians' View of the Evolving Nursing Profession," *Nursing Forum* 15, no. 2 (1976): 123–64.

94. See, for example, "President's Address," in *Transactions of the North Carolina Hospital Association*, April 20, 1920, Charlotte, N.C., NCC, 8. A physician is quoted as saying, "Don't make a poor doctor and spoil a good nurse."

95. W. Gilman Thompson, "Overtrained Nurse," 848.

96. Packard, "On the Training of Nurses," 577.

97. See, for example, Goodnow, *First-Year Nursing*, 197, and Solis-Cohen, "How to Observe Symptoms," 8.

98. Gladys M. Bayne, "Patients or Charts?," *Hospital Management* 31, no. 10 (1931): 34–38 (quotes on p. 35).

99. This is a fine but critical distinction drawn between nursing observation and medical diagnosis by Cortney Davis, in "Poetry about Patients: Hearing the Nurse's Voice," *Journal of Medical Humanities* 18, no. 2 (1997): 111–25 (specific information on p. 121).

100. Johns and Pfefferkorn, *Activity Analysis*, 21.

101. Wunderlich, *On the Temperature*, 74.

102. Seguin, *Medical Thermometry*, 281.

103. Wunderlich, *On the Temperature*, 75.

104. Seguin, *Medical Thermometry*, 281.

105. Wunderlich, *On the Temperature*, 75.

106. See, for example, Reiser, "Test Tube as Oracle" and "Technology and the Eclipse of Individualism." On the use and abuse of laboratory diagnosis (with an emphasis on the debate in North Carolina), see also, for example, Richard C. Cabot, "The Historical Development and Relative Value of Laboratory and Clinical Methods of Diagnosis," *Boston Medical and Surgical Journal* 157, no. 5 (1907): 150–53; Robert H. Lafferty, "The Importance of Chemistry and Physiology to the General Practitioner," *Transactions of the Medical Society of the State of North Carolina* 59 (June 18–20, 1912): 498–501; W. H. Prioleau, "What Laboratory Work Should Be Done by the Physician Himself?," *Transactions of the Medical Society of the State of North Carolina* 51 (May 24–26, 1904): 324–27; Paul H. Ringer, "Abuse of the Laboratory from the Viewpoint of the Laboratory Worker," *Transactions of the Medical Society of the State of North Carolina* 57 (June 21–23, 1910): 377–81; S. A. Stevens, "The Relation of the Specialist to the General Practitioner," *Transactions of the Medical Society of the State of North Carolina* 58 (June 20–22, 1911): 172–77; and John H. Tucker, "What Aid Is the Laboratory in Diagnosis?," *Transactions of the Medical Society of the State of North Carolina* 58 (June 20–22, 1911): 532–36.

107. Elizabeth Connolly, "The Nurse and the Fractional Ewald Meal by the Rehfus Method," in *Transactions of the Sixth Annual Meeting of the North Carolina Hospital Association*, April 16, 1923, Asheville, N.C., NCC, 80–84.

108. In addition to the literature cited in n. 28, above, and Howell, *Tech-*

nology in the Hospital, see Audrey B. Davis, Medicine and Its Technology: An Introduction to the History of Medical Instrumentation (Westport, Conn.: Greenwood Press, 1981) and "American Medicine in the Gilded Age: The First Technological Era," Annals of Science 47, no. 2 (1990): 111–25; Joel D. Howell, "Early Use of X-ray Machines and Electrocardiographs at the Pennsylvania Hospital, 1897 through 1927," Journal of the American Medical Association 255, no. 17 (1986): 2320–23; Howell, Technology and American Medical Practice, 1880–1930: Anthology of Sources (New York: Garland, 1988); and Howell, "Machines and Medicine: Technology Transforms the American Hospital," in The American General Hospital: Communities and Social Contexts, ed. Diana Elizabeth Long and Janet Golden (Ithaca, N.Y.: Cornell University Press, 1990), 109–34.

109. For the growing importance of science in this period, the association of new diagnostic instrumentation with science, and physicians' effective use of the rhetoric of science, see Borell, "Training the Senses"; Charles E. Rosenberg, No Other Gods: On Science and American Social Thought, rev. and exp. ed. (Baltimore: Johns Hopkins University Press, 1997); S. E. D. Shortt, "Physicians, Science, and Status: Issues in the Professionalization of Anglo-American Medicine in the Nineteenth Century," Medical History 27, no. 1 (1983): 51–68; and Ronald G. Walters, ed., Scientific Authority and Twentieth-Century America (Baltimore: Johns Hopkins University Press, 1997).

110. Evans, "Losing Touch," 799.

111. Warner, Therapeutic Perspective. See also Jens Lachmund, "Between Scrutiny and Treatment: Physical Diagnosis and the Restructuring of Nineteenth Century Medical Practice," Sociology of Health and Illness 20, no. 6 (1998): 779–801, on the "cultural innovations" (795) of physical and instrumental diagnosis in German-speaking countries.

112. Reiser, "Technology and the Eclipse of Individualism," 12. In his review of a draft of this book Christopher Crenner noted this paradox concerning subjectivity.

113. Jacalyn Duffin, To See with a Better Eye: A Life of R. T. H. Laennec (Princeton: Princeton University Press, 1998), 151.

114. Rosemary Stevens, In Sickness and in Wealth. According to Stevens, nurses were "captured by the hospital and institutionally subsumed" (12).

115. Anselm Strauss, Shizuko Fagerhaugh, Barbara Suczek, and Carolyn Wiener, "Sentimental Work in the Technologized Hospital," Sociology of Health and Illness 4, no. 3 (1982): 254–77.

116. See Malcolm T. MacEachern, foreword to Agnes B. Meade, Manual of Clinical Charting, 2nd ed. (Philadelphia: Lippincott, 1938), vii.

117. Malcolm T. MacEachern, "Nurses' Clinical Records," Trained Nurse and Hospital Review 86, no. 6 (1931): 760–63 (quote on p. 761).

118. Mary A. Merrill, "The Role of the Student Nurse in the 'Clinical Record,'" Trained Nurse and Hospital Review 86, no. 1 (1931): 84–86.

119. Carl Mitcham, Thinking through Technology: The Path between Engineering and Phi-

losophy (Chicago: University of Chicago Press, 1994), 209. What is often forgotten is that most physicians also did not bring technologies into existence but, rather, put them into use. We tend to valorize invention over application and to see physicians (males) as inventors and nurses (females) as only users. Moreover, we tend not to see the creativity involved in using technology that we see in invention, or to see use as continuous with invention as users redesign technologies in use.

120. Eva Gamarnikow, "Nurse or Woman: Gender and Professionalism in Reformed Nursing, 1860–1923," in *Anthropology and Nursing*, ed. Pat Holden and Jenny Littlewood (London: Routledge, 1986), 110–29 (quote on p. 119). Gamarnikow studied British nursing.

121. See, for example, "Laboratory Diagnosis," *RN* 2, no. 10 (1939), 20–24, 42. This article lists twenty-eight tests with their normal values and what conditions increase and decrease values. But there are no implications for nursing appraisal; instead, there are only cautions about how to collect specimens properly.

122. Clare Dennison, "Nursing Service in the Emergency," *American Journal of Nursing* 42, no. 7 (1942): 774–84. Print advertisements and early-twentieth-century promotional campaigns to bring patients into hospitals also blurred the lines between hospital and hotel, and hospital and home. For example, the ad for Simmons furniture in *Bulletin of the American Hospital Association* 1, no. 2 (1927), 121, emphasized the "homelike" feel of the hospital room, toward which Simmons furniture contributed. A nurse is shown opening the window. Nurses were thus linked to the hospital-as-home, where they were to be at the beck and call of patients. Hospitals were to have a "hotel air." See, for example, Raymond P. Sloan, "A Hospital That Is Known by Its Hotel Air," *Modern Hospital* 42, no. 5 (1934): 70–74. Hospitals promoted the telephones, signal lights, or other call/intercom systems that allowed patients continuous access to nurses. In a sense these devices were part of the technology of nursing observation and hospital administration. As nurses increasingly had to care for patients out of their immediate sight—that is, in private rooms instead of wards—these utilities linked patients to nurses. Call systems not only allowed nurses to watch their patients, however, but also to be watched by their superiors. These systems were a quality control mechanism that allowed supervisors to monitor how quickly nurses responded to patient calls, like hotel managers monitored their bell-hops. Some systems maintained a graphic record of the interval between patient call and nurse response in order to settle disputes with patients and to check on nurses. See, for example, Bryant Electric Company, *Bryant Silent Call Signal System for Hospitals*, Bridgeport, Conn., 1914, MTEC; the ad "You Certainly Are Prompt, Nurse," from Holtzer-Cabot Electric Company, in *Hospital Progress* 1, no. 8 (1920); and the ad "Where Seconds Count," from Chicago Signal Company, in *Hospital Management* 21, no. 1 (1926).

123. See Chapter 5 in this book.

124. Blanche Pfefferkorn and Marian Rottman, *Clinical Education in Nursing* (New York: Macmillan, 1932), 51–52.

125. Corlann Gee Bush, "Women and the Assessment of Technology: To Think, to Be; to Unthink, to Free," in *Machina ex Dea: Feminist Perspectives on Technology*, ed. Joan Rothschild (New York: Pergamon Press, 1983), 151–70 (quote on p. 155).

126. Davina Allen, "The Nursing-Medical Boundary: A Negotiated Order?," *Sociology of Health and Illness* 19, no. 4 (1997): 498–520.

127. Dramatic increases in surgery, exclusively in the physician's domain, also brought people into hospitals. See, for example, Rosemary Stevens, *In Sickness and in Wealth*.

128. Rosenberg, *Care of Strangers*, 153.

129. Crenner, "Professional Measurement," 126.

130. Andrew Abbott, "Status and Status Strain in the Professions," *American Journal of Sociology* 86, no. 4 (1981): 819–35 (quotes on pp. 824, 829). I am indebted to Nancy Tomes for this reference.

131. John Pickstone, "Objects and Objectives: Notes on the Material Cultures of Medicine," in *Technologies of Modern Medicine*, ed. Ghislaine Lawrence (London: Science Museum, 1994), 13–24 (quote on p. 19).

132. Susan M. Reverby, "A Legitimate Relationship: Nursing, Hospitals, and Science in the Twentieth Century," in Long and Golden, *American General Hospital*, 135–56.

133. Charles P. Emerson, "The Accuracy of Certain Clinical Methods," *Johns Hopkins Hospital Bulletin* 14, no. 42 (1903): 9–18 (quotes on p. 18).

134. The emergence of the nursing diagnosis movement in the 1960s was, in part, an effort to let physicians claim *medical* diagnosis while renaming and claiming the diagnostic work nurses actually performed as *nursing* diagnosis. Nursing diagnoses were generally not dependent on equipment-embodied technology. See, for example, Marjory Gordon, *Nursing Diagnosis: Process and Application*, 3rd ed. (St. Louis: C. V. Mosby, 1994).

135. Judy Wajcman, "Patriarchy, Technology, and Conceptions of Skill," *Work and Occupations* 18, no. 1 (1991): 29–45 (quote on p. 37).

Chapter 5

1. David Wagner, "The Proletarianization of Nursing in the United States, 1932–1946," *International Journal of Health Services* 10, no. 2 (1980): 271–90. Robert L. Brannon argued that proletarianization and professionalization are complex social processes that are not necessarily mutually exclusive. See Brannon, *Intensifying Care: The Hospital Industry, Professionalization, and the Reorganization of the Nursing Labor Process* (Amityville, N.Y.: Baywood, 1994). I use "proletarianization" here to refer to the transformation of nurses into laborers in hospitals, subordinate to both managerial and medical interests.

2. Joan E. Lynaugh and Barbara L. Brush, *American Nursing: From Hospitals to Health Systems* (Malden, Mass.: Blackwell, 1996), 1–25.

3. *Health Manpower Source Book 9: Physicians, Dentists, and Professional Nurses* (Washington, D.C.: U.S. Department of Health, Education, and Welfare, 1959), 70.

4. Virginia H. Walker, "Observations on the Nursing Service Department," in *Change and Dilemma in the Nursing Profession: Studies of Nursing Services in a Large General Hospital*, ed. Leonard Reissman and John H. Rohrer (New York: Putnam's, 1957), 18–59 (quote on p. 43), and Leonard Reissman and John H. Rohrer, "The Changing Role of the Professional Nurse," in Reissman and Rohrer, *Change and Dilemma*, 3–17 (quote on p. 14).

5. Ella L. Rothweiler, *Nursing in Pictures* (Philadelphia: F. A. Davis, 1945).

6. John H. Rohrer, "Methods for Studying Nursing Services," in Reissman and Rohrer, *Change and Dilemma*, 283–92 (quote on p. 286).

7. "Twenty Studies of Nursing Functions," *American Journal of Nursing* 54, no. 11 (1954): 1378–82.

8. *A Study of Nursing Functions* (Seattle: Washington State Nurses Association, 1953), app. A, tab. 30.

9. Thomas R. Ford and Diane D. Stephenson, *Institutional Nurses: Roles, Relationships, and Attitudes in Three Alabama Hospitals* (University: University of Alabama Press, 1954), 29. As the primary technology in these studies was the stopwatch, nurses were "subjugated to time" not only in their work but in how their work was perceived.

10. See, for example, Faye G. Abdellah and Eugene Levine, "Work-Sampling Applied to the Study of Nursing Personnel," *Nursing Research* 3 (June 1954): 11–16; Everett C. Hughes, Helen McGill, and Irwin Deutscher, *Twenty Thousand Nurses Tell Their Story: A Report on Studies of Nursing Functions Sponsored by the ANA* (Philadelphia: Lippincott, 1958); and Donald D. Stewart and Christine E. Needham, *The General Duty Nurse* (Fayetteville: University of Arkansas, 1955).

11. Hughes, McGill, and Deutscher, *Twenty Thousand Nurses*, 131.

12. Lynaugh and Brush, *American Nursing*, 1; Morris J. Vogel, *The Invention of the Modern Hospital: Boston, 1870–1930* (Chicago: University of Chicago Press, 1980), 77; and Rosemary Stevens, *In Sickness and in Wealth: American Hospitals in the Twentieth Century* (New York: Basic Books, 1989), 4.

13. See, for example, "The Biennial," *American Journal of Nursing* 46, no. 11 (1946): 728–46; Virginia Henderson, "The Nature of Nursing," *American Journal of Nursing* 64, no. 8 (1964): 62–68; Frances Reiter Kreuter, "What Is Good Nursing Care?," *Nursing Outlook* 5, no. 5 (1957): 302–4; and Mary Kelly Mullane, "Has Nursing Changed?," *Nursing Outlook* 6, no. 6 (1958): 323.

14. Dorothy E. Johnson, "A Philosophy of Nursing," *Nursing Outlook* 7, no. 4 (1959): 198–200 (quote on p. 199); Genevieve Rogge Meyer, *Tenderness and Technique: Nursing Values in Transition* (Los Angeles: University of California Institute of Industrial Relations, 1960).

15. "Medicine and Nursing," *Trained Nurse* 2, no. 3 (1889): 116.

16. Ibid.

17. Isabel M. Stewart, "The Science and Art of Nursing," *Nursing Education Bulletin* 2, no. 1 (1929): 1–4; Effie J. Taylor, "Of What Is the Nature of Nursing?," *American Journal of Nursing* 34, no. 5 (1934): 473–76.

18. Faye G. Abdellah, "Method of Identifying Covert Aspects of Nursing Problems: A Key to Improving Clinical Teaching," *Nursing Research* 6, no. 1 (1957): 4–23, and Faye G. Abdellah, Irene L. Beland, Almeda Martin, and Ruth V. Matheney, *Patient-Centered Approaches to Nursing* (New York: Macmillan, 1960), 2–4.

19. Ford and Stephenson, *Institutional Nurses*, 3.

20. Doris Carnevali and Nola Smith Sheldon, "How Early Ambulation Affects Nursing Service," *American Journal of Nursing* 52, no. 8 (1952): 954–56.

21. Lecture no. 13, ca. 1904, Chautauqua School of Nursing Lecture Notes, Center for the Study of the History of Nursing, School of Nursing, University of Pennsylvania, Philadelphia (hereafter cited as CSHN), 4, and Bertha Harmer, *Textbook of the Principles and Practice of Nursing* (New York: Macmillan, 1922), 33.

22. Temple Burling, Edith M. Lentz, and Robert N. Wilson, eds., *The Give and Take in Hospitals: A Study of Human Organization in Hospitals* (New York: Putnam's, 1956), 246.

23. Mary Daly, in *Gyn/Ecology: The Metaethics of Radical Feminism* (Boston: Beacon Press, 1978), 277, described nurses (among other women caregivers) as "token torturers" of patients on physicians' behalf by virtue of their high visibility administering painful therapies. Physicians tend to inflict pain from a distance and when patients are asleep. Giving injections was a duty nurses often dreaded, and it continues to confront nurses with the paradox of giving pain to relieve pain. See, for example, Josephine Hughes, "Hypodermic Injection," *American Journal of Nursing* 16, no. 2 (1916): 198–200, and Peggy Ann Field, "A Phenomenological Look at Giving an Injection," *Journal of Advanced Nursing* 6, no. 4 (1981): 291–96.

24. See, for example, Olive J. Rich, "Hospital Routines as Rites of Passage in Developing Maternal Identity," *Nursing Clinics of North America* 4, no. 1 (1969): 101–8, and Gladys Denny Shultz, "Journal Mothers Report on Cruelty in Maternity Wards," *Ladies Home Journal*, May 1958, 44–45, 152–55. See also Judith Walzer Leavitt, "'Strange Young Women on Errands': Obstetric Nursing between Two Worlds," *Nursing History Review* 6 (1998): 3–24, and Margarete Sandelowski, *Pain, Pleasure, and American Childbirth: From the Twilight Sleep to the Read Method, 1914–1960* (Westport, Conn.: Greenwood Press, 1984), 67–71. For more on obstetric nursing, see Chapter 6 of this book.

25. Lynaugh and Brush, *American Nursing*, 13.

26. Brannon, *Intensifying Care*, 3.

27. Marion Lesser and Vera Keane, *Nurse-Patient Relationships in a Maternity Service* (St. Louis: C. V. Mosby, 1956) and "Nursing and Bodily Care," *American Journal of*

Nursing 55, no. 7 (1955): 804–6 (quote on p. 804). See also Ellen D. Davis, "Give a Bath?," *American Journal of Nursing* 70, no. 11 (1970): 2366–67. Renee C. Fox, Linda H. Aiken, and Carla M. Messikomer, "The Culture of Caring: AIDS and the Nursing Profession," *Milbank Quarterly* 68, suppl. 2 (1990): 230, described bathing the patient as a "highly structured, expressive enactment of some of the cardinal values and meanings of nursing care." Most recently Lynne M. Hektor and Theris A. Touhy mourned the neglect of the "aesthetics aspects of the bath" and the loss of the bath as a "therapeutic art," in "The History of the Bath: From Art to Task?," *Journal of Geronotological Nursing* 23, no. 5 (1997): 13, 14.

28. See, for example, *Nursing Practice in California Hospitals* (n.p.: California State Nurses Association, 1953), 2.

29. See, for example, the complexity of bathing in the early twentieth century in E. M. Simpson, "The Bath as a Healing Agent," *American Journal of Nursing* 3, no. 5 (1903): 333–37, and (written by an unnamed "graduate") "Typhoid Baths," *American Journal of Nursing* 3, no. 5 (1903): 338–43. As indicated in these articles, bathing was also a stimulus for nurse invention.

30. See, for example, Robert W. Habenstein and Edwin A. Christ, *Professionalizer, Traditionalizer, and Utilizer* (Columbia: University of Missouri, 1955), and Meyer, *Tenderness and Technique*.

31. Lesser and Keane, "Nursing and Bodily Care," 805.

32. Meyer, *Tenderness and Technique*, 29 n. 4. Meyer suggested that "quickhand" or "thoroughhand" were more appropriate labels for this type, named "ironhand" by the respondents in her study. Yet "ironhand" better captures the increasing importance of technology (symbolized by iron) as extension of the hand and the discipline, order, and iron rule long associated with trained nursing.

33. Burling, Lentz, and Wilson, *Give and Take in Hospitals*, 224.

34. Ibid., 245, 246.

35. Edwin A. Christ, *Nurses At Work* (Columbia: University of Missouri, Institute for Research in the Social Sciences, 1956), 47.

36. Alice W. Goodwin, "Hospital Inhospitality," *American Journal of Nursing* 32, no. 9 (1932): 937–39 (quote on p. 939).

37. Esther Lucille Brown, *Nursing for the Future: A Report Prepared for the National Nursing Council* (New York: Russell Sage Foundation, 1948), 78–83.

38. Isabel M. Stewart, *The Education of Nurses: Historical Foundations and Modern Trends* (New York: Macmillan, 1943), 148–50.

39. Marian Randall and Mabel Reid, "Hypodermic Injections," *Public Health Nursing* 42, no. 1 (1950): 3–5.

40. Mildred L. Montag, *The Education of Nursing Technicians* (New York: Putnam's, 1951).

41. "American Nurses' Association's First Position on Education for Nursing," *American Journal of Nursing* 65, no. 12 (1965): 106–11.

42. Thomas G. Orr, "Continuous Intravenous Infusion: A Consideration of Its Possible Dangers," *Minnesota Medicine* 18, no. 12 (1935): 778–82 (quotes on p. 778).

43. Clare Dennison, "Maintaining the Quality of Nursing Service in the Emergency," *American Journal of Nursing* 42, no. 7 (1942): 774–84 (specific information on p. 777).

44. "Changes in Nursing from the 1930s to 1953," *Nursing Research* 5, no. 2 (1956): 85–86.

45. See, for example, Bertha Harmer and Virginia Henderson, *Textbook of the Principles and Practice of Nursing*, 5th ed. (New York: Macmillan, 1955), 739–59; Margaret A. Tracy, *Nursing: An Art and Science* (St. Louis: C. V. Mosby, 1942); and Mary C. Wheeler and Amalia Metzker, *Nursing Technic*, 3rd ed. (Philadelphia: Lippincott, 1930).

46. "Nursing Practice and Intravenous Therapy," *American Journal of Nursing* 56, no. 5 (1956): 572–73 (quote on p. 572).

47. Audrey D. London, Hedwig T. Bystrowski, and Charles M. Barbour, "Intravenous Therapy Is Work for Nurse Specialists," *Hospitals* 21, no. 4 (1947): 41–42.

48. Diane Hamilton, "The Cost of Caring: The Metropolitan Life Insurance Company's Visiting Nurse Service, 1909–1953," *Bulletin of the History of Medicine* 63, no. 3 (1989): 414–34. On p. 428 Hamilton cites a physician who objected to nurses taking blood pressures, doing urinalyses, and giving intramuscular injections.

49. "Should Nurses Do Venipunctures?," *American Journal of Nursing* 51, no. 10 (1951): 603–4 (quote on p. 603).

50. Jules K. Joseph, "Should We Permit Qualified Nurses to Administer Intravenous Therapy?," *Hospital Management* 64, no. 1 (1947): 65–68.

51. See Chapter 4 of this book.

52. Isabel A. Hampton, *Nursing: Its Principles and Practice* (Philadelphia: Saunders, 1893), 50.

53. See, for example, London, Bystrowski, and Barbour, "Intravenous Therapy," 41, and Ann H. Shanck, "The Nurse in an Intravenous Therapy Program," *American Journal of Nursing* 57, no. 8 (1957): 1012–13.

54. Barbara P. Levenstein, "Intravenous Therapy: A Nursing Specialty," *Nursing Clinics of North America* 1, no. 2 (1966): 259–67 (quote on p. 259); Anna L. Seal, "Symposium on Injection Therapy: The Nurse's Responsibilities," *Nursing Clinics of North America* 1, no. 2 (1966): 257–58 (quote on p. 257).

55. Levenstein, "Intravenous Therapy," 259; Seal, "Symposium on Injection Therapy," 257.

56. Marie Imperiale and Theodora Krebs, "The Intravenous Therapy Nurses," *American Journal of Nursing* 61, no. 5 (1961): 53–54.

57. See, for example, Sr. M. Rosalind, "We Plan to Teach Intravenous Administration of Fluids," *American Journal of Nursing* 54, no. 12 (1954): 1513–14, and

Emma K. Flinner, "The Decision Was No," *American Journal of Nursing* 60, no. 4 (1960): 518–20.

58. James A. Willan, "How the States Stand on IV Administration by Nurses," *Hospital Topics* 40, no. 7 (1962): 41–45 (quote on p. 41).

59. See, for example, Diane Hamilton, "Constructing the Mind of Nursing," *Nursing History Review* 2 (1994): 3–28.

60. Janice R. Anderzon, "Emerging Nursing Techniques: Venipuncture," *Nursing Clinics of North America* 3, no. 1 (1968): 165–78 (quote on p. 176).

61. Margaret A. Bergin, "All Our Nurses Give I.V.s!" *RN* 28, no. 11 (1965): 47–51.

62. Nathan Hershey, "Scope of Nursing Practice," *American Journal of Nursing* 66, no. 1 (1966): 117–20.

63. "Should Nurses Do Venipunctures?," 603.

64. Ibid.

65. Ibid., 604.

66. Andrew Abbott, *The System of Professions: An Essay on the Division of Expert Labor* (Chicago: University of Chicago Press, 1988), 71.

67. Ibid., 72.

68. Ibid.

69. Ada Lawrence Plumer, *Principles and Practice of Intravenous Therapy*, 2nd ed. (Boston: Little, Brown, 1975), 5–17.

70. John B. Richardson, "Intravenous Therapy Team: A New Nursing Service," *Hospitals* 36, no. 16 (1962): 80–90.

71. See, for example, Keith Grint and Rosalind Gill, "The Gender-Technology Relation: Contemporary Theory and Research," in *The Gender-Technology Relation: Contemporary Theory and Research*, ed Keith Grint and Rosalind Gill (London: Taylor and Francis, 1995), 1–28, and Judy Wajcman, "Patriarchy, Technology, and Conceptions of Skill," *Work and Occupations* 18, no. 1 (1991): 29–45.

72. Anne Phillips and Barbara Taylor, "Sex and Skill: Notes towards a Feminist Economics," *Feminist Review* 6 (1980): 79–88 (quote on p. 85).

73. Abbott, *System of Professions*, 92.

74. Frances Ginsberg and Barbara Clarke, "O.R. Nurse's Responsibility Extends outside the O.R.," *Modern Hospital* 118, no. 1 (1972): 108. These nurses refer to the state of affairs that characterized OR nursing "for many years."

75. See, for example, Anna M. Fullerton, *Surgical Nursing* (Philadelphia: P. Blakiston's Son, 1899); Minnie Goodnow, *First-Year Nursing: A Textbook for Pupils during Their First Year of Hospital Work*, 2nd ed. (Philadelphia: Saunders, 1919), 226–41, 310–20; Rose Marie Lee, "Early Operating Room Nursing," *AORN Journal* 24, no. 1 (1976): 124, 126–28, 131–32, 134, 136, 138; Ruth S. Metzger, "The Beginnings of OR Nursing Education," *AORN Journal* 24, no. 1 (1976): 73, 76–77, 80–81, 84–85, 88, 90; R. G. Schroth, *Instructions for Nurses* (Chicago: Illinois Post Graduate and Training School for Nurses, 1913); and Emily A. M. Stoney, *Bacteriology and Surgical Technique for Nurses* (Philadelphia: Saunders, 1900).

76. For histories of nurse anesthesia, see Marianne Bankert, *Watchful Care: A History of America's Nurse Anesthetists* (New York: Continuum, 1989); Virginia S. Thatcher, *History of Anesthesia, with Emphasis on the Nurse Specialist* (Philadelphia: Lippincott, 1953); and Committee on Education of the National League of Nursing Education, *Standard Curriculum for Schools of Nursing* (New York: National League of Nursing Education, 1919), 117.

77. See, for example, "Operating Room Nursing: Is It Professional Nursing?," *American Journal of Nursing* 65, no. 8 (1965): 58–63.

78. See, for example, Frances Ginsberg, "The Attitude of Nursing Educators Contributes to O.R. Nursing Shortage," *Modern Hospital* 108, no. 1 (1967): 102–4, and Caroline Rogers, "Phoenix Seminar: Keynote Speech," *AORN Journal* 16, no. 4 (1972): 165–70 (quote on p. 166).

79. Ford and Stephenson, *Institutional Nurses*, 60.

80. See, for example, Frances J. Braceland, "Psychiatry: Psychosomatic Medicine and the General Practitioner," *Medical Clinics of North America* (July 1950): 939–55; Flanders Dunbar, *Emotions and Bodily Changes: A Survey of Literature on Psychosomatic Interrelations, 1910–1953*, 4th ed. (New York: Columbia University Press, 1954); and Gerald N. Grob, "Psychiatry's Holy Grail: The Search for the Mechanisms of Mental Diseases," *Bulletin of the History of Medicine* 72, no. 2 (1998): 189–219.

81. Many of these nursing leaders were in psychiatric nursing. Tom Olson suggested that some nursing leaders chose psychiatry, a field with few technical procedures, to offset the discomfort they felt performing such procedures. See Tom Olson, "Fundamental and Special: The Dilemma of Psychiatric–Mental Health Nursing," *Archives of Psychiatric Nursing* 10, no. 1 (1996): 3–15 (including discussion).

82. See, for example, Dorothy Ellison, "The Need for Operating Room Experience in the Education of a Professional Nurse," *AORN Journal* 3, no. 2 (1965): 57–64, and Lucie S. Young, "O.R. Experience for Students," *Nursing Outlook* 12, no. 12 (1964): 47–49.

83. Lucie S. Young, "O.R. Experience," 49.

84. Lois C. Crooks, "The OR Technician: Assistant or Adversary?," *AORN Journal* 7, no. 5 (1968): 41–43.

85. Young questioned whether the turn to technicians as scrub nurses led to the reduced numbers of nurses in ORs or whether the decreased exposure of student nurses to the OR led to the decreased numbers of OR nurses and increased numbers of technicians. These factors likely operated together.

86. Ernest A. Gould, "The Operating Room Nurse . . . Is She a Dying Species?," *AORN Journal* 1, no. 2 (1963): 47–48; Geza De Takats, "The Scrub Nurse: A Vanishing Species," *Surgery, Gynecology, and Obstetrics* 112, no. 4 (1961): 494–96; Frances Elder, "Is the O.R. Nurse Still Necessary?," *RN* 22, no. 11 (1959): 48–53, 72–75.

87. Eleanor C. Lambertsen, "Does Education Mean Exodus?," *AORN Journal* 6,

no. 6 (1967): 48–49 (quote on p. 48). Lambertsen cited the Joint Commission on Accreditation of Hospitals, *Hospital Accreditation Reference* (Chicago: American Hospital Association, 1965), 91–92.

88. Frances A. Wollner, "The Disappearing Operating Room Nurse," *AORN Journal* 8, no. 3 (1968): 61–64; Kenneth J. Pickrell, "Requiem for the Scrub Nurse," *AORN Journal* 1, no. 1 (1963): 42–44.

89. See, for example, Frances Ginsberg, "A Problem of People: O.R. Aide and R.N.," *Modern Hospital* 108, no. 3 (1967): 142.

90. Vernita L. Cantlin, "O.R. Nursing Is a Professional Specialty," *Nursing Outlook* 8, no. 7 (1960): 376–78.

91. Frances Ginsberg, "The Case for Operating Room Technicians," *Nursing Clinics of North America* 3, no. 4 (1968): 613–20 (quote on p. 618).

92. "Operating Room Nursing," 58–63.

93. Merlyn Maillian, "Improving O.R. Experience for the Student Nurse," *Hospital Topics* 37, no. 11 (1959): 96–98 (quote on p. 96).

94. Dorothy Ellison, "Let's Stop Sacrificing the Clinical Laboratory to Expediency," *AORN Journal* 4, no. 2 (1966): 78–87.

95. Sr. Mary Luke, "How the Operating Room Nurse Can Help to Personalize Patient Care," *Modern Hospital* 105, no. 6 (1965): 90–92.

96. Frances Ginsberg, "Providing Emotional Support Is Part of O.R. Nurse's Job," *Modern Hospital* 118, no. 2 (1972): 118.

97. Edith Dee Hall, "What Does the Future Hold for the Specialty of Operating Room Nursing?," *Hospital Management* 100, no. 11 (1965): 72, 75–76.

98. Marilyn Yanick and Nancy Smith Podobnikar, "Don't You Miss Patient Care?," *American Journal of Nursing* 67, no. 6 (1967): 1260–62.

99. Lillian Sholtis Brunner, foreword, *Nursing Clinics of North America* 3, no. 4 (1968): 557–59.

100. William A. Ryan, "The Courts Look at O.R. Nursing," *RN* 26, no. 1 (1963): 33–36, 83–89.

101. "Role of the Professional Nurse in the O.R.: Four Viewpoints," *Hospital Topics* 44, no. 5 (1966): 128–30 (quote on p. 128).

102. William W. Monafo, "The Instrument Nurse and the Future," *AORN Journal* 6, no. 3 (1967): 56–58 (quote on p. 56).

103. Well into the nineteenth century, physicians aspiring to establish medicine as an intellectual endeavor had an "anti-technological" and "anti-manual" bias and, as a result, sought to separate themselves from surgeons. Surgeons were to them more like mechanics and carpenters; they were not true physicians. Physicians who established manual contact with patients were "derisively" called "body physicians." What tainted the surgeon, in addition to the barbarity and bloodiness of early surgery, was his use of instruments and the predominance of handwork. In a complete turnabout surgeons now enjoy even greater prestige than nonsurgeon physicians by virtue, in part, of the predominance of technology in their work. See Stanley Joel Reiser, "The Machine

at the Bedside: Technological Transformations of Practices and Values," in *The Machine at the Bedside: Strategies for Using Technology in Patient Care*, ed. Stanley Joel Reiser and Michael Anbar (Cambridge: Cambridge University Press, 1984), 3–19 (quotes on p. 7). See also Reiser, *Medicine and the Reign of Technology* (Cambridge: Cambridge University Press, 1978).

104. Frances Ginsberg, "Average O.R. Staff Nurse Called a Vanishing Breed," *Hospital Topics* 47, no. 4 (1969): 108–10.

105. See Irene Beland's comment on p. 241 in the discussion on pp. 237–47 following Florence S. Downs, "Technical Innovation and the Future of the Nurse-Patient Relationship," in *ANA Clinical Sessions* (New York: Appleton-Century-Croft, 1967), 232–37.

106. From an interview cited in Jacqueline Zalumas, *Caring in Crisis: An Oral History of Critical Care Nursing* (Philadelphia: University of Pennsylvania Press, 1995), 57–58.

107. Stella Goostray, *Memoirs: Half a Century in Nursing* (North Conway, N.H.: Reporter Press, 1969), 6–7.

108. Downs, "Technical Innovation," 232.

109. See, for example, Frances K. Brady, "A Head Nurse's Viewpoint of Automation," *ANA Regional Clinical Conferences* (New York: Appleton-Century-Croft, 1968), 46–50 (with discussion); Ruth R. Edelstein, "Automation: Its Effect on the Nurse," *American Journal of Nursing* 66, no. 10 (1966): 2194–98; Betty Jane Tarrant, "Automation: Its Effect on the Patient," *American Journal of Nursing* 66, no. 10 (1966): 2190–94; the special issue "The Nurse and the New Machinery," *Nursing Clinics of North America* 1, no. 4 (1966); and the special feature "Machines in Perspective," *American Journal of Nursing* 65, no. 2 (1965). Nurses did not typically use the word "technology" until the late 1970s.

110. Hildegard E. Peplau, "Automation: Will It Change Nurses, Nursing, or Both?," in *Technical Innovations in Health Care: Nursing Implications* (New York: American Nurses' Association, 1962), 37–53 (with discussion) (quote on p. 38).

111. Edelstein, "Automation," 2194.

112. Carl Mitcham identified "ancient skepticism," "enlightened optimism," and "romantic uneasiness" as three "ways of being-with technology." Nurses also fell into these camps. See Mitcham, *Thinking through Technology: The Path between Engineering and Philosophy* (Chicago: University of Chicago Press, 1994), 275–99.

113. A reference to the New Frontier of John F. Kennedy and to intensive care nursing as frontier nursing. Most of the new machinery of care was first located only in intensive or special care units. See Anselm Strauss, "The Intensive Care Unit: Its Characteristics and Social Relationships," *Nursing Clinics of North America* 3, no. 1 (1968): 7–15 (quote on p. 10).

114. Rita Chow, "Patient Monitoring Is More Than Just a Dream," *American Journal of Nursing* 61, no. 11 (1961): 60–62 (quotes on p. 60).

115. Ruby M. Harris, "Symposium on the Nurse and the New Machinery," *Nursing Clinics of North America* 1, no. 4 (1966), 535–36 (quote on p. 535).

116. Adeline C. Jenkins, "Successful Cardiac Monitoring," *Nursing Clinics of North America* 1, no. 4 (1966): 537–47 (quote on p. 539).

117. See, for example, Julie Fairman and Joan Lynaugh, *Critical Care Nursing: A History* (Philadelphia: University of Pennsylvania Press, 1998).

118. Barbara B. Minckley, "The Multiphasic Human-to-Human Monitor (ICU Model): Nursing Observation in the Intensive Care Unit," *Nursing Clinics of North America* 3, no. 1 (1968): 29–39 (drawing on p. 30).

119. Joyce Holmes George, "Electronic Monitoring of Vital Signs," *American Journal of Nursing* 65, no. 2 (1965): 68–71 (quote on p. 68).

120. Jenkins, "Successful Cardiac Monitoring," 546.

121. Rose Pinneo, "Nursing in a Coronary Care Unit," *American Journal of Nursing* 65, no. 2 (1965): 76–79 (quote on p. 79).

122. Margaret A. Bergin, "Monitoring the Fetal Heart," *Nursing Clinics of North America* 1, no. 4 (1966): 559–67 (quote on p. 559); Delores B. Carriker and Mervin Rosenberg, "Automation: A Facilitator of Nursing Practice," in *ANA Clinical Sessions*, 83–89.

123. Barbara G. Schutt, "Mastering the Mysteries," *American Journal of Nursing* 65, no. 2 (1965): unpaginated. This is an editorial preceding the special issue "Machines in Perspective."

124. Julie Fairman, "Watchful Vigilance: Nursing Care, Technology, and the Development of Intensive Care Units," *Nursing Research* 41, no. 1 (1992): 56–61; Carol Williams Trusk, "Hemodialysis for Acute Renal Failure," *American Journal of Nursing* 65, no. 2 (1965): 80–85 (quote on p. 82).

125. Henry Pratt, "The Doctor's View of the Changing Nurse-Physician Relationship," *Journal of Medical Education* 40, no. 8 (1965): 767–71.

126. Interview with Jo Ann Albers, *American Nephrology Nurses Association Oral History Project*, 1986–1987, CSHN. Albers described the beginnings of the renal dialysis program at the University of Washington and the Seattle Artificial Kidney Center from 1961 to 1970.

127. See, for example, Robert M. Farrier, "Problems of Electronic Patient Monitoring," *Hospitals* 37, no. 7 (1963): 50, 53–54, and Jenkins, "Successful Cardiac Monitoring," 540.

128. Margaret A. Bean, Frances Ann Krahn, Barbara L. Anderson, and Mabel T. Yoshida, "Monitoring Patients through Electronics," *American Journal of Nursing* 63, no. 4 (1963): 65–69 (quote on p. 67).

129. Ruby M. Harris, "Laying the Right Lines for Electronic Monitoring," *Nursing Outlook* 11, no. 8 (1963): 573–76 (quote on p. 573).

130. Schutt, "Mastering the Mysteries"; Strauss, "Intensive Care Unit," 10. The eminent sociologist, who both studied nursing and taught nurses, noted that intensive care nurses felt elite among nurses and shared a sense of camaraderie with physicians.

131. Advertisers picked up this view of intensive care nurses as special by

virtue of the machinery they worked with and the new power it gave them. A 1970 ad declared the coronary care unit nurse as "different" and as "transcending the traditional nursing role." See the ad for ROCOM CCU Multimedia Instruction System in *Nursing Outlook* 18, no. 1 (1970): 9–11.

132. Edelstein, "Automation," 2196.

133. From an interview with Gloria Kundrat, cited in Fairman, "Watchful Vigilance," 58.

134. From an interview with Margarite Kinney, cited in ibid., 58.

135. Harris, "Laying the Right Lines," 573.

136. Ibid.

137. Bean et al., "Monitoring Patients," 65.

138. Ibid., 68.

139. Downs, "Technical Innovation," 233–34.

140. "Untouched by Human Hands," *Nursing Forum* 1, no. 2 (1962): 12–20.

141. Eleanor C. Lambertsen, "The Nature and Objectives of Intensive Care Nursing," *Nursing Clinics of North America* 3, no. 1 (1968): 3–6 (quote on p. 4); Bean et al., "Monitoring Patients," 66.

142. Downs, "Technical Innovation," 235.

143. Jenkins, "Successful Cardiac Monitoring," 565.

144. Downs, "Technical Innovation," 234.

145. Donna Zschoche and Lillian E. Brown, "Intensive Care Nursing: Specialism, Junior Doctoring, or Just Nursing?," *American Journal of Nursing* 69, no. 11 (1969): 2370–74.

146. Peplau, "Automation."

147. Hildegard E. Peplau, *Interpersonal Relations in Nursing* (New York: Putnam's, 1952). In a 1995 interview Peplau recalled how preoccupied nurses were with doing. See "Hildegard Peplau in a Conversation with Mark Welch," pt. 1, *Nursing Inquiry* 2, no. 1 (1995): 53–56. Peplau's work exemplified nurse theorists' efforts to move the core of nursing to mental and away from manual labor.

148. Peplau, "Automation," 37.

149. Ibid., 39, 41, 42, 43, 48.

150. Annette Wollowick, "Will the Nursing Profession Become Extinct?," *Nursing Forum* 9, no. 4 (1970): 408–13.

151. Dorothy J. Walker, "Our Changing World: Its Implications for Nursing," *Nursing Forum* 9, no. 4 (1970): 328–39 (quotes on pp. 332, 334, 335).

152. Gertrud B. Ujhely, "Current Technological Advances and the Nurse-Patient Relationship," *Journal of the New York State Nurses Association* 5, no. 3 (1974): 25–28.

153. James Dickoff and Patricia James, "Highly Technical but Yet Not Impure: Varieties of Basic Knowledge," in *Perspectives on Nursing Theory*, 2nd ed., ed. Leslie H. Nicoll (Philadelphia: Lippincott, 1992), 572–75 (quotes on p. 573). See also, by the same authors and in the same anthology, "Taking Concepts as

Guides to Action: Exploring Kinds of Know-How," 576–80. Dickoff and James were key philosophers who participated in the Nursing Theory Movement in the 1960s.

154. Loretta Macon Birckhead, "Nursing and the Technetronic Age," *Journal of Nursing Administration* 8, no. 2 (1978): 16–19.

155. Ibid., 26; Leland R. Bennett, "This I Believe . . . That Nurses May Become Extinct," *AORN Journal* 11, no. 4 (1970): 57–63. Bennet's essay was first published in *Nursing Outlook* 18, no. 1 (1970): 28–32.

156. June C. Abbey, "Bioinstrumentation: Twentieth Century Slave," *Nursing Clinics of North America* 13, no. 4 (1978): 631–41.

157. Bennett, "This I Believe," 58.

158. Marcia Pope, "Thoughts from an Artificial Nurse," *American Journal of Nursing* 75, no. 2 (1975): 248–49.

159. Margaret J. Dunlop, "Is a Science of Caring Possible?," *Journal of Advanced Nursing* 11, no. 5 (1986): 661–70 (quote on p. 665).

Chapter 6

1. See Chapter 4 of this book.

2. See Chapter 2 of this book.

3. Simon J. Williams, "Modern Medicine and the 'Uncertain Body': From Corporeality to Hyperreality?," *Social Science and Medicine* 45, no. 7 (1997): 1041–49.

4. Carl Mitcham, *Thinking through Technology: The Path between Engineering and Philosophy* (Chicago: University of Chicago Press, 1994), 191.

5. Knowing the patient also entailed noninstrumentally mediated extensions of nursing observation into the inner life of patients as private subjects, involving the mind, emotions, spirit, and overall personhood of the patient. Nurses generally have not referred to this kind of knowing—by listening to patients talk—as surveillance, even though this practice is so designated in critical studies of medicine and health care. See, for example, William Ray Arney, *Power and the Profession of Obstetrics* (Chicago: University of Chicago Press, 1982).

6. Anthea Symonds, "Angels and Interfering Busybodies: The Social Construction of Two Occupations," *Sociology of Health and Illness* 13, no. 2 (1991): 249–64 (quote on p. 258).

7. See Chapter 3 of this book.

8. See Chapter 4 of this book.

9. Albert B. Robillard, "Communication Problems in the Intensive Care Unit," in *Reflexivity and Voice*, ed. Rosanna Hertz (Thousand Oaks, Calif.: Sage, 1997), 252–64 (quotes on p. 253).

10. As art historian Barbara Maria Stafford described the problem in another historical context. See "Voyeur or Observer? Enlightenment Thoughts on the

Dilemmas of Display," *Configurations: A Journal of Literature, Science, and Technology* 1, no. 1 (1993): 95–128.

11. Arney, *Power and the Profession*, 90.

12. Anne Balsamo, *Technologies of the Gendered Body: Reading Cyborg Women* (Durham, N.C.: Duke University Press, 1997), 5.

13. Michel Foucault, *Discipline and Punish: The Birth of the Prison*, trans. Alan Sheridan (New York: Pantheon, 1977). See also Julianne Cheek and Trudy Rudge, "The Panopticon Revisited? An Exploration of the Social and Political Dimensions of Contemporary Health Care and Nursing Practice," *International Journal of Nursing Studies* 31, no. 6 (1994): 583–91.

14. David Armstrong, "The Rise of Surveillance Medicine," *Sociology of Health and Illness* 17, no. 3 (1995): 393–404; Regina H. Kenen, "The At-Risk Health Status and Technology: A Diagnostic Invitation and the 'Gift' of Knowing," *Social Science and Medicine* 42, no. 11 (1996): 1545–53; Olav Helge Forde, "Is Imposing Risk Awareness Cultural Imperialism?," *Social Science and Medicine* 47, no. 9 (1998): 1155–59 (quote on p. 1155).

15. Armstrong, "Rise of Surveillance Medicine," 395.

16. See, for example, Margarete Sandelowski, "Channel of Desire: Fetal Ultrasonography in Two Use-Contexts," *Qualitative Health Research* 4, no. 3 (1994): 262–80, and Tjeerd Tymstra, "The Imperative Character of Medical Technology and the Meaning of 'Anticipated Decision Regret,'" *International Journal of Technology Assessment in Health Care* 5, no. 2 (1989): 207–13.

17. Balsamo, *Technologies of the Gendered Body*, 6.

18. Arney, *Power and the Profession*, 150.

19. Ibid., 100.

20. Judith Parker and John Wiltshire, "The Handover: Three Modes of Nursing Practice Knowledge," in *Scholarship in the Discipline of Nursing*, ed. Genevieve Gray and Rosalie Pratt (Melbourne: Churchill Livingstone, 1995), 151–68 (quote on p. 156). These Australian scholars contrasted this medical-like gaze with (1) "reconnoitre," or "the nursing scan," which nurses use to survey the terrain of their work, and the "spatial organization" and "features of the environment [that] constrain or facilitate effective nursing" (157), and with (2) "connaissance," or "the nursing look" (156), which involves the concrete knowledge of actual persons. Connaissance is the "embodied situated caring attentiveness" (163–64) that is said to distinguish nursing from medical practice. Nursing "reconnaissance" is the "reflective integration" (165) of these three kinds of observation that characterize the expert nurse.

21. Joan Liaschenko, "The Moral Geography of Home Care," *Advances in Nursing Science* 17, no. 2 (1994): 16–26 (quote on p. 23).

22. Lisa Cartwright, "Women, X-rays, and the Public Culture of Prophylactic Imaging," *Camera Obscura* 29 (1992): 18–54 (quote on p. 49).

23. See, for example, Judith Walzer Leavitt and Whitney Walton, "'Down to Death's Door': Women's Perceptions of Childbirth in America," in *Women*

and Health in America, ed. Judith Walzer Leavitt (Madison: University of Wisconsin Press, 1984), 155–65, and Margarete Sandelowski, *Pain, Pleasure, and American Childbirth: From the Twilight Sleep to the Read Method, 1914–1960* (Westport, Conn.: Greenwood Press, 1984).

24. See, for example, Paul De Kruif, "Why Should Mothers Die?," *Ladies Home Journal*, March 1936, 8, and Louise E. Zabriskie, "Maternity Nursing in Hospital and Home," *American Journal of Nursing* 29, no. 10 (1929): 1157–65 (quote on p. 1157).

25. See, for example, Monroe Lerner and Odin W. Anderson, *Health Progress in the United States, 1900–1960* (Chicago: University of Chicago Press, 1963), 32–33; George Clark Mosher, "Maternal Morbidity and Mortality in the United States," *American Journal of Obstetrics and Gynecology* 7, no. 3 (1924): 294–98; and U.S. Department of Health and Human Services, National Center for Health Statistics, *Vital Statistics of the United States, 1977*, vol. 1, *Natality* (Washington, D.C.: Government Printing Office, 1981).

26. New York Academy of Medicine, Committee on Public Health Relations, *Maternal Mortality in New York City: A Study of All Puerperal Deaths, 1930–1932* (New York: Commonwealth Fund, 1933), 113–27. See also Joyce Antler and Daniel M. Fox, "The Movement toward a Safe Maternity: Physician Accountability in New York City, 1915–1940," in *Sickness and Health in America: Readings in the History of Medicine and Public Health*, 2nd ed., ed. Judith Walzer Leavitt and Ronald L. Numbers (Madison: University of Wisconsin Press, 1985), 490–506, and Neal Devitt, "The Transition from Home to Hospital Birth in the United States, 1930–1960," *Birth and the Family Journal* 4, no. 2 (1977): 47–58.

27. On the duties of the obstetric nurse, see, for example, Nell V. Beeby, "Where and What Shall We Teach? An Analysis of the Situations in Which the Nurse Functions in Obstetrical Nursing," *American Journal of Nursing* 37, no. 1 (1937): 64–79; Mae M. Bookmiller and George L. Bowen, *Textbook of Obstetrics and Obstetric Nursing*, 4th ed. (Philadelphia: Saunders, 1963); M. Edward Davis and Mabel C. Carmon, *De Lee's Obstetrics for Nurses*, 13th ed. (Philadelphia: Saunders, 1944); Joseph B. Cooke, *A Manual of Obstetrical Technique*, 3rd ed. (Philadelphia: Lippincott, 1902), and *A Nurse's Handbook of Obstetrics*, 10th ed., rev. Carolyn E. Gray and Philip F. Williams (Philadelphia: Lippincott, 1924); M. Edward Davis and Catherine E. Sheckler, *De Lee's Obstetrics for Nurses*, 16th ed. (Philadelphia: Saunders, 1957); M. Edward Davis and Reva Rubin, *De Lee's Obstetrics for Nurses*, 17th, 18th eds. (Philadelphia: Saunders, 1962, 1966); Joseph B. De Lee, *Obstetrics for Nurses*, 3rd, 4th, 9th eds. (Philadelphia: Saunders, 1909, 1913, 1930); Joseph B. De Lee and Mabel C. Carmon, *Obstetrics for Nurses*, 11th ed. (Philadelphia: Saunders, 1937); Elise Fitzpatrick and Nicholson J. Eastman, *Zabriskie's Obstetrics for Nurses*, 10th ed. (Philadelphia: Lippincott, 1960); Elise Fitzpatrick, Sharon R. Reeder, and Luigi Mastroianni, *Maternity Nursing*, 12th ed. (Philadelphia: Lippincott, 1971); Dorothy E. House, "The Patient in Labor: The Nurse's Part in Her Care," *American Journal of Nursing* 39, no. 12 (1939): 1328–33; Sharon R.

Reeder, Luigi Mastroianni, Leonide L. Martin, and Elise Fitzpatrick, *Maternity Nursing*, 13th ed. (Philadelphia: Lippincott, 1976); Carolyn C. Van Blarcom, *Obstetrical Nursing: A Textbook on the Nursing Care of the Expectant Mother, the Woman in Labor, the Young Mother and Her Baby*, 1st, 3rd eds. (New York: Macmillan, 1922, 1933), and *Obstetrical Nursing*, 4th ed., rev. Erna Ziegel (New York: Macmillan, 1957); Ernestine Wiedenbach, *Family-Centered Maternity Nursing*, 1st, 2nd eds. (New York: Putnam's, 1958, 1967); Henry L. Woodward and Bernice Gardner, *Obstetric Management and Nursing* (Philadelphia: F. A. Davis, 1936); Henry L. Woodward, Bernice Gardner, Richard D. Bryant, and Anna E. Overland, *Obstetric Management and Nursing*, 5th ed. (Philadelphia: F. A. Davis, 1957); and Louise Zabriskie and Nicholson J. Eastman, *Nurses' Handbook of Obstetrics*, 7th ed. (Philadelphia: Lippincott, 1943). See also Sandelowski, *Pain, Pleasure*, 60–71.

28. A. Worcester, "Obstetrical Nursing," *Boston Medical and Surgical Journal* 150, no. 1 (1904): 1–5; De Lee and Carmon, *Obstetrics for Nurses*, 158.

29. De Lee and Carmon, *Obstetrics for Nurses*, 135.

30. Elizabeth Fishback, "Obstetrical Nursing as a Specialty," *American Journal of Nursing* 14, no. 10 (1914): 806–11 (quote on p. 807). Although Fishback used this phrase in the context of the postpartum period, it applies as well to nurses' intrapartal duties.

31. Sandelowski, *Pain, Pleasure*, chaps. 1, 2.

32. De Lee and Carmon, *Obstetrics for Nurses*, 19.

33. All quoted words and phrases in this chapter, if not referenced to any text, were spoken by the nurses I interviewed concerning fetal monitoring. They are described in Chapter 1 of this book.

34. Jane R. McLaughlin, "Teaching Obstetrics to Nurses," *American Journal of Nursing* 28, no. 6 (1928): 605–7 (quote on p. 607).

35. See, for example, ibid., 607, and Wiedenbach, *Family-Centered Maternity Nursing*, 1st ed., 214–39.

36. See, for example, Davis and Rubin, *De Lee's Obstetrics for Nurses*, 17th ed., 202; Phyllis A. Tryon, "Assessing the Progress of Labor through Observation of Patients' Behavior," *Nursing Clinics of North America* 3, no. 2 (1968): 315–26; and Wiedenbach, *Family-Centered Maternity Nursing*, 1st ed., 236–37, and 2nd ed., 256–59.

37. Frederick H. Falls and Jane R. McLaughlin, *Obstetric Nursing* (St. Louis: C. V. Mosby, 1946), 9.

38. See, for example, Judith Walzer Leavitt, *Brought to Bed: Childbearing in America, 1750–1950* (New York: Oxford University Press, 1986), and Judy Barrett Litoff, *American Midwives: 1860 to the Present* (Westport, Conn.: Greenwood Press, 1978).

39. See Chapter 4 of this book.

40. For a history of fetal auscultation, see Robert C. Goodlin, "History of Fetal Monitoring," *American Journal of Obstetrics and Gynecology* 133, no. 3 (1979): 323–52 (specific information on pp. 323–27).

41. Sandelowski, *Pain, Pleasure*, chap. 4.

42. See, for example, Janet G. Brown and Wayne L. Johnson, "A Fetal Intensive Care Nursing Program," *Journal of Obstetric, Gynecologic, and Neonatal Nursing* 5, no. 3 (1976): 23–25; Irene Matousek, "Fetal Nursing during Labor," *Nursing Clinics of North America* 3, no. 2 (1968): 307–14; and Jack A. Pritchard and Paul C. Macdonald, *Williams Obstetrics*, 15th ed. (New York: Appleton-Century-Croft, 1976).

43. Report of Consensus Development Conference, National Institute of Child Health and Human Development, *Antenatal Diagnosis, III: Predictors of Intrapartum Fetal Distress* (Bethesda, Md.: National Institutes of Health Pub. No. 80-1973, 1979), 46.

44. See, for example, Arney, *Power and the Profession*; "Corometrics Medical Systems, Inc.," *Wall Street Transcript*, May 7, December 3, 1973, 32,873–74, 35,217; Robert C. Goodlin, *Care of the Fetus* (New York: Masson, 1979), 102–4; and Judith R. Kunisch, "Electronic Fetal Monitors: Marketing Forces and the Resulting Controversy," in *Healing Technology: Feminist Perspectives*, ed. Kathryn Strother Ratcliff (Ann Arbor: University of Michigan Press, 1989), 41–60. Physician Goodlin found fetal monitors enjoyable and fetal monitoring intellectually satisfying. He admitted he was "unwilling to believe"—against the findings of a controlled study indicating no benefit from fetal monitoring—that all of his and other people's efforts in this area had "all been for nothing" (104).

45. Edward H. Hon, "The Electronic Evaluation of the Fetal Heart Rate: Preliminary Report," *American Journal of Obstetrics and Gynecology* 75, no. 6 (1958): 1215–30. This article was selected as a journal classic and was reprinted in 1996. See the comment in *American Journal of Obstetrics and Gynecology* 175, no. 3 (1996): 748.

46. "Corometrics Medical Systems," May 7, 1973, 32,874. See also Goodlin, *Care of the Fetus*, 102–3, and Kunisch, "Electronic Fetal Monitors." Hon was a major stockholder in and medical director of this company and received engineering and funding support from Corometrics for his research at Yale University and, later, at the University of Southern California. As one nurse who worked with him put it, he "was Corometrics."

47. Roger K. Freeman and Thomas J. Garite, *Fetal Heart Rate Monitoring* (Baltimore: Williams and Wilkins, 1981), vii.

48. Davis and Rubin, *De Lee's Obstetrics for Nurses*, 17th ed., 154.

49. Shelly Allen, "Nurse Attendance during Labor," *American Journal of Nursing* 64, no. 7 (1964): 70–74 (quotes on p. 70).

50. Benjamin Kendall and David M. Farell, "Uses of Fetal Electrocardiography," *American Journal of Nursing* 64, no. 7 (1964): 75–78.

51. Mildred E. Grever, "Fetal Heart Monitoring," *Hospital Topics* 44, no. 5 (1966): 116–17.

52. Margaret A. Bergin, "Monitoring the Fetal Heart," *Nursing Clinics of North*

America 1, no. 4 (1966): 559–67. In the early years of monitoring it is hard to distinguish purely clinical from research uses.

53. These parameters were based on classifications developed by Edward Hon and Uruguayan physician Roberto Caldeyro-Barcia. Clinicians were not as yet so concerned with more sophisticated parameters of assessment such as heart rate variability, in part, because of the limitations of monitors themselves to display them. See, for example, the workbook by Edward H. Hon, *An Introduction to Fetal Heart Rate Monitoring*, 2nd ed. (n.p., 1975). For a review of changes in assessment parameters and their definitions, see Sze-Ya Yeh, "Changing Trends of Fetal Heart Rate Monitoring in the United States," in *Fetal Heart Rate Monitoring: Clinical Practice and Pathophysiology*, ed. W. Kunzel (Berlin: Springer-Verlag, 1985), 22–33.

54. See, for example, the workbook by Marshall Klavan, Arthur T. Laver, and Mary Ann Boscola, *Clinical Concepts of Fetal Heart Rate Monitoring* (Waltham, Mass.: Hewlett-Packard, 1977); Sasi K. Pillay, Lawrence Chik, Robert J. Sokol, and Ivan E. Zador, "Fetal Monitoring: A Guide to Understanding the Equipment," *Clinical Obstetrics and Gynecology* 22, no. 3 (1979): 571–82; and Susan Martin Tucker, *Fetal Monitoring and Fetal Assessment in High-Risk Pregnancy* (St. Louis: C. V. Mosby, 1978), 72.

55. See, for example, J. M. Butler and J. T. Parer, "Is Intensive Intrapartum Monitoring Necessary?," *Journal of Obstetric, Gynecologic, and Neonatal Nursing* 5, no. 5 (supplement) (1976): 4s–6s (quote on p. 6s); Edward G. Hon, "Direct Monitoring of the Fetal Heart," *Hospital Practice* 5, no. 9 (1970): 91–97; and Richard Paul and Edward Hon, "A Clinical Fetal Monitor," *Obstetrics and Gynecology* 35, no. 2 (1970): 161–69.

56. As noted by Frederick P. Zuspan in the preface to the Report of Consensus Development Conference, *Antenatal Diagnosis*, perinatal and infant mortality rates had "symbolic importance" in that U.S. rates compared poorly with those of other industrialized countries and thus seemed to indict U.S. health care.

57. See, for example, Goodlin, *Care of the Fetus*, 114.

58. Barry S. Schifrin, *Workbook in Fetal Heart Rate Monitoring* (n.p., 1975), 6.

59. See, for example, Report of Consensus Development Conference, *Antenatal Diagnosis*, 23–24.

60. Hon, "Direct Monitoring of the Fetal Heart," 91.

61. See Don Ihde, *Instrumental Realism: The Interface between Philosophy of Science and Philosophy of Technology* (Bloomington: Indiana University Press, 1991), and Chapter 2 of this book.

62. Ralph C. Benson, Frank Shubeck, Jerome Deutsch Berger, William Weiss, and Heinz Berendes, "Fetal Heart Rate as a Predictor of Fetal Distress: A Report from the Collaborative Project," *Obstetrics and Gynecology* 32, no. 2 (1968): 259–66.

63. "Corometrics Medical Systems," May 7, 1973, 32,873.

64. See, for example, Hon, *Introduction to Fetal Heart Rate Monitoring*, 11.

65. See, for example, Butler and Parer, "Is Intensive Intrapartum Monitoring Necessary?," 5s, and Klavan, Laver, and Boscola, Clinical Concepts, viii.

66. Barbara L. Williams and Sharon F. Richards, "Fetal Monitoring during Labor," American Journal of Nursing 70, no. 11 (1970): 2384–88.

67. Richard H. Paul, "Clinical Fetal Monitoring: Experience on a Large Clinical Service," American Journal of Obstetrics and Gynecology 113, no. 5 (1972): 573–77.

68. "Corometrics Medical Systems," December 3, 1973, 35,217.

69. P. V. Dilts, "Current Practices in Antepartum and Intrapartum Fetal Monitoring," American Journal of Obstetrics and Gynecology 126, no. 4 (1976): 491–94.

70. See, for example, Janet S. Malinowski, "Interpreting Fetal Heart Rates," in Nursing Care of the Labor Patient, ed. Janet S. Malinowski, Carolyn P. Burdin, Regina P. Lederman, and Patricia S. Williams (Philadelphia: F. A. Davis, 1978), 19–30 (quote on p. 20).

71. Nurses' Association of the American College of Obstetricians and Gynecologists, Obstetric, Gynecologic, and Neonatal Nursing Functions and Standards (Chicago: the author, 1975).

72. Linda J. Chagnon and Cheryll L. Heldenbrand, "Nurses Undertake Direct and Indirect Fetal Monitoring at a Community Hospital," Journal of Obstetric, Gynecologic, and Neonatal Nursing 3, no. 5 (1974): 41–46 (quote on p. 41). Several of the nurses I interviewed also used the phrase "collecting dust" to describe the early lack of use of fetal monitors; one nurse said the machine needed a dust cover. Freeman and Garite, Fetal Heart Rate Monitoring, p. vii, also mentioned that at the close of the 1970s few obstetricians were trained to use monitors.

73. See the editorial preceding the special supplement "Intrapartum Evaluation of the Fetus," in the Journal of Obstetric, Gynecologic, and Neonatal Nursing 5, no. 5 (supplement) (1976): 7.

74. See, for example, Chagnon and Heldenbrand, "Nurses Undertake," and Mary F. Haire and Frank H. Boehm, "A Statewide Program to Teach Nurses the Use of Fetal Monitors," Journal of Obstetric, Gynecologic, and Neonatal Nursing 7, no. 3 (1978): 29–31. As one nurse recalled, anesthesiologists and lawyers also attended the seminars she conducted in the late 1970s. Nurses also contributed to the workbooks from which clinicians learned to monitor. See, for example, Klavan, Laver (both physicians), and Boscola (a nurse), Clinical Concepts.

75. Freeman and Garite, Fetal Heart Rate Monitoring, vii.

76. One nurse recalled that when machine monitoring first entered her practice, she too thought that a "flat and stable" tracing was a "good" tracing.

77. There was no consensus on whether and/or why electronic fetal monitoring raised Caesarean birth rates. See, for example, Report of Consensus Development Conference, Antenatal Diagnosis, and Paul and Hon, "Clinical Fetal Monitor," 166–67.

78. In his study of fetal monitoring in a rural Canadian Hospital in the early 1980s, physician Ken L. Bassett found that nurses used fetal monitoring to con-

trol doctors—that is, to keep them away in the first stage of labor in order to reduce unnecessary intervention. See Bassett, "Taming Chance and Taking Chances: The Electronic Fetal Heart Monitor in a Rural Canadian Hospital and Community" (Ph.D. diss., McGill University, Toronto, Ontario, 1993). Bassett subsequently published his findings as "Anthropology, Clinical Pathology, and the Electronic Fetal Monitor: Lessons from the Heart," *Social Science and Medicine* 42, no. 2 (1996): 281–92.

79. A historical prime directive for nurses was that they do not diagnose or treat; see Chapter 4 of this book. One of the nurses interviewed denied that nurses were doing anything diagnostic when they interpreted fetal heart tracings. To her, diagnosis was what the doctor did when he performed fetal blood sampling to verify an ominous fetal heart rate pattern typically identified by the nurse. Another nurse insisted that fetal monitoring was about surveillance, not diagnosis. These comments reflect both a reluctance on the part of nurses to claim "diagnosis" and current arguments about the technology itself in which sharp lines are drawn between surveillance and diagnosis. "Diagnosis" remains a contested term, and techniques such as electronic fetal monitoring have both illuminated and intensified the controversy.

80. Goodlin, *Care of the Fetus*, 104, recalled his initial belief that fetal monitoring would "reduce nursing requirements in the labor ward."

81. See, for example, Jody Applegate, Albert D. Haverkamp, Miriam Orleans, and Cherri Taylor, "Electronic Fetal Monitoring: Implications for Obstetrical Nursing," *Nursing Research* 28, no. 6 (1979): 369–71 (specific information on p. 370); William A. Check, "Electronic Fetal Monitoring: How Necessary?," *Journal of the American Medical Association* 241, no. 17 (1979): 1772–74 (specific information on p. 1774); and "Corometrics Medical Systems," December 3, 1973, 35,217. Advertising contributed to the idea that machine monitoring would allow fewer nurses to care for more patients. For example, the Minneapolis-Honeywell Regulator Company showed one nurse at one of its consoles monitoring the vital signs of twelve patients. See the photo in Rita Chow, "Patient Monitoring Is More Than Just a Dream," *American Journal of Nursing* 61, no. 11 (1961): 62.

82. See, for example, Report of Consensus Development Conference, *Antenatal Diagnosis*, 138. Leah L. Albers and Cara J. Krulewitch suggested that the nursing shortage was one factor contributing to the increase in the 1980s of fetal monitoring. See their "Electronic Fetal Monitoring in the United States in the 1980s," *Obstetrics and Gynecology* 82, no. 1 (1993): 8–10. Yet as Albert Haverkamp pointed out, if there were not enough nurses to be with laboring patients continuously, there were not enough nurses for continuous fetal monitoring. Haverkamp is cited in Ruth Watson Lubic, "The Impact of Technology on Health Care—The Childbearing Center: A Case for Technology's Appropriate Use," *Journal of Nurse-Midwifery* 24, no. 1 (1979): 6–10 (specific information on p. 8).

83. Shelly Allen, "Nurse Attendance," 71, 74.

84. Obstetrics was often referred to as the Cinderella or stepchild specialty. For an overview of obstetricians' efforts to reverse this image, which included the incorporation of technology, see Pamela S. Summey and Marsha Hurst, "Ob/Gyn on the Rise: The Evolution of Professional Ideology in the Twentieth Century," pts. 1 and 2, *Women and Health* 11, nos. 1, 2 (1986): 133–45, 103–22. Goodlin, in *Care of the Fetus*, 125, observed that fetal monitoring had brought obstetrics in the United States a "certain degree of scientific respectability."

85. See, for example, Temple Burling, Edith M. Lentz, and Robert N. Wilson, eds., *The Give and Take in Hospitals: A Study of Human Organization in Hospitals* (New York: Putnam's, 1956), 224.

86. Childbearing women and their infants in hospitals were (and remain) typically cared for by different nurses: labor and delivery, postpartum, and nursery nurses. Labor and delivery nurses were considered the most knowledgeable and skilled because of the acute, intensive, surgical, and "technical" milieu of the labor and delivery unit. While labor nurses floated to postpartum units in times of short staffing, postpartum nurses were not similarly floated to labor, as they were deemed less capable of functioning there. Few nurses were (or are) cross-trained to function in all maternity settings equally well.

87. Brown and Johnson, "Fetal Intensive Care Nursing Program," 25.

88. See, for example, Carol Lasater, "Electronic Monitoring of Mother and Fetus," *American Journal of Nursing* 72, no. 4 (1972): 728–30 (specific information on pp. 729–30).

89. See, for example, Christine Sullivan Cranston, "Obstetrical Nurses' Attitudes toward Fetal Monitoring," *Journal of Obstetric, Gynecologic, and Neonatal Nursing* 9, no. 6 (1980): 344–47 (specific information on p. 346).

90. If she had her hand on the woman's abdomen, a nurse could also feel a contraction begin before the woman sensed it.

91. See, for example, Lasater, "Electronic Monitoring," 730.

92. See, for example, Williams and Richards, "Fetal Monitoring," 2386. Two psychologists also concluded that fetal monitoring could be used as a feedback device to increase women's "preparation" for contractions in "prepared childbirth." See William S. Brasted and Edward J. Callahan, "An Evaluation of the Electronic Fetal Monitor as a Feedback Device during Labor," *Journal of Applied Behavior Analysis* 17, no. 2 (1984): 261–66.

93. Cranston, "Obstetrical Nurses' Attitudes," 346.

94. See Chapter 3 of this book.

95. Shizuko Y. Fagerhaugh, Anselm Strauss, Barbara Suczek, and Carolyn L. Wiener, *Hazards in Hospital Care: Ensuring Patient Safety* (San Francisco: Jossey-Bass, 1987), 81–82.

96. "Corometrics Medical Systems," May 7, 1973, 32,874.

97. As nurses generally recalled, fetal monitors were initially seen and used to improve "quality of care." Only later, by the end of the 1970s, were they

used to provide evidence in lawsuits. As one nurse suggested, at first the moni-tor was "for us," but by the end of the 1970s it began to be used "against us." The "us" here shows some nurses' identification with physicians. Physi-cians and hospitals were more likely to be sued than nurses both because of the typical view of the nurse as following doctor's orders and because nurses did not have—as one nurse put it—"deep pockets." An Institute of Medicine study showed that almost 50 percent of liability claims against obstetricians involved fetal monitoring. See *Medical Professional Liability and the Delivery of Obstetri-cal Care*, vol. 1 (Washington, D.C.: National Academy Press, 1989), 151. H. David Banta and Stephen B. Thacker reported in 1979 that more than ten malprac-tice suits had been brought against physicians and hospitals in cases where a baby had been born mentally retarded or died and fetal monitoring had not been used. At least one suit was brought against a physician for using fetal monitoring, which was alleged to have caused a fatal maternal infection. See Banta and Thacker, "Policies Toward Medical Technology: The Case of Elec-tronic Fetal Monitoring," *American Journal of Public Health* 69, no. 9 (1979): 931–35 (specific information on p. 934). See also Jerry Wiley, "The Nurse's Legal Re-sponsibility in Obstetric Monitoring," *Journal of Obstetric, Gynecologic, and Neonatal Nursing* 5, no. 5 (supplement) (1967): 77s–78s.

98. Elizabeth Cartwright, "The Logic of Heartbeats: Electronic Fetal Moni-toring and Biomedically Constructed Birth," in *Cyborg Babies: From Techno-Sex to Techno-Tots*, ed. Robbie Davis-Floyd and Joseph Dumit (New York: Routledge, 1998): 240–54 (quote on p. 249). Cartwright, an obstetric nurse and anthro-pologist, pointed out that clinicians were oriented less to the fetus per se than to the "strip of paper" representing the fetus. That is, their attention was di-rected toward the quality of the strip as standing for the quality of the fetus. Accordingly, it was a "bad strip" that required "cure." The strip is thus in-vested with the power to exonerate clinicians from charges of malpractice, or to implicate them.

99. This nurse left labor and delivery after monitoring was adopted and because it interfered with the kind of care she believed women should have.

100. Helen L. Dulock and Marie Herron, "Women's Responses to Fetal Monitoring," *Journal of Obstetric, Gynecologic, and Neonatal Nursing* 5, no. 5 (supple-ment) (1976): 68s–70s.

101. Ann Woolbert Russin, Joan E. O'Gureck, and Jacques F. Roux, "Elec-tronic Monitoring of the Fetus," *American Journal of Nursing* 74, no. 7 (1974): 1294–99 (quote on p. 1295).

102. Sandelowski, *Pain, Pleasure*, chap. 1.

103. Arney, *Power and the Profession*, 90, 88.

104. Elizabeth Cartwright, in "Logic of Heartbeats," also emphasized the Foucauldian dimensions of electronic fetal monitoring.

105. Dulock and Herron, "Women's Responses."

106. Spiral electrodes placed on the fetal scalp or buttocks were a source

of trauma and infection to the fetus. See, for example, Carol Lang Gee and William J. Ledger, "Maternal and Fetal Morbidity Associated with Intrapartum Monitoring," *Journal of Obstetric, Gynecologic, and Neonatal Nursing* 5, no. 5 (supplement) (1976): 65s–67s.

107. Monica N. Starkman, "Psychological Responses to the Use of the Fetal Monitor during Labor," *Psychosomatic Medicine* 38, no. 4 (1976): 269–77. This physician published the results of her study also as "Fetal Monitoring: Psychologic Consequences and Management Recommendations," *Obstetrics and Gynecology* 50, no. 4 (1977): 500–504 (quote on p. 502).

108. See, for example, Cheryl Tatano Beck, "Patient Acceptance of Fetal Monitoring as a Helpful Tool," *Journal of Obstetric, Gynecologic, and Neonatal Nursing* 9, no. 6 (1980): 350–53; Dulock and Herron, "Women's Responses"; Katherine Rubin, "Fetal Monitoring" (letter to editor in response to Beck's study), *Journal of Obstetric, Gynecologic, and Neonatal Nursing* 10, no. 3 (1981): 237; Donna Shields, "Maternal Reactions to Fetal Monitoring," *American Journal of Nursing* 78, no. 12 (1978): 2110–12; and Starkman, "Psychological Responses" and "Fetal Monitoring."

109. Williams and Richards, "Fetal Monitoring," 2388.

110. See, for example, Reeder et al., *Maternity Nursing*, 13th ed., 352.

111. Klavan, Laver, and Boscola, *Clinical Concepts*, 7.

112. Marie D. Strickland, "Fetal Assessment Techniques: A Challenge to the Nurse Practitioner," in *Current Concepts in Clinical Nursing*, vol. 3, ed. Margery Duffy, Edith H. Anderson, Betty S. Bergersen, Mary Lohr, and Marion H. Rose (St. Louis: C. V. Mosby, 1971), 179–88 (quote on p. 186).

113. False-positive readings tended to be more of a problem. See, for example, David Banta and Stephen Thacker, "Electronic Fetal Monitoring: Is It of Benefit?," *Birth and the Family Journal* 6, no. 4 (1979): 237–50.

114. See, for example, Cindy Afriat and Barry S. Schifrin, "Sources of Error in Fetal Heart Rate Monitoring," *Journal of Obstetric, Gynecologic, and Neonatal Nursing* 5, no. 5 (supplement) (1976): 11s–15s.

115. As later studies would show, machine monitoring was no more objective than fetal auscultation. See, for example, Alan R. Cohen, Henry Klapholz, and Mark S. Thompson, "Electronic Fetal Monitoring and Clinical Practice: A Survey of Obstetric Opinion," *Medical Decision Making* 2, no. 1 (1982): 79–95, and P. V. Nielsen, B. Stigsby, C. Nickelson, and J. Nim, "Intra- and Inter-Observer Variability in the Assessment of Intrapartum Cardiotocograms," *Acta Obstetricia Gynecologica Scandinavica* 66, no. 5 (1987): 421–24. Herbert F. Sandmire, in "Whither Electronic Fetal Monitoring?," *Obstetrics and Gynecology* 76, no. 6 (1990): 1131, observed that because the fetal monitor "leaves a permanent record for hindsight interpretation by expert witnesses," and because this record is open to so much variation in interpretation, machine monitoring "substantially increased the plaintiff's chances of prevailing" in claims of preventable infant brain damage.

116. One nurse strongly in favor of fetal monitoring admitted not liking bedside nursing at all. Although most nurses saw fetal monitoring as a way to improve bedside obstetric nursing, this nurse's admission suggests that fetal monitoring could also be used to escape it.

117. These nurses are referring here to Patricia Benner's differentiation between novice and expert; see Benner, *From Novice to Expert: Excellence and Power in Clinical Nursing Practice* (Menlo Park, Calif.: Addison-Wesley, 1984).

118. See, for example, Sr. Jeanne Meurer, "Intrapartal Fetal Distress," *Journal of Obstetric, Gynecologic, and Neonatal Nursing* 2, no. 1 (1973): 80, a letter to the editor in response to Gail Taylor Rice, "Recognition and Treatment of Intrapartal Fetal Distress," *Journal of Obstetric, Gynecologic, and Neonatal Nursing* 1, no. 2 (1972): 15–22, which featured machine monitoring.

119. Reeder et al., *Maternity Nursing*, 13th ed., 323.

120. See, for example, Lois J. Vice, "Touching the High-Risk Obstetrical Patient," *Journal of Obstetric, Gynecologic, and Neonatal Nursing* 8, no. 5 (1979): 294–95.

121. Whether electronic fetal monitoring delivered or defaulted on its promises was and is a highly controversial subject, and the debate has generated a vast literature. Contributing to the controversy is the difficulty mounting studies, and the lack of comparability among studies, to warrant conclusions. In general, electronic fetal monitoring has not emerged as superior to intermittent fetal auscultation in improving perinatal outcomes. Moreover, expert nursing care, including intermittent fetal auscultation, was found to yield outcomes at least equal to machine monitoring. For reviews of research evaluating electronic fetal heart rate monitoring, see, for example, H. David Banta and Stephen B. Thacker, "Assessing the Costs and Benefits of Electronic Fetal Monitoring," *Obstetrical and Gynecological Survey* 34, no. 8 (1979): 627–42; Adrian Grant, "Monitoring the Fetus during Labor," in *Effective Care in Pregnancy and Childbirth*, vol. 2, *Childbirth*, ed. Iain Chalmers, Murray Enkin, and Marc J. N. C. Keirse (Oxford: Oxford University Press, 1989), 846–82; and Report of Consensus Development Conference, *Antenatal Diagnosis*. For the results of clinical trials conducted between 1973 and 1987, see Albert D. Haverkamp, Miriam Orleans, S. Langendoerfer, John McFee, J. Murphy, and Horace E. Thompson, "A Controlled Trial of the Differential Effects of Intrapartum Fetal Monitoring," *American Journal of Obstetrics and Gynecology* 134, no. 4 (1979): 399–408; Albert D. Haverkamp, Horace E. Thompson, John G. McFee, and Curtis Cetrulo, "The Evaluation of Continuous Fetal Heart Rate Monitoring in High-Risk Pregnancy," *American Journal of Obstetrics and Gynecology* 125, no. 3 (1976): 310–17; Ian M. Kelso, R. John Parsons, Gordon F. Lawrence, Shyam S. Arora, D. Keith Edmonds, and Ian D. Cooke, "An Assessment of Continuous Fetal Heart Rate Monitoring in Labor: A Randomized Trial," *American Journal of Obstetrics and Gynecology* 131, no. 5 (1978): 526–32; Kenneth J. Leveno, F. Gary Cunningham, Sheryl Nelson, Micki Roark, M. Lynne Williams, David Guzick, Sharon Dowling, Charles R. Rosenfeld, and Ann Buckley, "A Prospec-

tive Comparison of Selective and Universal Electronic Fetal Monitoring in 34,995 Pregnancies," *New England Journal of Medicine* 315, no. 10 (1986): 615–19; David A. Luthy, Kirkwood K. Shy, Gerald Van Belle, Eric B. Larson, James P. Hughes, Thomas J. Benedetti, Zane A. Brown, Sydney Effer, James F. King, and Morton A. Stenchever, "A Randomized Trial of Electronic Fetal Monitoring in Preterm Labor," *Obstetrics and Gynecology* 69, no. 5 (1987): 687–95; Dermot MacDonald, Adrian Grant, Margaret Sheridan-Pereira, Peter Boylan, and Iain Chalmers, "The Dublin Randomized Controlled Trial of Intrapartum Fetal Heart Rate Monitoring," *American Journal of Obstetrics and Gynecology* 152, no. 5 (1985): 524–39; Steen Neldham, Mogens Osler, Peder Kern Hansen, Jette Nim, Soren Friis Smith, and Jens Hertel, "Intrapartum Fetal Heart Rate Monitoring in a Combined Low- and High-Risk Population: A Controlled Trial," *European Journal of Obstetrics, Gynecology, and Reproductive Biology* 23, no. 1/2 (1986): 1–11; Peter Renou, Allan Chang, Ian Anderson, and Carl Wood, "Controlled Trial of Fetal Intensive Care," *American Journal of Obstetrics and Gynecology* 126, no. 4 (1976): 470–76; and C. Wood, P. Renou, J. Oats, E. Farrell, N. Beischer, and I. Anderson, "A Controlled Trial .of Fetal Heart Rate Monitoring in a Low-Risk Obstetric Population," *American Journal of Obstetrics and Gynecology* 141, no. 5 (1981): 527–34.

122. See, for example, "The Childbirth Educator: Certified to Represent the Hospital or the Parents?," pt. 2, "A Wide Spectrum of Views of 6 Nurses," *Birth and the Family Journal* 7, no. 2 (1980): 75–80.

123. See Margot Edwards's letter to the editor in response to Beck's article, in *Journal of Obstetric, Gynecologic, and Neonatal Nursing* 11, no. 4 (1982): 254.

124. John C. Hobbins, Roger Freeman, and John T. Queenan, "The Fetal Monitoring Debate," *Obstetrics and Gynecology* 54, no. 1 (1979): 103–9 (quote on p. 108).

125. Mortimer G. Rosen and Janet C. Dickinson, "The Paradox of Electronic Fetal Monitoring: More Data May Not Enable Us to Predict or Prevent Infant Neurologic Morbidity," *American Journal of Obstetrics and Gynecology* 168, no. 3 (1993): 745–51.

126. See, for example, National Institute of Child Health and Human Development Research Planning Workshop, "Electronic Fetal Heart Rate Monitoring: Research Guidelines for Interpretation," *Journal of Obstetric, Gynecologic, and Neonatal Nursing* 26, no. 6 (1997): 635–40.

127. See, for example, "Electronic Fetal Monitoring Competency—To Validate or Not to Validate: The Opinions of Experts," *Journal of Perinatal and Neonatal Nursing* 8, no. 3 (1994): 1–15; Susan D. Guild, "A Comprehensive Fetal Monitoring Program for Nursing Practice and Education," *Journal of Obstetric, Gynecologic, and Neonatal Nursing* 23, no. 1 (1994): 34–41; and Virginia Gramzow Kinnick, "A National Survey about Fetal Monitoring Skills Acquired by Nursing Students in Baccalaureate Programs," *Journal of Obstetric, Gynecologic, and Neonatal Nursing* 18, no. 1 (1989): 57–58.

128. In addition to the trials and review of trials listed in n. 121, see also Kirkwood K. Shy, David A. Luthy, Forrest C. Bennett, Michael Whitfield, Eric B. Larson, Gerald Van Belle, James P. Hughes, Judith A. Wilson, and Morton A. Stenchever, "Effects of Electronic Fetal Heart Rate Monitoring, as Compared with Periodic Auscultation, on the Neurologic Development of Premature Infants," *New England Journal of Medicine* 322, no. 9 (1990): 588–93, and Anthony M. Vintzileos, Aris Antsaklis, Ioannis Varvarigos, Costas Papas, Ioannis Sofatzis, and Jane T. Montgomery, "A Randomized Trial of Intrapartum Electronic Fetal Heart Rate Monitoring versus Intermittent Auscultation," *Obstetrics and Gynecology* 81, no. 6 (1993): 899–907. Controversy also exists about the validity of these trials and their ability to show the "true" benefits of fetal monitoring. See, for example, Anthony M. Vintzileos, David J. Nochimson, Edwin R. Guzman, Robert A. Knuppel, Marian Lake, and Barry S. Schifrin, "Intrapartum Electronic Fetal Heart Rate Monitoring versus Intermittent Auscultation: A Meta-Analysis," *Obstetrics and Gynecology* 85, no. 1 (1995): 149–55. This meta-analysis of nine clinical trials indicated that electronic fetal monitoring was associated with increased rates of surgical intervention but with decreased rates of perinatal mortality due to fetal hypoxia.

129. American Academy of Pediatrics and American College of Obstetricians and Gynecologists, *Guidelines for Perinatal Care*, 2nd ed. (Washington, D.C.: the author, 1988). See also American College of Obstetricians and Gynecologists, *Intrapartum Fetal Heart Rate Monitoring* (Washington, D.C., ACOG Technical Bulletin no. 132, 1989).

130. Roger Freeman, "Intrapartum Fetal Monitoring: A Disappointing Story" (editorial), *New England Journal of Medicine* 322, no. 9 (1990): 624–26; Stefan Timmermans, "High Touch in High Tech: The Presence of Relatives and Friends during Resuscitation Efforts," *Scholarly Inquiry for Nursing Practice* 11, no. 2 (1997): 153–68 (quote on p. 156).

131. Barry S. Schifrin, "Polemics in Perinatology: The Electronic Fetal Monitoring Guidelines," *Journal of Perinatology* 10, no. 2 (1990): 188–92 (quotes on p. 189). Three arguments advanced were (1) that clinical trials of machine monitoring came too soon, before standardization of fetal heart rate patterns was achieved and unambiguous definitions were agreed to; (2) that these trials were methodologically deficient; and (3) that while continuous machine monitoring had been compared in these trials to intermittent auscultation with a fetoscope, intermittent auscultation itself had never been compared to no auscultation of the fetal heart. See also Julian T. Parer, *Handbook of Fetal Heart Rate Monitoring*, 2nd ed. (Philadelphia: Saunders, 1990), chap. 15.

132. See the Association of Women's Health, Obstetric, and Neonatal Nurses (AWHONN) 1992 Position Statement, *Nursing Responsibilities in Implementing Intrapartum Fetal Heart Rate Monitoring*, available from AWHONN in Washington, D.C. The findings of one study indicated that these more stringent protocols for fetal auscultation were generally not feasible unless 1:1 nursing care was avail-

able. The authors of this study therefore still saw machine monitoring as superior, ignoring the fact that such monitoring also required 1:1 attendance if its benefits were to be harnessed: namely, the immediate detection of actionable fetal heart rate patterns. See John C. Morrison, Bonnie F. Chez, Ivory D. Davis, Rick W. Martin, William E. Roberts, James N. Martin, and Randall C. Floyd, "Intrapartum Fetal Heart Rate Assessment: Monitoring by Auscultation or Electronic Means," *American Journal of Obstetrics and Gynecology* 168, no. 1 (1993): 63–66. Schifrin, in "Polemics in Perinatology," 189, claimed that fetal auscultation "requires no experience [and] boasts no experts."

133. Davina Allen, "The Nursing-Medical Boundary: A Negotiated Order?," *Sociology of Health and Illness* 19, no. 4 (1997): 498–520.

134. Advertisements from manufacturers of fetal monitoring systems, prinicipally Corometrics, have appeared in nearly every issue of the *Journal of Obstetric, Gynecologic, and Neonatal Nursing* since its inception in 1972. The journal is the major communication channel for the Association of Women's Health, Obstetric and Neonatal Nurses (formerly, the Nurses' Association of the American College of Obstetricians and Gynecologists). Advertisers place ads in outlets aimed at audiences who influence the purchasing of their products. See Penny P. Smith and Margarete Sandelowski, "Agenda-Setting through Fetal Monitoring System Advertisements for a Nursing Audience" (paper presented at International Communications Association Conference, Chicago, Ill., 1996). Several of the nurses I interviewed mentioned offers by Corometrics to employ them in these capacities; one nurse worked for Corometrics.

135. As one nurse recalled, however, physicians still received the most · lucrative attention from companies. She was amazed at the kinds of "free" merchandise and services these companies offered to physicians at their conventions, in contrast to the free items of lesser value offered to nurses at their conferences.

136. Since nurses might be identified by explicit reference to companies, I have omitted company names here.

137. In one reported case, a company's engineers failed to listen to nurses' advice about a new design feature, and the product subsequently languished in the marketplace.

138. Bassett, in "Anthropology," 287, argued—from the Canadian perspective—that the nurses he observed gained an explicit diagnostic role but lost the private and "embodied authority" for the condition of the laboring woman, as machine monitoring made labor progress public and open to everyone's scrutiny. I argue that although nurses always had the responsibility for diagnosis and care in the first stage of labor, they never had the authority for them. Fetal monitoring did not significantly alter the responsibility-authority calculus for nurses.

139. Technologies, such as machine surveillance, require patients' work in addition to clinicians' work. See Anselm Strauss, Shizuko Fagerhaugh, Barbara

Suczek, and Carolyn Wiener, "The Work of Hospitalized Patients," *Social Science and Medicine* 16, no. 9 (1982): 977–86.

140. See, for example, Banta and Thacker, "Policies toward Medical Technology."

141. "Corometrics Medical Systems," May 7, 1973, 32,874.

142. Bassett, in "Taming Chance," 54, referred to tracings as "ambiguous facts [and] precise fictions."

143. Michel Callon and John Law, "On Interests and Their Transformation: Enrolment and Counter-Enrolment," *Social Studies of Science* 12 (1982): 615–25. I am indebted to Joanna Latimer for the reference to "enrolment." See also Joanna Latimer, "The Nursing Process Re-Examined: Enrolment and Translation," *Journal of Advanced Nursing* 22, no. 2 (1995): 213–20.

144. See Chapter 2 of this book.

145. This nurse recalled one nurse colleague saying that if she liked a particular product, then that was good enough for her. She also noted that the company that employed her to teach classes used the promise of education to enter hospitals. Company representatives would leave flyers advertising seminars on fetal monitoring and, as a "carrot," offer "free" classes and workbooks for nurses in those hospitals buying their product.

146. Andrew Abbott, "Status and Status Strain in the Professions," *American Journal of Sociology* 86, no. 4 (1981): 819–35 (quotes on pp. 824, 829); *The System of Professions: An Essay on the Division of Expert Labor* (Chicago: University of Chicago Press, 1988), 72.

147. Abbott, *System of Professions*, 59.

148. Anselm L. Strauss, Shizuko Fagerhaugh, Barbara Suczek, and Carolyn Wiener, *Social Organization of Medical Work* (New Brunswick, N.J.: Transaction, 1997), chap. 7. This text was originally published in 1985 by the University of Chicago Press. See also Susan Leigh Star, "The Sociology of the Invisible: The Primacy of Work in the Writings of Anselm Strauss," in *Social Organization and Social Process: Essays in Honor of Anselm Strauss*, ed. David R. Maines (New York: Aldine De Gruyten, 1991), 265–83, and "Invisible Work and Silenced Dialogues in Knowledge Representation," in *Women, Work, and Computerization: Understanding and Overcoming Bias in Work and Education*, ed. Inger V. Eriksson, Barbara A. Kitchenham, and Kea G. Tijdens (New York: North-Holland, 1991), 81–92.

149. Liaschenko, "Moral Geography of Home Care," 16–26 (quote on p. 18). Liaschenko referred to the vision of nursing as "stereoscopic" in having to accommodate both gazes.

150. Edith Wyschogrod, in "Empathy and Sympathy as Tactile Encounter," *Journal of Medicine and Philosophy* 6, no. 1 (1981): 25–43, differentiated between touching patients to diagnose disease, where "tactility is deployed in the manner of seeing" (41), and touching as a "tactile encounter" to convey "empathy and sympathy."

151. See, for example, Margaret Busche, "Concerning Charting," *American*

Journal of Nursing 28, no. 1 (1928): 17–20. As Busche observed, "in spite of the apparent importance of charting, it probably is one of the greatest 'hates' of nurses" (17). As nursing began to be seen legally as the "proximate cause" (Maureen J. McRae, "Litigation, Electronic Fetal Monitoring, and the Obstetric Nurse," *Journal of Obstetric, Gynecologic, and Neonatal Nursing* 22, no. 5 (1993): 414) of poor fetal outcomes in cases involving fetal monitoring, documentation became even more important. A common inference was that if an event was not charted, it did not happen. Nurses were thus cautioned to be sure to engage in "defensive charting" as the only evidence that could show they had provided appropriate care. See, for example, Linda Chagnon and Beverly Easterwood, "Managing the Risks of Obstetrical Nursing," *MCN: American Journal of Maternal Child Nursing* 11, no. 5 (1986): 303–10, and McRae, "Litigation," 410–19. For descriptions of cases involving alleged nurse liability, see, for example, "Failure to Monitor Fetal Heart Rate: Catastrophic Results," *Regan Report on Nursing Law* 33, no. 7 (1992): 1; "Failure to Use Fetal Monitor and Timely Call Physician," *Regan Report on Nursing Law* 31, no. 12 (1991): 4; and "Fetal Monitor Delay: 'Proximate Cause' Issue," *Regan Report on Nursing Law* 31, no. 10 (1991): 1. Other cases are cited in McRae, "Litigation."

152. "Childbirth Educator," 80.

153. See, for example, Gladys Denny Shultz, "Journal Mothers Report on Cruelty in Maternity Wards," *Ladies Home Journal*, May 1958, 44–45, 152–55. See also Judith Walzer Leavitt, "'Strange Young Women on Errands': Obstetric Nursing between Two Worlds," *Nursing History Review* 6 (1998): 3–24, and Sandelowski, *Pain, Pleasure*, 60–71.

154. "Childbirth Educator," 80.

155. Madeleine H. Shearer, "Some Deterrents to Objective Evaluation of Fetal Monitors," *Birth and the Family Journal* 2, no. 2 (1975): 58–62 (specific information on p. 59).

156. British scholars Kate Robinson, Hugh Robinson, and Hilary Davis used these terms to describe nurses' responses to information technology in "Towards a Social Constructionist Analysis of Nursing Informatics," *Health Informatics* 2, no. 4 (1996): 179–87.

157. Similarly, and contrary to common notions of technology as dehumanizing, Stefan Timmermans showed how resuscitation technology can be used to ensure a dignified death. See his "Resuscitation Technology in the Emergency Department: Towards a Dignified Death," *Sociology of Health and Illness* 20, no. 2 (1998): 144–67.

158. Mitcham differentiated between these two kinds of engagements with technology, whereby invention is viewed as creative but application is viewed as repetitive and routine. See Mitcham, *Thinking through Technology*, 231.

159. H. Tristram Engelhardt, "Physicians, Patients, Health Care Institutions—and the People in Between: Nurses," in *Caring, Curing, Coping: Nurse, Physician,*

Patient Relationships, ed. Anne H. Bishop and John R. Scudder (University: University of Alabama Press, 1983), 62–79.

160. Nurses are often referred to as the glue or cement that holds health care together. See, for example, Donald M. Sledz, "Nursing an Old Wound in Medicine," *Wall Street Journal*, February 6, 1997.

161. Anja Hiddinga and Stuart S. Blume, "Technology, Science, and Obstetric Practice: The Origins and Transformation of Cephalopelvimetry," *Science, Technology, and Human Values* 17, no. 2 (1992): 154–79 (quote on p. 176); Diana E. Forsythe, "New Bottles, Old Wine: Hidden Cultural Assumptions in a Computerized Explanation System for Migraine Sufferers," *Medical Anthropology Quarterly* 10, no. 4 (1996): 551–74.

Chapter 7

1. Anne Balsamo, *Technologies of the Gendered Body: Reading Cyborg Women* (Durham, N.C.: Duke University Press, 1997), 32.

2. Irma Van Der Ploeg, "Hermaphrodite Patients: In Vitro Fertilization and the Transformation of Male Infertility," *Science, Technology, and Human Values* 20, no. 4 (1995): 460–81; Judith Halberstam and Ira Livingston, eds., *Posthuman Bodies* (Bloomington: Indiana University Press, 1995); David F. Channell, *The Vital Machine: A Study of Technology and Organic Life* (New York: Oxford University Press, 1991).

3. Balsamo, *Technologies of the Gendered Body*, 33; Donna J. Haraway, "A Cyborg Manifesto: Science, Technology, and Socialist-Feminism in the Late Twentieth Century," in *Simians, Cyborgs, and Women: The Reinvention of Nature*, by Donna J. Haraway (New York: Routledge, 1991), 177.

4. Haraway, "Cyborg Manifesto," 150.

5. Simon J. Williams proposed that rather than transcending "gendered forms of embodiment," cyborg technology "upholds" it. Rather than challenging mind/body divisions, "postmodern" medi(c)a(l) technologies reinforce these "modern" divisions. See his "Modern Medicine and the 'Uncertain Body': From Corporeality to Hyperreality?," *Social Science and Medicine* 45, no. 7 (1997): 1041–49. Gary Lee Downey and Joseph Dumit, in "Locating and Intervening: An Introduction," in *Cyborgs and Citadels: Anthropological Interventions in Emerging Sciences and Technologies*, ed. Gary Lee Downey and Joseph Dumit (Santa Fee, N.M.: School of American Research Press, 1997), 8, observed "the cyborg risks becoming essentialized as a fad."

6. Michel Callon and John Law, "On Interests and Their Transformation: Enrolment and Counter-Enrolment," *Social Studies of Science* 12 (1982): 615–25. I am indebted to Joanna Latimer for the reference to "enrolment." See Joanna Latimer, "The Nursing Process Re-Examined: Enrolment and Translation," *Journal of Advanced Nursing* 22, no. 2 (1995): 213–20.

7. Balsamo, *Technologies of the Gendered Body*, 160.

8. Carl May and Christine Fleming, "The Professional Imagination: Narrative and the Symbolic Boundaries between Medicine and Nursing," *Journal of Advanced Nursing* 25, no. 5 (1997): 1094–1100.

9. Stefan Timmermans, Geoffrey C. Bowker, and Susan Leigh Star, "The Architecture of Difference: Visibility, Control, and Comparability in Building a Nursing Interventions Classification," in *Differences in Medicine: Unraveling Practices, Techniques, and Bodies*, ed. Marc Berg and Annemarie Mol (Durham, N.C.: Duke University Press, 1998), 202–25 (quote on p. 221).

10. Judith Parker, "The Body as Text and the Body as Living Flesh: Metaphors of the Body and Nursing in Postmodernity," in *The Body in Nursing*, ed. Jocalyn Lawler (Melbourne: Churchill Livingstone, 1997), 11–29 (quote on p. 22); H. Tristram Engelhardt, "Physicians, Patients, Health Care Institutions—and the People in Between: Nurses," in *Caring, Curing, Coping: Nurse, Physician, Patient Relationships*, ed. Anne H. Bishop and John R. Scudder (University: University of Alabama Press, 1983), 62–79; Jenny Littlewood, "Care and Ambiguity: Towards a Concept of Nursing," in *Anthropology in Nursing*, ed. Pat Holden and Jenny Littlewood (London: Routledge, 1986), 170–89 (quote on p. 185).

11. Littlewood, "Care and Ambiguity," 185.

12. Judith Parker, "Body as Text," 27.

13. See, for example, Linda M. Lacey and Michelle Beck-Warden, "Health Care Restructuring: Bitter Medicine or a Shot in the Arm for Nursing?," *Research in the Sociology of Health Care* 15 (1998): 187–201, and Susan Trossman, "Staffing Smart: A Difficult Proposition," *American Nurse*, January/February 1999, 1–2.

14. See, for example, anthropologists' ideas about cultural intervention, in Downey and Dumit, "Locating and Intervening."

15. Joan E. Lynaugh, "Narrow Passageways: Nurses and Physicians in Conflict and Concert since 1875," in *The Physician as Captain of the Ship: A Critical Reappraisal*, ed. Nancy M. P. King, Larry R. Churchill, and A. W. Cross (Dordrecht: D. Reidel, 1988), 23–37.

16. Joan Liaschenko, "Ethics and the Geography of the Nurse-Patient Relationship: Spatial Vulnerabilities and Gendered Space," *Scholarly Inquiry for Nursing Practice* 11, no. 1 (1997): 45–59 (quote on p. 47).

17. See, for example, Joan L. Bottorff, "A Methodological Review and Evaluation of Research on Nurse-Patient Touch," in *Anthology on Caring*, ed. Peggy L. Chinn (New York: National League for Nursing Press, 1991), 303–43. The hand here is an instrument for therapeutic touch.

18. Jocalyn Lawler, "Knowing the Body and Embodiment: Methodologies, Discourses, and Nursing," in Lawler, *Body in Nursing*, 31–51 (quote on p. 44). See also Margaret J. Dunlop, "Is a Science of Caring Possible?," *Journal of Advanced Nursing* 11, no. 5 (1986): 661–70.

19. Mary Jo Arndt, "Caring as Everydayness," *Journal of Holistic Nursing* 10, no. 4 (1992): 285–93; Judith Parker and Glenn Gardner, "The Silence and the Silenc-

ing of the Nurse's Voice: A Reading of Patient Progress Notes," *Australian Journal of Advanced Nursing* 9, no. 2 (1992): 3–9 (quotes on pp. 6, 8).

20. Susan Reverby, "A Caring Dilemma: Womanhood and Nursing in Historical Perspective," *Nursing Research* 36, no. 1 (1987): 5–11 (specific information on p. 10).

21. Andrew Abbott, *The System of Professions: An Essay on the Division of Expert Labor* (Chicago: University of Chicago Press, 1988), 71.

22. Robert L. Brannon, *Intensifying Care: The Hospital Industry, Professionalization, and the Reorganization of the Nursing Labor Process* (Amityville, N.Y.: Baywood, 1994), 170.

23. In the 1970s and 1980s nurses tried to offset these losses by taking these tasks back in the form of primary nursing, a mode of nursing care that revived the one-nurse-to-one-patient model of care. But, as Brannon argued, it was difficult for nurses to go back to an earlier form of nursing as they remained accountable for the medical tasks increasingly delegated to them. Primary nursing, or total patient care, simply added to the labor of the nurse and forced her to find means to reduce her burden, including transferring some of her work to patients and, ultimately, again to ancillary nurses.

24. According to Abbott's notion of "professional regression" in *System of Professions*, professional status is advanced by movement away from direct and routine client involvement and toward the profession's knowledge base. Yet nurses have always been divided on whether this is the right way to move, and some have pondered whether prevailing notions of professionalism are not forms of imperialism that themselves divide nurses. See, for example, Boston Nurses' Group, "The False Promise: Professionalism in Nursing," *Science for the People*, May–June, July–August 1978, 20–34, 23–33, and Margarete Sandelowski, *Women, Health, and Choice* (Englewood Cliffs, N.J.: Prentice-Hall, 1981), 164–68.

25. Nursing care has been described as crossing temporal and spatial boundaries, as mediating between cultures, and as managing ambiguity. See, for example, Liaschenko, "Ethics and Geography"; Littlewood, "Care and Ambiguity"; Judith Parker, "Body as Text"; and Helle Samuelson, "Nurses between Disease and Illness," in Holden and Littlewood, *Anthropology in Nursing*, 190–202.

26. Liaschenko, "Ethics and Geography," 52.

27. Judith Parker, "Body as Text," 27. One of my doctoral students, Vivian West, is studying the new/old role of the nurse as "presenter" of the patient in telemedicine. The nurse here holds a device (for example, a stethoscope) in place so that a physician in a distant location can appraise a part of the patient's body as it is visually or acoustically transmitted electronically. Although ostensibly new, such diagnosis by telemedicine simply reprises a long-standing function of the nurse: to hold a patient and instrument in place for physician examination. The nurse here is literally between patient and physician, and between one device (the instrument placed on or into the patient's body) and

another device (the equipment that transmits images and sounds of that body to a physician at another location). Indeed, in this form of telemedicine, the nurse's body is again a tool and a component of a network linking devices and people to one another.

28. See, for example, Dunlop, "Is a Science of Caring Possible?" For an overview of nursing theories comprising the Nursing Theory Movement, see, for example, Afaf I. Meleis, *Theoretical Nursing: Development and Progress*, 3rd ed. (Philadelphia: Lippincott, 1998).

29. Kim Walker, "On What It Might Mean to Be a Nurse: A Discursive Ethnography" (Ph.D. diss., Latrobe University, Bundoora, Victoria, Australia, 1993), 94.

30. See, for example, Lynn M. Stearney, "Sex Control Technology and Reproductive 'Choice': The Conflation of Technical and Political Argument in the New Science of Human Reproduction," *Communication Theory* 6, no. 4 (1996): 388–405.

31. May and Fleming, "Professional Imagination."

32. According to Nancy S. Jecker and Donnie J. Self, there are four models of caring in the health professions: (1) those who care for and about their patients, (2) those who care for but not about their patients, (3) those who care about but not for their patients, and (4) those who care neither for nor about their patients. See Jecker and Self, "Separating Care and Cure: An Analysis of Historical and Contemporary Images of Nursing and Medicine," *Journal of Medicine and Philosophy* 16, no. 3 (1991): 285–306 (specific information on p. 301).

33. Sally A. Gadow, "Nurse and Patient: The Caring Relationship," in Bishop and Scudder, *Caring, Curing, Coping*, 31–43 (quote on p. 31).

34. Sally Gadow, "Covenant without Cure: Letting Go and Holding On in Chronic Illness," in *The Ethics of Care and the Ethics of Cure: Synthesis in Chronicity*, ed. Jean Watson and Marilyn Ray (New York: National League for Nursing, 1988), 5–14.

35. Renee C. Fox, Linda H. Aiken, and Carla M. Messikomer, "The Culture of Caring: AIDS and the Nursing Profession," *Milbank Quarterly* 68, suppl. 2 (1990): 226–56.

36. Ibid., 229.

37. Rita Fahrner, "Nursing Interventions," in *Nursing Care of the Person with AIDS/ARC*, ed. Angie Lewis (Rockville, Md.: Aspen, 1988), 115–30 (quote on p. 115). Until recently AIDS was also an invisible disease by virtue of the people seen to be affected by it, namely, homosexuals, drug addicts, and other groups of persons we do not wish to acknowledge. That is, AIDS is a disease we have not wanted to see, engendering the same kind of discomfort as nurses' body/dirty work. Nurses, in what Timmermans, Bowker, and Star referred to in "Architecture of Difference," 218, as the "quintessentially invisible" profession of nursing, have thus allied themselves with a disease that still stirs the impulse to avert the eyes.

38. Marion J. Ball, Kathryn J. Hannah, Susan K. Newbold, and Judith V. Douglas, eds., *Nursing Informatics: Where Caring and Technology Meet*, 2nd ed. (New York: Springer-Verlag, 1995).

39. The Association of Nurses in AIDS Care now has forty-nine active chapters and publishes the *Journal of the Association of Nurses in AIDS Care*. There are several graduate programs in HIV/AIDS nursing. See the association's Web site at http://www.anacnet.org. There are several graduate programs in nursing informatics. The American Nurses' Association published *The Scope of Practice for Nursing Informatics* in 1994. For information on the American Nurses Informatics Association, see http://www.ania.org.

40. Connie Delaney, Peg Mehmert, and Dickey Johnson, "The Evolving Role of the Informatics Nurse," in *Nursing Roles: Evolving or Recycled?*, ed. Sue Moorhead (Thousand Oaks, Calif.: Sage, 1997), 59–77; Ronald A. Jydstrup and Malvern J. Gross, "Continuity of Information Handling in Hospitals," *Health Services Research* 1, no. 3 (1966): 235–71.

41. Delaney, Mehmert, and Johnson, "Evolving Role," 60. See also American Nurses' Association, *The Scope of Practice for Nursing Informatics* (Washington, D.C.: American Nurses' Association, 1994).

42. Timmermans, Bowker, and Star, "Architecture of Difference," 204.

43. See, for example, Lynda J. Carpenito, *Nursing Diagnosis: Application to Clinical Practice* (Philadelphia: Lippincott, 1997); Marjory Gordon, *Nursing Diagnosis: Process and Applications*, 3rd ed. (St. Louis: C. V. Mosby, 1994); Gertrude K. McFarland and Elizabeth T. McFarlane, eds., *Nursing Diagnosis and Intervention: Planning for Patient Care* (St. Louis: C. V. Mosby, 1997); North American Nursing Diagnosis Association, *Nursing Diagnosis: Definitions and Classification, 1999–2000* (Philadelphia: NANDA, 1999); Joanne C. McCloskey and Gloria M. Bulechek, eds., *Nursing Interventions Classification (NIC)*, 2nd ed. (St. Louis: C. V. Mosby, 1996); Marion Johnson and Meridean Maas, eds., *Nursing Outcomes Classification (NOC)* (St. Louis: C. V. Mosby, 1997); and Timmermans, Bowker, and Star, "Architecture of Difference," 204–5.

44. Timmermans, Bowker, and Star, "Architecture of Difference," 211.

45. Ibid., 222.

46. Suzanne Poirier, Lorie Rosenblum, Lioness Ayres, Daniel J. Brauner, Barbara F. Sharf, and Ann Folwell Stanford, "Charting the Chart: An Exercise in Interpretation(s)," *Literature and Medicine* 11, no. 1 (1992): 1–22 (quote on p. 9).

47. Parker and Gardner, "Silence and the Silencing," 8.

48. Kathryn Montgomery Hunter, *Doctors' Stories: The Narrative Structure of Medical Knowledge* (Princeton: Princeton University Press, 1991), 85.

49. Marc Berg and Geoffrey Bowker, "The Multiple Bodies of the Medical Record: Toward a Sociology of an Artifact," *Sociological Quarterly* 38, no. 3 (1997): 513–37 (quotes on pp. 524–25).

50. See, for example, Carole A. Estabrooks, "Will Evidence-Based Nursing Practice Make Practice Perfect?," *Canadian Journal of Nursing Research* 30, no. 4

(1999): 273–94, and Peter French, "The Development of Evidence-Based Nursing," *Journal of Advanced Nursing* 29, no. 1 (1999): 72–78. These words now comprise the language of and arguably the latest fad in talking about modern Western health care. When, for example, was any nursing or medical practice not based on evidence? Clinicians always used what they deemed the best evidence to care for their patients, no matter what we may think of their approaches now. The appeal to evidence-based practice today is, in part, a device to exclude and/or to diminish the value of any evidence that is not produced from randomized clinical trials. By emphasizing evidence-based nursing practice, nurses move themselves both into and out of the mainstream of health care discourse, as they exclude the kinds of evidence practicing nurses (and many physicians) have always prized, such as intuition, tacit knowledge, and other forms not readily verbalized or measured.

51. Lawler, "Knowing the Body," 45.

52. Ibid., 34, 41, 43.

53. Ibid., 48.

54. Ina Wagner, "Women's Voice: The Case of Nursing Information Systems," *AI and Society* 7 (1993): 295–310 (quote on p. 306).

55. Lawler, "Knowing the Body," 48.

56. Timmermans, Bowker, and Star, "Architecture of Difference," 217.

57. Lawler, "Knowing the Body," 43.

58. See, for example, Anne H. Bishop and John R. Scudder, "Applied Science, Practice, and Intervention Technology," in *In Search of Nursing Science*, ed. Anna Omery, Christine E. Kasper, and Gayle G. Page (Thousand Oaks, Calif.: Sage, 1995), 263–90, and Gail J. Mitchell, "Nursing Diagnosis: An Ethical Analysis," *Image: Journal of Nursing Scholarship* 23, no. 2 (1991): 99–103. An important constituency of Australian, Canadian, and European scholars worry about the undue influence of U.S. nursing on nursing in their countries. In his address titled "Don't Worry, Be Happy: Reflections on Caring," given on April 8, 1999, during the Fifth International Qualitative Health Research Conference in Newcastle, New South Wales, Australia, educator and philosopher Max Van Manen told the story of a nurse leaning over her patient, who was on a ventilator, to tell him that she was leaving for the day but that "you are on my mind." Weeks later, when the patient had recovered, he told this nurse, "You do not know how much you helped me." In the current era of managed care, nurses indeed feel pressed to determine *how much* help was provided in this situation and how much it cost to provide it. Moreover, they feel obliged to convert this help into a classifiable intervention. This moment in the nurse/patient relationship illustrates both the essence of true nursing and the futility of efforts to capture it in a data base.

59. See, for example, Diana E. Forsythe, "New Bottles, Old Wine: Hidden Cultural Assumptions in a Computerized Explanation System for Migraine Sufferers," *Medical Anthropology Quarterly* 10, no. 4 (1996): 551–74, and Suzanne

Bakken Henry and Charles N. Mead, "Nursing Classification Systems: Necessary but Not Sufficient for Representing 'What Nurses Do' for Inclusion in Computer-Based Patient Record Systems," *Journal of the American Medical Informatics Association* 4, no. 3 (1997): 222–32.

60. See, for example, M. Theobald, "Formalizing Nursing Knowledge," in *Nursing Informatics*, ed. Paul Wainwright (Edinburgh: Churchill Livingstone, 1994), 29–40. See also Gro Bjerknes and Tone Bratteteig, "Florence in Wonderland: System Development with Nurses," in *Computers and Democracy: A Scandinavian Challenge*, ed. Gro Bjerknes, Pelle Ehn, and Morten Kyng (Aldershot: Avebury, 1987), 279–95.

61. See, for example, Laurel E. Radwin, "Conceptualizations of Decision Making in Nursing: Analytic Models and 'Knowing the Patient,' " *Nursing Diagnosis* 6, no. 1 (1995): 16–22.

62. Susan Leigh Star, "From Hesta to Home Page: Feminism and the Concept of Home in Cyberspace," in *Between Monsters, Goddesses, and Cyborgs*, ed. Nina Lykke and Rosi Braidotti (London: Zed Books, 1996), 30–46 (quote on p. 33).

63. Ina Wagner, "Women's Voice," 304–5. Wagner, an Austrian, cited Rosalyn Feldberg, "Computers in Hospital Care: An Overview of Developments in the USA," in *Computers in Hospital Care*, ed. E. Dimitz (Vienna: Proceedings of International Colloquium, 1990), 43.

64. Geoffrey C. Bowker, Stefan Timmermans, and Susan Leigh Star, "Infrastructure and Organizational Transformation: Classifying Nurses' Work," in *Information Technology and Changes in Organizational Work*, ed. Wanda Orlikowski, Geoff Walsham, Matthew R. Jones, and Janice DeGross (London: Chapman and Hall, 1995), 344–70 (quote on p. 345).

65. Susan Leigh Star cited poet Adrienne Rich's "Cartographies of Silence" (in *The Dream of a Common Language* [New York: Norton, 1978], 17) in "Invisible Work and Silenced Dialogues in Knowledge Representation," in *Women, Work, and Computerization: Understanding and Overcoming Bias in Work and Education*, ed. Inger V. Eriksson, Barbara A. Kitchenham, and Ken G. Tijdens (New York: North-Holland, 1991), 81–92 (citation on p. 83).

66. Judith Parker, "Body as Text," 26.

67. Kate Robinson, Hugh Robinson, and Hilary Davis, "Towards a Social Constructionist Analysis of Nursing Informatics," *Health Informatics* 2, no. 4 (1996): 179–87 (quote on p. 186).

68. Ina Wagner, "Women's Voice," 308.

69. Littlewood, "Care and Ambiguity," 185.

70. See, for example, Mary Jamila Cairo, "Emergency Physicians' Attitudes toward the Emergency Nurse Practitioner Role: Validation versus Rejection," *Journal of the American Academy of Nurse Practitioners* 8, no. 9 (1996): 411–17; Colleen Conway-Welch and A. Harshman-Green, "At the Table: Nursing in Managed Care," *Nursing Policy Forum* 1, no. 5 (1995): 10–16; Linda Dunn, "A Literature Review of Advanced Clinical Nursing Practice in the United States of America,"

Journal of Advanced Nursing 25, no. 4 (1997): 814–19; Larry W. Koch, S. H. Pazaki, and James D. Campbell, "The First Twenty Years of Nurse Practitioner Literature: An Evolution of Joint Practice Issues," Nurse Practitioner 17, no. 2 (1992): 62–71; and Walter O. Spitzer, "The Nurse Practitioner Revisited: Slow Death of a Good Idea," New England Journal of Medicine 310, no. 16 (1984): 1049–51.

71. Lois M. Raday, "Nurse Practitioner: Just What the Doctor Ordered?," in ANA Clinical Sessions, 1974 (New York: Appleton-Century-Croft, 1975), 379–82, and see, for example, Barbara L. Brush and Elizabeth A. Capezuti, "Revisiting 'A Nurse for All Settings': The Nurse Practitioner Movement, 1965–1995," Journal of the American Academy of Nurse Practitioners 8, no. 1 (1996): 5–11; Anne Keane and Therese Richmond, "Tertiary Nurse Practitioners," Image: Journal of Nursing Scholarship 25, no. 4 (1993): 281–84; and James R. Knickman, Mack Lipkin, Steven A. Finkler, Warren G. Thompson, and Joan Kiel, "The Potential for Using Non-Physicians to Compensate for the Reduced Availability of Residents," Academic Medicine 67, no. 7 (1992): 429–38.

72. See, for example, Loretta C. Ford, "Nurse Practitioners: History of a New Idea and Predictions for the Future," in Nursing in the 1980s: Crises, Opportunities, Challenges, ed. Linda H. Aiken (Philadelphia: Lippincott, 1982), 231–47, and Eileen Hayes, "The Nurse Practitioner: History, Current Conflicts, and Future Survival," Journal of American College Health 34, no. 3 (1985): 144–47.

73. The nurse practitioner is also viewed as a technologist. See, for example, Office of Technology Assessment, Nurse Practitioners, Physician Assistants, and Certified Nurse-Midwives: A Policy Analysis (Washington, D.C.: U.S. Government Printing Office, 1986). But I see the role as differentiated, in large part, by nurses' new use of technology, especially diagnostic technology.

74. Nurse Loretta Ford and physician Henry Silver developed the nurse practitioner role—in pediatrics—in 1967. See, for example, Loretta C. Ford and Henry K. Silver, "The Expanded Role of the Nurse in Child Care," Nursing Outlook 15, no. 9 (1967): 43–45; Koch, Pazaki, and Campbell, "First Twenty Years"; and Henry K. Silver, Loretta C. Ford, and Lewis R. Day, "The Pediatric Nurse-Practitioner Program," Journal of the American Medical Association 204, no. 4 (1968): 298–303.

75. American College of Physicians, "Physician Assistants and Nurse Practitioners," Annals of Internal Medicine 121, no. 9 (1994): 714–16.

76. Martha E. Rogers, "Nursing: To Be or Not to Be?," Nursing Outlook 20, no. 1 (1972): 42–46.

77. See, for example, Linda Dunn, "A Literature Review of Advanced Clinical Nursing Practice in the United States of America," Journal of Advanced Nursing 25, no. 4 (1997): 814–19, and Loretta C. Ford, "Nurse Practitioners." The "traitors to nursing" quote is from Joan E. Lynaugh, Barbara Medoff-Cooper, Ann L. O'Sullivan, Henry L. Barnett, Marianne W. Reilly, Elizabeth A. Kuehne, Jo Anne Staats, Jane K. Butler, and William Kavesh, "Introduction: The Practice Paradigm," in Nurses, Nurse Practitioners: Evolution to Advanced Practice, ed. Mathy D.

Mezey and Diane O. McGivern (New York: Springer, 1993): 119–27 (quote on p. 126). See also Chapter 5 of this book.

78. "NPs in Neonatalogy," *NEWSLine for Nurse Practitioners* 1 (1995): 4–7 (quote on p. 5).

79. Barbara J. Daly, "Introduction: A Vision for the Acute Care Nurse Practitioner Role," in *The Acute Care Nurse Practitioner,* ed. Barbara J. Daly (New York: Springer, 1997), 1–11 (quote on p. 6).

80. Cecily Lynn Betz, "Is Nursing Selling Itself Short? The Shift to Educate More Nurse Practitioners" (editorial), *Journal of Pediatric Nursing* 9, no. 3 (1994): 139–40 (quote on p. 140).

81. Nurses and nursing have recurringly been referred to as fillers of voids and bridgers of gaps.

82. Barbara J. Daly, "Introduction," 5.

83. Studies of nurse practitioners have shown them to perform at least as well as, and often even better than, physicians. See, for example, Marilyn A. Chard, Barbara Dunn, and JonnaLynn Mandelbaum, *Nurse Practitioners: A Review of the Literature, 1965–1982* (Kansas City: American Nurses' Association, 1983), and Office of Technology Assessment, *Nurse Practitioners.*

84. Barbara L. Brush and Elizabeth A. Capezuti, "Professional Autonomy: Essential for Nurse Practitioner Survival in the Twenty-first Century," *Journal of the American Academy of Nurse Practitioners* 9, no. 6 (1997): 265–70 (quote on p. 266). See also Kathleen Martin, "Nurse Practitioners' Use of Nursing Diagnosis," *Nursing Diagnosis* 6, no. 1 (1995): 9–15. Martin reported that nurse practitioners rarely used nursing diagnoses, as they found them largely irrelevant. Medical diagnoses remain the model for "diagnosis" and the currency for services rendered. As Martin noted, "Services that generate charges paid by insurers are generally tied to medical diagnoses" (14). Services tied to nursing diagnoses are more time consuming than those tied to medical diagnoses and thus run against the mandate to limit the time spent in any one primary care provider/patient encounter.

85. Brush and Capezuti, "Professional Autonomy," 268.

86. "Perspectives 20 Years Later: From the Pioneers of the NP Movement," *Nurse Practitioner* 10, no. 1 (1985): 17, 18.

87. Mary F. Kohnke, "The Nurse's Responsibility to the Consumer," *American Journal of Nursing* 78, no. 3 (1978): 440–42 (quotes on p. 442).

88. Barbara J. Daly, "Introduction," 5, 6.

89. See, for example, the editorial by Edith P. Lewis, "A Role by Any Other Name," *Nursing Outlook* 22, no. 2 (1974): 89.

90. Betz, "Is Nursing Selling Itself Short?"

91. See Chapter 4 of this book, and William Forrest Maule, "Screening for Colorectal Cancer by Nurse Endoscopists," *New England Journal of Medicine* 330, no. 3 (1994): 183–87. Maule believed that allowing nurses to perform such procedures would increase their "professional satisfaction." See Maule's response

to commentary in "Nurse Practitioners as Endoscopists," *New England Journal of Medicine* 330, no. 21 (1994): 1535.

92. See, for example, Richard A. Cooper, Tim Henderson, and Craig L. Dietrich, "Roles of Nonphysician Clinicians as Autonomous Providers of Patient Care," *Journal of the American Medical Association* 280, no. 9 (1998): 795–802; Richard A. Cooper, Prakash Laud, and Craig L. Dietrich, "Current and Projected Workforce of Nonphysician Clinicians," *Journal of the American Medical Association*, 280, no. 9 (1998): 788–94; and the editorial by Kevin Grumbach and Janet Coffman, "Physicians and Nonphysician Clinicians: Complements or Competitors?," *Journal of the American Medical Association* 280, no. 9 (1998): 825–26.

93. Koch, Pazaki, and Campbell, "First Twenty Years," 62.

94. Abbott, *System of Professions*, 72.

95. See, for example, ibid., 53–54, and Nancy Campbell-Heider and Donald Pollock, "Barriers to Physician-Nurse Collegiality: An Anthropological Perspective," *Social Science and Medicine* 25, no. 5 (1987): 421–25 (quote on p. 422).

96. See, for example, Audrey B. Davis, "Anesthetist and Anesthesiologist: Technology in the Social Context of a Medical and Nursing Specialty," *Transactions and Studies of the College of Physicians of Philadelphia*, 5th ser, 11, no. 2 (1989): 123–34, and Maureen Searle, "The Professionalization of Anesthesiology—Again," *Social Science and Medicine* 18, no. 4 (1984): 323–27.

97. James Bryant, "Nurse Practitioners as Endoscopists," *New England Journal of Medicine* 330, no. 21 (1994): 1534. Bryant is responding here to Maule's call for nurse endoscopists in "Screening for Colorectal Cancer." As he put it, if a nurse could do these tasks, a third-year medical student could do them.

98. See, for example, Campbell-Heider and Pollock, "Barriers to Physician-Nurse Collegiality."

99. See, for example, C. K. Buppert, "Justifying Nurse Practitioner Existence: Hard Facts to Hard Figures," *Nurse Practitioner* 20, no. 8 (1995): 43–44, 46–48, and May and Fleming, "Professional Imagination," 1097.

Studying the relationship between nursing and technology requires an eclectic combination of, and ecumenical approach to, sources of information, as it entails two phenomena that are both there and not there: ubiquitous but invisible, at hand's end but also belonging to the embodied eye and the mind's eye.

Nursing, Medical, and Hospital Books and Periodicals

The major sources of information about the nursing/technology relationship are nursing textbooks and periodicals, including not only the text they contain but also photographs, drawings, and advertisements. These sources include prescriptions for practice and, just as frequently, personal and even impassioned descriptions of nurses' experiences with patients, procedures, and devices. In these works are nurses who became well known for their writing and nurses who wrote only one or two articles.

Most invaluable in finding relevant texts featuring practice is Virginia Henderson's 3-volume *Nursing Studies Index* (1963), an annotated guide to English-language periodicals, books, and pamphlets covering the period between 1900 and 1959. The *Cumulative Index to Nursing and Allied Health Literature* covers the period from 1956 to the present, with on-line entries beginning in 1982. Additional sources for nursing books include *Health Science Books, 1876–1982* (1982) and Alice Thompson's *A Bibliography of Nursing Literature*, vol. 1, 1859–1960 (1968). Key journals of nursing covering the period of study include the *Trained Nurse* and, later, the *Trained Nurse and Hospital Review* and the *American Journal of Nursing*, which began publication in 1888 and 1900, respectively. A special feature of the *American Journal of Nursing* is the "trading post," an "exchange for ingenious ideas about nursing." Key hospital journals include the *Bulletin of the American Hospital Association* (1916), *Modern Hospital* (1913), *Hospital Management* (1916), *Hospital Progress* (1920), and *Hospital Topics* (1922). To capture the range of entities conceived of as technology over the last century, and because the word "technology" was rarely used by nurses or as a term in these indexes before the 1970s, I searched under keywords such as "nursing arts," "nursing care," "procedures," "equipment," and "technics" in addition to such terms as "thermometer," "blood pressure," and "oxygen" for information on specific devices and procedures.

An especially useful way to discern continuity and change in practice is to read successive editions of key nursing texts or a cross section of texts in a field of practice over a period of time. Most notable here are the series of fundamentals of nursing textbooks Bertha Harmer and Virginia Henderson authored between 1922 and 1978 and successive editions of specialty texts, such as Joseph B. De Lee's *Obstetrics for Nurses*, published between 1908 and 1966. Major late-nineteenth- and early-twentieth-century nursing texts include Isabel A. Hampton's (later Isabel Hampton Robb's) *Nursing: Its Principles and Practice*, first published in 1893; Clara S. Weeks's (later Clara Weeks-Shaw's) *A Textbook of Nursing: For the Use of Training Schools, Families, and Private Students*, first published in 1885; *A Handbook of Nursing for Family and General Use* and *A Manual of Nursing Prepared for the Training School for Nurses Attached to Bellevue Hospital*, both first published by the Connecticut Training School for Nurses in 1878; and of course, Florence Nightingale's *Notes on Nursing: What It Is and What It Is Not*, first published in 1859.

Medical literature provides an important context for these nursing texts. Among the most important sources for this study are Edouard Seguin's *Family Thermometry: A Manual of Thermometry for Mothers, Nurses, Hospitalers, Etc., and All Those Who Have Charge of the Sick and the Young* (1873) and *Medical Thermometry and Human Temperature* (1876), S. Weir Mitchell's *The Early History of Instrumental Precision in Medicine* (1891), and Carl A. Wunderlich's *On the Temperature in Diseases: A Manual of Medical Thermometry* (1871).

I found the journals and texts I used for this study in libraries at the University of North Carolina at Chapel Hill, the University of Pennsylvania, the College of Physicians of Philadelphia, and the National Library of Medicine.

Archival Collections

One of the best archival collections for the study of technology in nursing is at the Center for the Study of the History of Nursing at the University of Pennsylvania School of Nursing in Philadelphia. Especially relevant to this study was the center's collection of student lecture notes, annual hospital reports, hospital procedure manuals, and oral history transcripts and a photographic collection of equipment trays. An unexpectedly rich and delightful source of information was medical trade ephemera, including instrument and equipment catalogs and other promotional material, that I discovered by chance during a visit to the Library of the College of Physicians of Philadelphia. This material offers information on what devices looked like and the claims made for them. In addition to owning one of the largest collections of medical trade ephemera, the College's Mutter Museum has an excellent collection of various medical artifacts to look at and hold.

Another major archival collection in the history of nursing is the Adelaide Nutting Historical Nursing Collection and the Archives of the Department of Nursing Education, at Teachers College, Columbia University, and on microfiche. The collection, indexed in two volumes, includes documents on medicine, nursing, and hospitals dating from the fifteenth century but covers primarily the late nineteenth and twentieth centuries. Most valuable is the inclusion of entire texts of journal articles and books.

Local archives, such as the North Carolina Collection at the University of North Carolina at Chapel Hill and the North Carolina State Archives in Raleigh, contain useful materials such as annual hospital reports, convention proceedings, and photographs of devices (including incubators and iron lungs), area hospital nurseries, and operating and hospital rooms.

Histories of Hospitals and Schools of Nursing and Autobiographies of Nurses

Histories of hospitals and schools of nursing also offer relevant information about practice and lead to other sources. Notable examples of such histories include T. J. Berry's *The Bryn Mawr Hospital, 1893–1968* (1969); Dorothy Giles's *A Candle in Her Hand: A Story of the Nursing Schools of Bellevue Hospital* (1949); Ethel Johns and Blanche Pfefferkorn's *The Johns Hopkins Hospital School of Nursing, 1889–1949* (1954); Eleanor Lee's *Neighbors, 1892–1967* (a 1967 history of the Presbyterian Hospital School of Nursing and, later, Columbia University Department of Nursing, in New York); and Mary Lewis Wyche's *The History of Nursing in North Carolina* (1938). Memoirs written by nurses are also useful for discerning what things nurses used in their practice and what they thought about them. Most notable for my purposes were Stella Goostray's *Memoirs: Half a Century in Nursing* (1969), Daisy Barnwell Jones's *My First Eighty Years* (1986), and *Reminiscences of Linda Richards: America's First Trained Nurse* (1911).

Period Studies of Nursing

Important period evaluations of the structure, function, and future of nursing include Jo Ann Ashley's *Hospitals, Paternalism, and the Role of the Nurse* (1976); Esther Lucille Brown's *Nursing for the Future* (1948); Temple Burling, Edith M. Lentz, and Robert N. Wilson's anthology *The Give and Take in Hospitals: A Study of Human Organization in Hospitals* (1956); Edwin A. Christ's *Nurses at Work* (1956); Fred Davis's anthology *The Nursing Profession: Five Sociological Essays* (1966); Thomas R. Ford and Diane D. Stephenson's *Institutional Nurses: Roles, Relationships, and Attitudes in Three Alabama Hospitals* (1954); Robert W. Habenstein and Edwin A. Christ's *Professionalizer, Traditionalizer, and Utilizer* (1955); Everett C. Hughes, Helen McGill, and Irwin Deutscher's *Twenty Thousand Nurses Tell Their Story: A Report on Studies of*

Nursing Functions Sponsored by the ANA (1958); Ethel Johns and Blanche Pfefferkorn's An Activity Analysis of Nursing (1934); Marion S. Lesser and Vera R. Keane's Nurse-Patient Relationships in a Maternity Service (1956); Genevieve Rogge Meyer's Tenderness and Technique: Nursing Values in Transition (1960); Leonard Reissman and John H. Rohrer's Change and Dilemma in the Nursing Profession: Studies of Nursing Services in a Large General Hospital (1957); and Donald D. Stewart and Christine E. Needham's The General Duty Nurse (1955).

Contemporary Studies of Nursing

Contemporary studies of nursing provide an important context for interpreting the nursing/technology relationship. These studies offer historical, sociological, ethnographic, and philosophical interpretations of nursing. Most notable here are Davina Allen's "The Nursing-Medical Boundary: A Negotiated Order?" Sociology of Health and Illness 19, no. 4 (1997): 498–520; David Armstrong's "The Fabrication of Nurse-Patient Relationships," Social Science and Medicine 17, no. 8 (1983): 457–60; Marianne Bankert's Watchful Care: A History of America's Nurse Anesthetists (1989); Anne H. Bishop and John R. Scudder's anthology Caring, Curing, Coping: Nurse, Physician, Patient Relationships (1983); Robert L. Brannon's Intensifying Care: The Hospital Industry, Professionalization, and the Reorganization of the Nursing Labor Process (1994); Julianne Cheek and Trudy Rudge's "The Panopticon Revisited? An Exploration of the Social and Political Dimensions of Contemporary Health Care and Nursing Practice," International Journal of Nursing Studies 31, no. 6 (1994): 583–91; Julie Fairman and Joan Lynaugh's Critical Care Nursing: A History (1998); Pat Holden and Jenny Littlewood's Anthropology in Nursing (1986); Jocalyn Lawler's Behind the Screens: Nursing, Somology, and the Problem of the Body (1991); Joan E. Lynaugh's "Narrow Passageways: Nurses and Physicians in Conflict and Concert since 1875," in Nancy M. P. King, Larry R. Churchill, and A. W. Cross's anthology The Physician as Captain of the Ship: A Critical Reappraisal (1988); Joan E. Lynaugh and Barbara L. Brush's American Nursing: From Hospitals to Health Systems (1996); Carl May and Christine Fleming's "The Professional Imagination: Narrative and the Symbolic Boundaries between Medicine and Nursing," Journal of Advanced Nursing 25, no. 5 (1997): 1094–1100; Barbara Melosh's "The Physician's Hand": Work Culture and Conflict in American Nursing (1982); Judith Parker and John Wiltshire's "The Handover: Three Modes of Nursing Practice Knowledge," in Genevieve Gray and Rosalie Pratt's anthology Scholarship in the Discipline of Nursing (1995); Susan M. Reverby's Ordered to Care: The Dilemma of American Nursing, 1850–1945 (1987); David Wagner's "The Proletarianization of Nursing in the United States, 1932–1946," International Journal of Health Services 10, no. 2 (1980): 271–90; Zane Robinson Wolf's Nurses' Work: The Sacred and the Profane (1988); and Jacqueline Zalumas's Caring in Crisis: An Oral History of Critical Care Nursing (1995).

Studies of the American Hospital

A most important secondary source of information and context for this book was studies of the American hospital, including Diana Elizabeth Long and Janet Golden's *The American General Hospital: Communities and Social Contexts* (1990); Charles E. Rosenberg's *The Care of Strangers: The Rise of America's Hospital System* (1987); Rosemary Stevens's *In Sickness and in Wealth: American Hospitals in the Twentieth Century* (1989); and John D. Thompson and Grace Goldin's *The Hospital: A Social and Architectural History* (1975).

Studies of Medical Technology

One of the most important secondary sources for any exploration of medical/health care technology is the increasing array of studies of specific technologies crossing the disciplines of primarily history and sociology. These studies are especially useful in showing the application of various conceptualizations of technology to empirical cases. Most important to this book were Jeffrey Baker's *The Machine in the Nursery: Incubator Technology and the Origins of Newborn Intensive Care* (1996); Marc Berg's "Practices of Reading and Writing: The Constitutive Role of the Patient Record in Medical Work," *Sociology of Health and Illness* 18, no. 4 (1996): 499–524; Berg's "Of Forms, Containers, and the Electronic Medical Record: Some Tools for a Sociology of the Formal," *Science, Technology, and Human Values* 22, no. 4 (1997): 403–33; Berg's "Medical Work and the Computer-Based Patient Record: A Sociological Perspective," *Methods of Information in Medicine* 37 (1998): 294–301; Christopher William Crenner's "Professional Measurement: Quantifying Health and Disease in American Medical Practice, 1880–1920" (Ph.D. dissertation, 1993); Hughes Evans "Losing Touch: The Controversy over the Introduction of Blood Pressure Instruments into Medicine," *Technology and Culture* 34, no. 4 (1993): 784–807; Diana E. Forsythe's "New Bottles, Old Wine: Hidden Cultural Assumptions in a Computerized Explanation System for Migraine Sufferers," *Medical Anthropology Quarterly* 10, no. 4 (1996): 551–74; Anja Hiddinga and Stuart S. Blume's "Technology, Science, and Obstetric Practice: The Origins and Transformation of Cephalopelvimetry," *Science, Technology, and Human Values* 17, no. 2 (1992): 154–79; Joel D. Howell's *Technology in the Hospital: Transforming Patient Care in the Early Twentieth Century* (1995); Alan Prout's "Actor-Network Theory, Technology, and Medical Sociology: An Illustrative Analysis of the Metered Dose Inhaler," *Sociology of Health and Illness* 18, no. 2 (1996): 198–219; Stanley Joel Reiser's classic *Medicine and the Reign of Technology* (1978); and Stefan Timmermans's "Saving Lives or Saving Multiple Identities? The Double Dynamic of Resuscitation Scripts," *Social Studies of Science* 26, no. 4 (1996): 767–97, and "Resuscitation Technology in the Emergency Department: Towards a Dignified Death," *Sociology of Health and Illness* 20, no. 2 (1998): 144–67.

Most notable for attention to nursing/technology work is the sociological research of Shizuko Y. Fagerhaugh, Anselm Strauss, Barbara Suczek, and Carolyn L. Wiener, including (in variously ordered authorship) *Hazards in Hospital Care: Ensuring Patient Safety* (1987) and *Social Organization of Medical Work* (1985, 1997).

Another important literature in this domain concerns the senses and diagnostic techniques. Most notable are W. F. Bynum and Roy Porter's anthologies *Medicine and the Five Senses* (1993) and the *Companion Encyclopedia of the History of Medicine*, vol. 2 (1993).

Theory and Method in the Study of Technology, Especially Medical Technology

There is a large and important literature crossing the history and philosophy of Western technology; the history of medicine and medical technology; social, anthropological, and cultural/postmodern studies of technology; and material culture studies that addresses how we should define, think about, and study technology in general and medical technology in particular. Taken together, this literature provides much of the conceptual and methodologic context for this study. Among the most important works are Wiebe E. Bijker, Thomas P. Hughes, and Trevor J. Pinch's anthology *The Social Construction of Technological Systems: New Directions in the Sociology and History of Technology* (1987); Monica J. Casper and Marc Berg's "Constructivist Perspectives on Medical Work: Medical Practices and Science and Technology Studies," *Science, Technology, and Human Values* 20, no. 4 (1995): 395–407; Monica J. Casper and Barbara A. Koenig's special edition "Biomedical Technologies: Reconfiguring Nature and Culture," *Medical Anthropology Quarterly* 10, no. 4 (1996); Ruth Schwartz Cowan's *A Social History of American Technology* (1997); Audrey Davis's "Historical Studies of Medical Instruments," *History of Science* 16 (1978): 107–33; Davis's *Medicine and Its Technology: An Introduction to the History of Medical Instrumentation* (1981); Davis's (with Mark S. Dreyfus) *The Finest Instruments Ever Made: A Bibliography of Medical, Dental, Optical, and Pharmaceutical Company Trade Literature, 1700–1939* (1986); Davis's "American Medicine in the Gilded Age: The First Technological Era," *Annals of Science* 47, no. 2 (1990): 111–25; Gary Lee Downey and Joseph Dumit's anthology *Cyborgs and Citadels: Anthropological Interventions in Emerging Sciences and Technologies* (1997); James M. Edmonson's "Learning from the Artifact: Surgical Instruments as Resources in the History of Medicine and Medical Technology," *Caduceus* 9, no. 2 (1993): 87–95; Joel D. Howell's *Technology and American Medical Practice, 1880–1930: Anthology of Sources* (1988); Don Ihde's *Technics and Praxis* (1979); Ihde's *Technology and the Lifeworld: From Garden to Earth* (1990); Ihde's *Instrumental Realism: The Interface between Philosophy of Science and Philosophy of Technology* (1991); W. David Kingery's *Learning from Things: Method and Theory of Material Cul-*

ture Studies (1996); Ghislaine Lawrence's "The Ambiguous Artifact: Surgical Instruments and the Surgical Past," in Christopher Lawrence's anthology *Medical Theory, Surgical Practice: Studies in the History of Surgery* (1992); Ghislaine Lawrence's anthology *Technologies of Modern Medicine* (1994); Hughie Mackay and Gareth Gillespie's "Extending the Social Shaping of Technology Approach: Ideology and Appropriation," *Social Studies of Science* 22, no. 4 (1992): 685–716; Donald MacKenzie and Judy Wajcman's anthology *The Social Shaping of Technology: How the Refrigerator Got Its Hum* (1985); Carl Mitcham's *Thinking through Technology: The Path between Engineering and Philosophy* (1994); Wanda J. Orlikowski's "The Duality of Technology: Rethinking the Concept of Technology in Organizations," *Organization Science* 3, no. 3 (1992): 398–427; Trevor J. Pinch and Wiebe E. Bijker's "The Social Construction of Facts and Artefacts: Or How the Sociology of Science and the Sociology of Technology Might Benefit Each Other," *Social Studies of Science* 14, no. 3 (1984): 399–441; Carroll Pursell's *The Machine in America: A Social History of Technology* (1995); Merritt Roe Smith and Leo Marx's anthology *Does Technology Drive History? The Dilemma of Technological Determinism* (1994); Simon J. Williams's "Modern Medicine and the 'Uncertain Body': From Corporeality to Hyperreality?" *Social Science and Medicine* 45, no. 7 (1997): 1041–49; and Gretchen Worden's "Steel Knives and Iron Lungs: Medical Instruments as Medical History," *Caduceus* 9, no. 2 (1993): 111–18.

Feminist Critique/Gender Studies of Technology

A special domain of scholarship within technology studies, but also a key shaper of it, is the burgeoning field of gender/technology studies. Included here are conceptualizations of the gender/technology relation and empirical studies and philosophical critiques of technologies of significance to women. Most recent scholarship shows a strong influence of postmodern/cultural studies. Among the texts most important to this book were Rima D. Apple's *Mothers and Medicine: A Social History of Infant Feeding, 1890–1950* (1987); Anne Balsamo's *Technologies of the Gendered Body: Reading Cyborg Women* (1997); Cynthia Cockburn's *Machinery of Dominance: Women, Men, and Technical Know-How* (1985); Ruth Schwartz Cowan's *More Work for Mother: The Ironies of Household Technology from the Open Hearth to the Microwave* (1983) and "Technology Is to Science as Female Is to Male: Musings on the History and Character of Our Discipline," *Technology and Culture* 37, no. 3 (1996): 572–82; Robbie Davis-Floyd and Joseph Dumit's anthology *Cyborg Babies: From Techno-Sex to Techno-Tots* (1998); Diane M. Douglas's "The Machine in the Parlor: A Dialectical Analysis of the Sewing Machine," *Journal of American Culture* 5, no. 1 (1982): 20–29; Dion Farquhar's *The Other Machine: Discourse and Reproductive Technologies* (1996); Sarah Franklin and Helena Ragone's anthology *Reproducing Reproduction: Kinship, Power, and Technological Innovation* (1998); Eileen Green, Jenny Owen, and Den Pain's anthology *Gendered by Design? Informa-*

tion *Technology and Office Systems* (1993); Keith Grint and Rosalind Gill's anthology *The Gender-Technology Relation: Contemporary Theory and Research* (1995); Donna J. Haraway's "A Cyborg Manifesto: Science, Technology, and Socialist-Feminism in the Late Twentieth Century," in her *Simians, Cyborgs, and Women: The Reinvention of Nature* (1991); Nina Lerman, Arwen Mohun, and Ruth Oldenziel's "Versatile Tools: Gender Analysis and the History of Technology," *Technology and Culture* 38, no. 1 (1997): 1–8; Judith A. McGaw's "Women and the History of American Technology," *Signs: Journal of Women in Culture and Society* 7, no. 4 (1982): 798–828; Maureen McNeil's anthology *Gender and Expertise* (1987); Ruth Oldenziel's *Making Technology Masculine: Men, Women, and Modern Machines in America, 1870–1945* (1999); Kathryn S. Ratcliff's anthology *Healing Technology: Feminist Perspectives* (1989); Joan Rothschild's anthology *Machina ex Dea: Feminist Perspectives on Technology* (1983); Autumn Stanley's *Mothers and Daughters of Invention: Notes for a Revised History of Technology* (1995); Michelle Stanworth's anthology *Reproductive Technologies: Gender, Motherhood, and Medicine* (1987); Paula Treichler and Lisa Cartwright's anthology "Imaging Technologies, Inscribing Science," *Camera Obscura* 28, 29 (1992); Irma Van Der Ploeg's "Hermaphrodite Patients: In Vitro Fertilization and the Transformation of Male Infertility," *Science, Technology, and Human Values* 20, no. 4 (1995): 460–81; and Judy Wajcman's *Feminism Confronts Technology* (1991).

Other Social Science and Historical Perspectives

Several additional works, not in the domain of technology studies, were also highly influential in framing this study, including Andrew Abbott's *The System of Professions: An Essay on the Division of Expert Labor* (1988); David Armstrong's "The Rise of Surveillance Medicine," *Sociology of Health and Illness* 17, no. 3 (1995): 393–404; William Ray Arney's *Power and the Profession of Obstetrics* (1982); Susan Leigh Star's "The Sociology of the Invisible: The Primacy of Work in the Writings of Anselm Strauss," in David R. Maines's *Social Organization and Social Process: Essays in Honor of Anselm Strauss* (1991), 265–83; and Candace West and Don H. Zimmerman's "Doing Gender," *Gender and Society* 1, no. 2 (1987): 125–51.

Photos and drawings of devices are important sources of information for any study of technology. Texts that contain photos and essays on their history and proper interpretation include Daniel M. Fox and Christopher Lawrence's *Photographing Medicine: Images and Power in Britain and America since 1840* (1988) and Janet Golden and Charles E. Rosenberg's *Picture of Health: A Photographic History of Health Care in Philadelphia, 1860–1945* (1991).

Personal Experience

Any nurse studying some aspect of nursing practice has her or his own experience from which to draw. My clinical encounters with technology began in the mid-1960s as a nursing student. I have utilized devices in use in nursing since the early decades of the twentieth century, including a range of metal, ceramic, glass, rubber, and cloth implements (bedpans, urinals, enema cans, needles and syringes, breast and abdominal binders, and surgical instruments) and contraptions (gastric suction and intravenous equipment, orthopedic traction, and crank beds). I have also used tools that did not enter nursing practice until the 1960s, including electronic fetal monitors. Handling these devices encompasses not only the knowledge and skill required to use them but also the knowledge obtained from this use—about the patient and about oneself. Entering patients' bodies with needles or enema tubing, for example, produces knowledge about the resistance of human tissue, the curvature of anatomy, the weight and flexibility of objects, and the range of human responses to such intrusions. Using these devices also generates knowledge about one's own psychomotor and perceptual skills, technical aptitudes and anxieties, and aesthetic inclinations. Practitioners have available to them an incredibly rich source of information in the implements they use to care for their patients. There is much to be learned from personal encounters with things outside ourselves, not the least of which is knowledge about ourselves.

This book contains material, in a revised and/or expanded form, that has
   been previously published by the author. These articles are listed in
   chronological order.

"Out of Eden: Philosophical Perspectives on Reproductive Technology."
   In *Women's Health Care: A Comprehensive Handbook*, edited by Catherine I.
   Fogel and Nancy F. Woods, 701–21. Thousand Oaks, Calif.: Sage, 1995. By
   permission of Sage Publications.

"Tools of the Trade: Analyzing Technology as Object in Nursing." *Scholarly
   Inquiry for Nursing Practice* 10, no. 1 (1996): 3–14. By permission of Springer
   Publishing.

"Exploring the Gender-Technology Relation in Nursing." *Nursing Inquiry* 4,
   no. 4 (1997): 219–28. By permission of Blackwell Science Asia.

"(Ir)Reconcilable Differences? The Debate Concerning Nursing and Technology." *Image: Journal of Nursing Scholarship* 29, no. 2 (1997): 169–74. By
   permission of Sigma Theta Tau International.

"Knowing and Forgetting: The Challenge of Technology for a Reflexive
   Practice Science of Nursing." In *Nursing Praxis: Knowledge and Action*, edited by
   Sally Thorne and Virginia E. Hayes, 69–85. Thousand Oaks, Calif.: Sage,
   1997). By permission of Sage Publications.

" 'Making the Best of Things': Technology in American Nursing, 1870–
   1940." *Nursing History Review* 5 (1997): 3–22. By permission of Springer
   Publishing.

"Looking to Care or Caring to Look? Technology and the Rise of Spectacular
   Nursing." *Holistic Nursing Practice* 12, no. 4 (1998): 1–11. Erratum in 13, no. 1
   (1998): 82–84. By permission of Aspen Publishers.

"Venous Envy: The Post–World War II Debate over IV Nursing." *Advances in
   Nursing Science* 22, no. 1 (1999): 52–62. By permission of Aspen Publishers.

"Troubling Distinctions: A Semiotics of the Nursing/Technology Relation." *Nursing Inquiry* 6, no. 3 (1999): 198–207. By permission of Blackwell
   Science Asia.

"The Physician's Eyes: American Nursing and the Diagnostic Revolution in

Medicine." *Nursing History Review* 8 (2000): 3–38. By permission of Springer Publishing.

"Retro-fitting Technology to Nursing: The Case of Electronic Fetal Monitoring," *Journal of Obstetric, Gynecologic, and Neonatal Nursing* 29, no. 3 (2000): 316–24. By permission of Lippincott Williams and Wilkins.

Charting, 16–17, 167, 172–73, 184;
defensive, 264 (n. 151)
Childbirth: and activists, 173; by
Caesarean section, 153, 158, 254
(n. 77); and embodied authority,
262 (n. 138); history of, 138–39; at
home, 49, 50, 51; at hospital, 52;
low-technology methods for, 167;
mortality in, 139; natural, 143,
157, 174; and neurological and
mental deficits, 148; "prepared,"
163–64
Classification, systems of, 183–84,
185–86, 270 (n. 58)
Communication, 153–54
Conception, 38–39, 40, 41–42
Contraception, 38–39, 40, 41
Corometrics Medical Systems, 149,
151, 152, 160, 169
Coronary care units, 126
CT scanners, 30
Culture: change in, 38–40; hierarchies in, 7–8; of risk, 137–38
"Cyborg manifesto," 176
Cyborgs: 265 (n. 5); imagery of, 176;
nurse practitioners as, 193; nurses
as, 177

Democratization of health care
functions, 177
Dental probes, 35–36
Design: of devices, 26; and gender,
27; of machine monitors, 127; and
nurses, 169; of stethoscopes for
nurses, 231 (n. 66)
Deskilling, 65, 225 (n. 117)
Devices: and nurses, 104–5, 179;
techniques mediated by, 92; and
patient care technology, 104–5;
and "world of the tool," 135–36
Diagnosis: assistive role of nurses
in, 86–91; and changing tasks
for nurses, 95–99; as collabora-

tive, 82; early, 72; versus effective
treatment, 97; and fetal monitoring, 255 (n. 79); hierarchy
of tasks for, 90; impact of technology in, 92; and "informatics
nurse," 183; Nightingale on, 68;
by nurse practitioners, 187–88,
191–92; processual versus episodic, 89; revolution in, 92–99,
237 (n. 134); rhetoric of, 96–99;
roles of nurses in, 82–83
Division of labor, 96
"Docile bodies," 137, 138
Dock, Lavinia, 173
Documentation by exception, 183–
84
"Domestication strategy," 27–28
Douche pan, 56
Doulas, 166
Drugs, 139, 162

Edwards, Margot, 173
Education, medical, 149, 152, 254
(n. 74). See also Nursing—educa-
tion for
EKG monitors, 121
Electronic fetal monitoring. See
Monitoring—electronic fetal
E-mail, 29–30
Embodiment relations, 35–36
Emotional support, 118, 129
Endoscopy, examinations using, 192
Enemas, 50, 60
Equipment, 50, 53–54; pneumatic
and hydraulic, 133; problems
with, 58–62; promotional lit-
erature for, 53–58; specialized
trays for, 62, 77; and thermome-
ters, 77; for laboratory and x-ray
diagnosis, 83. See also Instruments;
Machines; Monitoring; specific
equipment names
Eroticism, 215 (n. 143)

123–24, 129, 133. *See also* Equipment; Instruments
—electronic fetal, 144–49; advertising for, 262 (n. 134); benign tracings in, 164–65; clinical trials of, 167–68, 170; criteria for using, 149–50; critics of, 173; debate over, 259 (n. 121), 261 (nn. 128, 131); defensive charting in, 264 (n. 151); diagnosis by nurses in, 255 (n. 79); diverts attention from patient, 166; early systems for, 145; early usage of, 143–44; errors in, 165; and essence of nursing, 164; versus fetal auscultation, 171; internal and external, 147, 162, 163, 172; interpretation by nurses of, 159; introduction of, 144–45, 252 (n. 44); and intuition, 154; language of, 159; learning to use, 150–52; as legal evidence, 256–57 (n. 97), 258 (n. 115); as means to control doctors, 254–55 (n. 78); measurements in, 145–47; as "mechanical monster," 163; nonneutrality of, 26; nurses as consumers of, 169, 171; and nurses versus physicians, 151–52; and nursing/technology relation, 170; ominous tracings in, 165; "paradox" of, 167, 175; "perfect patterns" in, 161, 162, 164, 172, 257 (n. 98); and physician/nurse relationship, 173–74; prestige of, 156; purity as clinical tool of, 171–72; resistance to, 151, 158; "seeing with sound" in, 30; significance of, 19; as subjective technique, 168–69; as symbol, 137, 144; as technology of nursing, 168; tending machines for, 160; as tool for coaching, 157, 256 (n. 92); usage of, 149; validates nursing knowl-

edge, 153–56; women's responses to, 163. *See also* Fetus
—by machines, 121–22; and articulation work, 172; and critical practice context, 169; as "crutch factor," 165; disadvantages of, 129; factors determining use of, 149; introduction of, 121–22; and "prepared" childbirth, 163–64; role of nurses in, 127; as social control, 137, 162; technical problems with, 128–30. *See also* Machines

Nature: related to science and technology, 33; versus technology, 34–35
NIC, 183, 184
Nightingale, Florence, 67–69, 226 (n. 5)
Nurse practitioners, 181, 182, 187–93; and diagnosis, 273 (n. 84); and instruments, 189; as physician extenders, 190–91, 273 (n. 83); role of, 188, 191, 272 (n. 73); as "traitors to nursing," 189
Nurse technicians, 106
Nurses: academic, 180–81, 188–89, 202 (n. 78); assistants to, 103; bags used by, 53–54; overtrained, 87–88; scrub, 117, 119, 243 (n. 85); as servants, 1, 8; technical, 106; as "undifferentiated other," 177; working hours of, 216 (n. 9)
—professional: ambivalence among, 180; distinctions within, 132–33; regression of, 267 (n. 24); tasks of, 106
—registered: as agents of physicians, 114; and functional nursing, 101; and IV therapy, 114; numbers of, 103
Nursing: aesthetics of, 76–77; as anomalous among professions,

256 (n. 84); prophylactic, 157; and social control, 138, 162, 173; surveillance and tensions and, 19

Operating rooms, 118

Overtraining of nurses, 87–88

Oxygen therapy, 58, 64

"Paper nursing," 172–73, 263–64 (n. 151)

Patients, for diagnostic testing, 95
—care of: administration of, 101; effects of automation on, 129–30; in OR nursing, 116; predictions of mechanization of, 129; in primary nursing, 267 (n. 23). See also "Knowing the patient"
—records of: contents of, 17; and nursing informatics, 184; as primary sources, 15, 202 (n. 82); in work and social relations, 17; secondary purposes of, 203 (n. 90)

Personnel, substitution of, 177

Physicians: authority and technology of, 92, 98; contemporary challenges to, 192; delegating functions of, 107, 113, 192; diagnosis reserved by, 87–90; early views of nursing by, 46; functional indispensability of, 63–64; and IV therapy, 112–13; and mastery of machine monitoring by nurses, 127–28; and maternal labor, 139, 140, 141; and nurse practitioners, 188; nurses as instruments or tools of, 3; on nurses in laboratory and x-ray fields, 85; nurses versus house, 85–86; and patient records, 184; prestige of, 171–72; and role of nurse in diagnosis, 87–90, 97; scopic devices of, 81–

82; separations from patients of, 93; special knowledge of, 64; and technology, 13; thermometer reading by, 48

Poultices, 54, 56, 221 (n. 74)

Power, 137, 173

"Practical knowledge," 224 (n. 114)

"Practice theories", 224 (n. 114)

Pregnancy. See Conception

Private rooms, 4

Professionalization, 104, 186

Prostheses, 25

Pulse, observation of, 71

Radio, 27, 28

Referent systems, 197 (n. 30)

Reproduction. See Conception

Resuscitation, technology for, 264 (n. 157)

Robots, 122, 123, 124

Science: dependency of technology on, 33; embodied in technology, 34; as new religion, 92; self-interested relationship of with technology, 212 (n. 97); symbols of, 4

Seguin, Edouard, 73, 74, 89

Semiotics, 197 (n. 26)

Sentimental work, 2. See also True nursing

Servants, nurses as, 1, 8

Shearer, Madeleine, 173

Skill: defining, 99; and enskilling and deskilling, 193; and IV therapy, 114; obsolescence of, 131

Specialization, 83; impact of technology on, 2. See also Nursing

Speculum, 42

Sphygmomanometers, 48, 93, 141

Steam tent apparatus, 120–21

Stethoscopes: designed for nurses,

231 (n. 66); fetal, 141–42, 158; maternal labor, 141–42; and nurse practitioners, 187; and physicians, 64, 96; as scientific, 93; as sense extenders, 48; usage by nurses of, 78, 80–81

Sterilizers: bedpan, 58; dressing, 58, 59

Stewart, Isabel, 65, 66, 105

Structuration model of technology, 43

Supplies, 62

Surgeons, 244 (n. 103)

Surveillance, 137, 138, 186. *See also* Observation

Symbols: electronic fetal monitoring as, 137, 144; hospitals as, 195–96 (n. 12); of science, 4; thermometer as, 77–78

Symptomatology, 71–72

Tape recorders, 31–32

Taxonomies, 183–84, 185–86

Technization, 208 (n. 37)

Technology: artifacts of, 25, 207 (n. 37); of care, 9; comfort, 26; concepts of, 18–19; "defining," 42–43; definitional issues of, 21–22, 23, 32; "deflective power" of, 42; dependence of on science, 33; depictions of, 23; displaying, 2–3; duality of, 43; effects of, 38–42; electronic, 24; engagements with, 264 (n. 158); and erosion of nursing, 131; and eroticism, 215 (n. 143); historical dimensions of, 22–23; and inequality among nurses, 127; invention versus use of, 236 (n. 119); knowing, 35–38; linked to nursing, 2; and masculinity, 14, 131; and narrative, 206 (n. 22); and nurse practitioners,

192–93; postwar innovations in, 102; public access to, 177; as science's Other, 8; screen(ing), 136–37; self-interested relationship of with science, 212 (n. 97); and skill and status, 179; social history of, 18; status quo of maintained, 174–75; and subordination of nursing to medicine, 13; technical problems with, 128–30; transfer of, 14–15; transportation, 28; women's role in, 12

—computer, 21; and AIDS, 181, 182–86; as "defining" technology, 42–43; and invisibility of nursing, 40; as second self, 42; as text, 42

—laboratory and x-ray: as diagnostic procedures, 90, 93; and nurse practitioners, 187; and role of nurses, 82–86, 90, 233 (n. 80)

"Technology of silence," 186

Telemedicine, 267–68 (n. 27)

"Tender loving care" (TLC), 178–79, 185

Thermometers, 73–78; advertising for, 56, 68; breakage of, 62, 76; dangers of, 60; early, 57; invention of, 73; and maternal labor, 141; as "prestige tool," 98; testimonials by nurses for, 54; as womanly craft, 73. *See also* Thermometry, clinical

Thermometry, clinical, 28, 73–78; delegation to nurses of, 73–74; feminized, 28; and hermeneutic relations, 36; and hierarchy of diagnostic tasks, 89–90, 96; instruction in, 74–76; interpretive readings of, 48, 219 (n. 30); time required for, 60–61. *See also* Thermometers

Thingness: of technology, 18, 23–25; and valence of things, 29–32
Time, management of, 50, 186
Tocodynamometer, 31
Tools. *See* Equipment; Instruments
True nursing: and fetal monitoring, 172; and machine monitoring, 128; new language of, 184; and new postwar machinery, 105, 133–34; versus nurse practioners, 190; OR nursing as, 115–16, 118–19; versus team nursing, 179–80; versus technological advances, 105, 130; and technology as care, 178; and TLC, 178–79
"Twilight sleep," 139, 162

Ultrasound machine, 25–26
University of Iowa Nursing Interventions Classification (NIC) System, 183, 184
Urine, drainage of, 50, 222 (n. 89)

Venipuncture. *See* Intravenous therapy

Weeks, Clara S., 70
"World of the screen," 135, 136–38
World War II, 109
Wunderlich, Carl, 73, 89, 90

X-rays. *See* Technology—laboratory and x-ray

Studies in Social Medicine

Nancy M. P. King, Gail E. Henderon, and Jane Stein, eds., *Beyond Regulations: Ethics in Human Subjects Research* (1999).

Laurie Zoloth, *Health Care and the Ethics of Encounter: A Jewish Discussion of Social Justice* (1999).

Susan M. Reverby, ed. *Tuskegee's Truths: Rethinking the Tuskegee Syphilis Study* (2000).

Margarete Sandelowski, *Devices and Desires: Gender, Technology, and American Nursing* (2000).

DEMCO